A NEW DEAL FOR CANCER

A NEW DEAL FOR CANCER

Lessons from a 50 Year War

EDITED BY

ABBE R. GLUCK &
CHARLES S. FUCHS

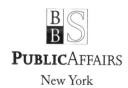

PUBLICAFFAIRS
New York

PublicAffairs
Hachette Book Group
1290 Avenue of the Americas, New York, NY 10104
www.publicaffairsbooks.com
@Public_Affairs

Printed in the United States of America

First Edition: November 2021

Published by PublicAffairs, an imprint of Perseus Books, LLC, a subsidiary of Hachette Book Group, Inc. The PublicAffairs name and logo is a trademark of the Hachette Book Group.

The Hachette Speakers Bureau provides a wide range of authors for speaking events. To find out more, go to www.hachettespeakersbureau.com or call (866) 376-6591.

The publisher is not responsible for websites (or their content) that are not owned by the publisher.

Editorial production by Christine Marra, *Marra*thon Production Services. www.marrathoneditorial.org

Print book interior design by Jane Raese
Set in 12-point Adobe Caslon

Library of Congress Cataloging-in-Publication Data has been applied for.

ISBNs: 978-1-5417-0061-1 (hardcover), 978-1-5417-0062-8 (e-book)

LSC-C

Printing 1, 2021

For my wife, Joanna Fuchs,
a proud cancer survivor who inspires me
and gives me strength every day.
—C. S. F.

For my extraordinary mother, Ruth Rubin Gluck,
who lost her war far too young, in 1999,
but remains with me always.
—A. R. G.

Contents

PART THREE
SCIENCE AND TREATMENT TRANSFORMED

PART FOUR
GOVERNING CANCER

A New Deal for Cancer

Charles S. Fuchs, Abbe R. Gluck, and Eugene Rusyn

When President Richard Nixon entered the White House state dining room just before noon on December 23, 1971, he was greeted by some 137 assembled guests hailing from the most powerful precincts of government, science, industry, and advocacy. They were there to witness the signing of the landmark National Cancer Act—the product of feverish debate and political jockeying extending over decades of committed advocacy. While what would later be called the "War on Cancer Act" was not the parlance of the day, Nixon set forth "a national commitment for the conquest of cancer" and reflected that "we may look back on this day and this action as being the most significant action taken during this administration."

According to a report submitted to Congress in 1970 by a group of experts tasked with studying the issue, cancer was the number

---

Charles S. Fuchs is the Senior Vice President and Global Head of Product Development for Oncology and Hematology at Roche and Genentech; Former Director of Yale Cancer Center.

Abbe R. Gluck is the Alfred M. Rankin Professor of Law and the founding Faculty Director of the Solomon Center for Health Law and Policy at Yale Law School; she is also Professor of Medicine at Yale School of Medicine.

Eugene Rusyn is a Senior Fellow, Solomon Center for Health Law and Policy, and Lecturer in Law at Yale Law School.

one health concern of the American people at the time—a facet of American life that remained unchanged even in a 2016 survey conducted by the Mayo Clinic. And yet, as of 1969, the US spent only $0.889 per person in America on cancer research. This has since risen to $20 per person. An important Senate committee report issued shortly before the act was signed into law opined, "There seems to be a consensus among cancer researchers that they are within striking distance of achieving the basic understanding of cancer cells which has eluded the most brilliant medical minds in the world." The prescription for government action was clear: "The development of a comprehensive national program for the conquest of cancer is now essential. Such a program will require three major ingredients that are not present today: effective administration with clearly defined authority and responsibility, a comprehensive national plan, and necessary financial resources."[1]

Looking back today on the fiftieth anniversary of the War, its achievements are clear in the enormous strides that have been made. Although the cancer death rate in the US continued to rise in the twenty years that followed passage of the bill, cancer mortality rates have declined 29 percent since 1991, translating into an estimated 2.9 million fewer cancer deaths than would have occurred if peak rates had persisted.[2] Efforts in cancer prevention, most notably reduction in the use of tobacco products, account for much of the mortality reductions, though recent advances in cancer therapeutics are now also contributing.

While we celebrate these achievements, we must also recognize the shortfalls. Cancer was not cured by 1976. The mission statement was too simple. And the 1971 law did not go far enough. Senator Ted Kennedy, standing mere feet from Nixon during the signing ceremony, was the chief sponsor of a more ambitious bill that would have created a National Cancer Authority—an independent agency responsible for cancer research—alongside a major expansion in federal funding for research itself. Championed and in many ways crafted by famed cancer advocate Mary Lasker, Kennedy's Conquest of Cancer was inspired by the Apollo 11 moon landing. The renowned December 1969 *New York Times* full-page ad—"Mr. Nixon: You Can Cure Cancer"—quoted Harvard's

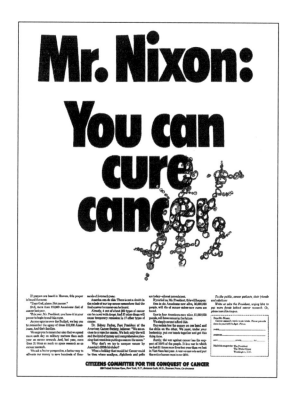

Sidney Farber as saying: "We lack only the will and the kind of money and comprehensive planning that went into putting a man on the moon . . . Why don't we try to conquer cancer by America's 200th birthday?" The vision was for cancer to have its own NASA—the first cancer moonshot had arrived, at least as an idea.

But that idea fell short in the House, which forced the compromise legislation enacted in 1971 that expanded the authority of the National Cancer Institute (NCI) but left it under the National Institutes of Health (NIH). The final version of the act was still intended to meet a towering five-year goal, which of course was not met: curing cancer by the nation's bicentennial in 1976.

But the War on Cancer might also have gotten ahead of itself. Experts worried at the time that the science of cancer was not sufficiently well understood to even come close to the goals set by the Nixon administration. As Sol Spiegelman, director of Columbia University's Institute of Cancer Research, pointedly noted, "An all-out effort at this time would be like trying to land a man on the moon without knowing Newton's laws of gravity."

Today, we recognize that cancer is not a single illness to be conquered, but hundreds of different, complex diseases requiring a deep understanding of each entity's unique biology, genetics, clinical characteristics, susceptibility to treatment, and ability to rapidly develop therapeutic resistance. Additionally, the notion of a truly comprehensive nationally run strategy for cancer was never fully realized. The 1971 act envisioned a key role for the federal government: one in which it had to play a central—perhaps *the* central—role in confronting cancer in America. This would require not just the power of the purse—through funding and appropriations—but all the might of the federal government, bringing to bear public organization, agency action, and presidential leadership.

But subsequent decades of slow, albeit persistent, progress and fragmented policies underscore a simple truth: we still do not have a clear and unified federal government–led approach that fully harnesses and focuses the vast talent and resources of this nation to tackle the panoply of challenges and steps needed to eliminate cancer—that is, a program that truly "lands a man on the moon."

The mission as conceived was not ambitious enough while also being too narrow in critical ways. The idea that a scientific cure was the only goal—the only barrier to eradicating the scourge of the disease—did not predict the enormous range of cancer as an "institution," as Siddhartha Mukherjee so aptly puts it in these pages, and the obligation of any government response to think about the world cancer inhabits more broadly so as to properly address it. The War was not against a single enemy but countless adversaries—and not just in the vast number of unique cancer subtypes we understand to exist today. On the battlefield are also the business and economics of cancer, the fragmented and often costly and inefficient regulatory landscape, intolerable problems of health justice and equity, crushing pressures on the everyday practice of cancer medicine, and lack of prevention and attention to public health—all alongside enduring questions about the proper role of our state and federal governments.

This book aims to tackle those issues and open a broader lens onto the War on Cancer. We seek to shift the metaphor—to advance a "New Deal for Cancer" that places the federal government at the center of a whole-of-nation response that recognizes the need to make progress not just on the science of cures but also with respect to the people and institutions that make up the system.

The book's goal is to explore "everything beyond the science"—but of course the science appears on every page because, fundamentally, the project of addressing cancer is about how policy on all levels—economic, social, medical, and regulatory—should interact with, support, and spread scientific developments. We aimed to fill a gap that we quickly discovered there was great hunger to fill; to examine the ways in which policy, politics, and law can and should advance our New Deal for Cancer and how obstacles they have helped to construct can be dismantled.

Today, national cancer costs are on track to reach $246 billion by 2030—having already hit $183 billion in 2015. The cost of cancer care has been growing considerably faster than the overall cost of health care—with the former expected to rise 34 percent by 2030 compared to 20 percent for the latter. It has emerged as a chronic condition, with 22.1 million cancer survivors anticipated in 2030 and a five-year survival rate greater than 70 percent.[3] We pay too much for it, and the economic structures of our cancer institutions are not rational. Cancer patients receive many high-value essential services—such as palliative care—that are underreimbursed, driving health-care providers to rely on highly reimbursed goods and services to make up for the shortfall—particularly pharmaceuticals. This phenomenon of what Ed Benz in this book aptly calls "cross-subsidization" creates perverse incentives for patients and providers, heavily skewing care toward some procedures and testing while undermining other key forms of medical intervention. Smaller cancer providers face pressure to consolidate; pricing structures remain uneven and nontransparent. Inadequate access to health insurance is still a primary driver of cancer outcomes, and there are also intolerably persistent disparities in cancer outcomes and treatment across racial groups. Prevention, despite years of evidence about its promise, remains underfunded and undervalued.

New breakthroughs that are cause for celebration also create new challenges. Physicians are under enormous pressure to absorb new therapeutic and technological innovations, adapt to electronic medical records, and tackle new problems, such as survivorship. Our legal and regulatory regimes have not yet caught up with precision medicine and the largely unfulfilled opportunity to fully mine the treasure trove of patient clinical and genomic data toward the next generation of transformative discoveries. For future research to flourish, genomic and clinical outcome data must be shared on a much larger scale than is currently taking place. This will require overcoming perceived privacy risks by modernizing the laws that govern the space and ensuring that there are robust legal protections against identifying patients whose data resides in de-identified registries. Research and development (R&D) remains costly, often ineffective, and marked by redundancy while needing to change to meet the challenge of precision medicine—a targeted approach to cancer that results in therapies that apply to fewer people.

Fragmentation remains an enormous problem. The main government agencies of cancer are siloed from one another and often create inefficiencies rather than accelerating progress. Our healthcare system remains fragmented both in terms of the provision of insurance and in the differences across the fifty states in how cancer is prevented and treated. Data sharing and other collaborations across government, academic institutions, and the private sector have been identified by most experts as key, and yet we have not found ways to break down existing silos and truly bring all sectors of the nation together to join forces.

The COVID-19 pandemic has been a wake-up call of sorts for cancer. It shows what the federal government can accomplish in short order when it harnesses *all* its power—as President Joseph Biden has put it, a "whole-of-government approach" that includes the private and public sectors, forces collaboration, breaks down inefficiencies, targets equity and access, and is coordinated from the top. This modern vision of a New Deal—one that also recognizes the federal government's critical role but insists that it cannot solve the problem alone—is what the authors in this book chart for the next fifty years.

Pulitzer Prize–winning author **Siddhartha Mukherjee**'s opening chapter sets the stage by capturing our present moment—one in which the extraordinary breakthroughs of the past fifty years have begun to pose new challenges of their own. This includes the pervasive feeling—thanks to advances in cancer surveillance—that we are all, in a sense, citizens of "Cancerland." Mukherjee urges an approach to the next fifty years in which the "balance between curative therapies and the condition of being mortal" wins out over anxiety about impending risk.

We then survey the landscape of cancer care—where it is delivered and who pays for it—including how the business has changed over the past half century. **Randall A. Oyer** and **Erin O. Aakhus** detail the benefits of expanded access that have accrued from the dispersion of cancer care from academic medical centers to community practices. At the same time, they raise more recent concerns about the risks of excessive industry consolidation for the future availability of cancer care nested within local communities—a theme echoed later by others. **K. Robin Yabroff** looks at finance from the patient side, describing a health insurance system that has greatly improved, but remains fragmented and incomplete. Health insurance coverage, she notes, is one of the strongest predictors of access to cancer care and health cancer outcomes, explaining why the continuing epidemic of undercoverage plays a central role in cancer disparities. Yabroff's theme of fragmentation reappears throughout the book: We see inefficiencies, costly redundancies, and obstacles caused by fragmentation across virtually every aspect of the cancer space.

Edward J. Benz Jr. takes us into an area rarely explored in writings about cancer policy: the business of cancer institutions, and how financial incentives and disincentives are misaligned to encourage overutilization of costly procedures while discouraging lower cost interventions as well as research. As noted, he emphasizes the phenomenon of "cross-subsidization," pointing out that many high-value and essential services for cancer patients, including research, are paid for by overreimbursed goods and services. The policy implications of recognizing this situation are profound—cutting drug prices as well as the cost of other cancer services cannot be achieved successfully without considering broader reforms to avoid the unintended consequences of losing underreimbursed services we care deeply about. Whereas Benz comes from the perspective of large cancer institutions, **Barbara McAneny** offers us a perspective from the physician-owned practice side, an area of cancer care at risk of disappearing thanks to the steamroller of consolidation. She argues that our health-care system "is stacked against community practices in many ways," including reimbursement models that favor large hospitals and cancer centers over smaller practices.

Part 2 opens with the broader lens demanded by our conception of a New Deal, looking at how cancer policy affects different communities and the role of patients in policy. **Matt K. Nguyen** and **Otis W. Brawley** reject the "flawed view that biological factors constitute a key driver of racial disparities in cancer," and instead target what they view as the "root causes of cancer disparities—namely structural barriers to high-quality prevention, screening, diagnosis, and treatment among populations of color." Like Yabroff, they highlight access to health insurance as a driver of disparities along with socioeconomic disparities that have not been linked to cancer as often as they should—pointing out, for example, the proven link between lack of access to education and cancer outcomes. These themes are picked up by **Blase N. Polite** and **Lindsay F. Wiley**, who offer concrete examples of state and local governments that have developed strategies to address cancer disparities—from proper screenings, to tackling financial burdens, to promoting concrete steps that support healthier living. They argue that it is a moral obligation of governments to address these inequities and work to dismantle the pillars of structural racism in the US health-care system.

Health inequities and poor cancer outcomes have been deepened by a failure to invest in public health, as **Melinda L. Irwin, Abigail S. Friedman, Nicole C. Deziel,** and **Linda M. Niccolai** detail. Looking at identifying modifiable risk factors that public health interventions can address and that are critical to cancer prevention, the authors use tobacco, obesity, environmental carcinogens, and human papillomavirus (HPV) as examples where we underperform because we do not equally invest in prevention alongside the scientific research.

In his address at the signing of the National Cancer Act, Nixon emphasized that "a total national commitment means more than government. It means all the voluntary activities must also continue." **Nancy Goodman** and **Sherry Lansing** offer a pair of chapters about their groundbreaking work as cancer advocates—a space both moved into after deeply personal cancer losses. Goodman's focus has been on childhood cancers, working to pass new laws through Congress that help incentivize pediatric cancer R&D despite the financial disincentives and other hurdles that have prevented adequate progress in that field. Lansing, a noted entertainment executive, cofounded Stand Up To Cancer, which uses its platform to harness the private sector to break down silos and fragmentation that impede R&D—for instance, the organization funds grants that explicitly require recipients to work across institutions.

New science brings new challenges for regulators and physicians alike. In Part 3, **Aphrothiti J. Hanrahan, Gurshan S. Gill,** and **David B. Solit** discuss the paradigm shift in cancer drug development toward targeted and immune-based therapies. These groundbreaking treatments are most effective in molecularly defined subsets of patients, with therapy selection increasingly guided by real-time testing for the genetic mutations or other molecular changes responsible for cancer development in individual patients. This approach, referred to as precision oncology, requires innovative clinical trial designs and regulatory flexibility to facilitate the testing of more personalized targeted, immune-based, and cellular therapies. And because drugs will be effective in only small subsets of cancer patients or even in a single individual, ensuring affordability while addressing the expenses of developing tailored treatments will be a pressing challenge in coming years.

For practicing physicians, all the developments discussed above have revolutionized the nature of clinical practice. **Neal J. Meropol** and **Eric P. Winer** describe the sea-change practitioners have experienced in recent decades. Whereas a cancer diagnosis was once a death sentence, oncology today is more multifaceted, with new emphases on shared decision-making between doctors and patients, the growing importance of survivorship, and the development of multimodal teams. New pressures have also emerged—including consolidation, the challenges of incorporating new innovations and technologies at a rapid clip, and the burdens placed on practicing doctors of having to implement even ultimately beneficial practices, such as electronic health records. On the research side, **Cynthia Jung, Kenna Shaw, Arjun Mody, Barrett J. Rollins,** and **Charles L. Sawyers** offer a deep look into new legal and regulatory challenges posed for research by precision oncology. Widespread adoption of tumor sequencing into current clinical oncology practice has provided the opportunity to create linked registries, but this has not happened at the scale and pace needed to power precision medicine. Fragmentation reemerges as a theme, with vital data currently scattered among the public, academic, and private sectors. Future reforms must meet the need to reinvent data and privacy protections to guard patients while still allowing clinical genomic data collection that spans all relevant sectors—from the public through the academic and private.

Finally, **Cary Gross, Stacie B. Dusetzina,** and **Ezekiel J. Emanuel** diagnose a slew of problems with how we pay for cancer, what we pay, and what we pay for. They highlight several vital areas, including underperformance in the prevention space, overly aggressive care and screening, conflicts of interest in clinical care, and the need to reshape the way we pay for drugs.

Part 4 returns to where the War on Cancer began—with the government. **Gideon Blumenthal** details the evolution of cancer R&D, highlighting pressing issues regarding costs and redundancy in drug development. Blumenthal looks ahead to new efforts from the Biden administration to fund high-risk, high-reward projects that aim to work with a variety of groups, including venture capitalists, academic researchers, and drug manufacturers to "de-risk" investments in future cures that might otherwise not be prioritized. He also calls for a further reduction in red tape within the clinical trials enterprise, including cutting out needless measures that add to burdens on patients and investigators while slowing down the development process.

Turning beyond the FDA to a broader view of the sweeping federal bureaucracy, **Shelagh Foster, Shimere Sherwood,** and

Richard L. Schilsky identify overlaps, silos, and fragmentation across the key US federal agencies engaged with cancer. They find that the large number of federal agencies involved in cancer research and treatment can present barriers to advancing cancer care by imposing regulatory roadblocks, engaging in uncoordinated efforts, or failing to keep pace with the breakneck speed at which cancer research is advancing. They argue that the first fifty years since the passage of the National Cancer Act saw the US build an expansive infrastructure to support cancer care and research, but that the next fifty should address how best to harness all its power.

Cary Gross and **Deborah Schrag** widen the lens even further, reminding us of the importance of state governments and the state regulatory landscape for cancer. States play a central role in areas ranging from insurance regulation to public health, and are given wide latitude to set cancer control priorities according to local needs, resources, and culture. This makes the states potentially powerful innovators for cancer policy, but it also raises concerns about profound inequity across the country depending on which state one resides in.

Congress, of course, remains a central player. As **Congresswoman Rosa L. DeLauro** and **Abbe R. Gluck** detail, federal legislation touches almost every aspect of cancer—from expanding insurance access, to protecting patient data privacy, to incentivizing the development of potentially lifesaving drugs. Congress makes big choices in this space, whether it's a choice to fund one specific cancer over another or to fund basic research over translational. And, perhaps most critically, Congress holds the purse strings. What Congress decides to fund—and what it decides to underfund, such as prevention—sets the programmatic priorities and signals to the nation what is most "important." But even as Congress engages with nearly all aspects of the cancer space, the authors argue that they must be viewed more holistically rather than as separate efforts—a 360-degree approach that views equity, prevention, access to insurance and the social safety net, R&D, pricing, and more as part of a single, coherent problem.

Finally, **Greg Simon** and **Allison Rabkin Golden** take us to another moonshot—the Obama-Biden administration's Cancer

Moonshot—while looking ahead to President Biden's renewed efforts to address cancer today. The 2016 Moonshot was not one rocket aimed at a single destination, or even an effort envisioned as driven by the federal government. Instead, the Obama-Biden Moonshot sought to harness the unique platform of the presidency to address fragmentation and lack of collaboration and data sharing, and convince actors from across the government and beyond to work together and share their efforts as never before. Looking ahead, Simon and Rabkin Golden see the government's response to the COVID-19 pandemic as a powerful example of what government can do—quickly and well—when agencies are coordinated and government uses its power to "remove barriers to the rapid development and testing of new therapies." They argue that continuing to expand on that effort in the service of cancer is essential—with presidential leadership vital to the effort. But they also argue, as does virtually every chapter of the book more broadly, that today's vision for the future of cancer policy must be wider and more ambitious. It should take into account not only the government, but also the private sector—and not only cancer science, but also the importance of socioeconomic factors as well as the pressing work of dismantling health inequities root and branch so that we may truly achieve what we set out to do.

"EVERYONE WHO IS BORN holds dual citizenship," Susan Sontag famously wrote, "in the kingdom of the well and in the kingdom of the sick."[4] We did not win the War on Cancer but the breakthroughs of the past fifty years have been extraordinary. We recognize the accomplishments in cancer biology, prevention, and treatment since passage of the National Cancer Act, but we remain a long way from declaring mission accomplished. With the great advances in the prevention and therapy of heart disease witnessed in the twentieth century, cancer is now the leading cause of mortality among Americans under the age of eighty. Our continuing commitment to scientific progress requires a parallel commitment to progress when it comes to people, institutions, providers, and regulators of cancer. It requires attention to public health and prevention; the economics for patients and providers alike; racial justice and health equity; fragmentation and siloing; and inefficiencies, redundancies, and waste.

In his 1962 speech on the original moonshot, President John F. Kennedy stated, "We set sail on this new sea because there is new knowledge to be gained, and new rights to be won, and they must be won and used for the progress of all people." Cancer is among the greatest medical challenges of the twenty-first century, and both its challenges and solutions reflect the larger, fundamental need to accelerate innovation and novel approaches across the gamut of biomedical research—while at the same time pushing us to think beyond the science to the myriad other structures and institutions that deliver those innovations to the sick.

It calls for a New Deal, all-hands-on-deck approach to a multimodal problem that reinvests in the nation for the general welfare of all its people.

Notes

1. US Congress, Senate, Committee on Labor and Public Welfare, *A National Program for the Conquest of Cancer: Report*, 91st Congress, 2nd sess., 1970, S. Rep. 91-1402.

2. Rebecca L. Siegel, Kimberly D. Miller, and Ahmedin Jemal, "Cancer Statistics, 2020," *CA: A Cancer Journal for Clinicians* 70, no. 1 (2020): 7–30, https://acsjournals.onlinelibrary.wiley.com/doi/10.3322/caac.21590.

3. American Cancer Society, *Cancer Treatment & Survivorship Facts & Figures 2019–2021* (Atlanta: American Cancer Society, 2019), https://www.cancer.org/content/dam/cancer-org/research/cancer-facts-and-statistics/cancer-treatment-and-survivorship-facts-and-figures/cancer-treatment-and-survivorship-facts-and-figures-2019-2021.pdf; National Academies of Sciences, Engineering, and Medicine, *Guiding Cancer Control: A Path to Transformation*, eds. Michael M. E. Johns et al. (Washington, DC: National Academies Press, 2019), https://doi.org/10.17226/25438.

4. Susan Sontag, "Illness as Metaphor," *New York Review of Books*, January 26, 1978, https://www.nybooks.com/articles/1978/01/26/illness-as-metaphor/.

PART ONE

CANCER CARE TODAY: WHERE WE ARE AND WHO PAYS

CHAPTER 1

The New Borders of Cancerland

Siddhartha Mukherjee

I was trained as an oncologist and cancer biologist in the 2000s. As that decade began, newspapers echoed the language of the early 1970s in articles about treatment advances. Cancer's Achilles' heel would be found as surely as we could create a "magic bullet" for cancer itself. And some of those magic bullet medicines have, indeed, arrived. For certain forms of breast cancer, for prostate cancer, some blood cancers, we are inhabiting a new era of medical therapy. But here, rather than concentrate on therapies alone, I want to turn to a different question. Cancer is appropriately perceived as a disease of risk—genetic or heritable risks, lifestyle risks, and the unknown risks of chance. How does this view of cancer as a looming risk alter our medical and cultural relationship with disease? What effect does a risk-based culture create? The oncologist David Scadden called his book *Cancerland*,[1] borrowing that word from popular culture (see, for instance, Barbara Ehrenreich's essay, "Welcome to Cancerland"[2]); it is a word that patients use as they countenance their diagnosis and all the medical, cultural, and social contours that change with the diagnosis.

Most of the chapters in this book think about how to reform the system—the structures of cancer access, research, and treatment. That is critical work. But we—the patients, policy makers,

Siddhartha Mukherjee is Assistant Professor of Medicine at Columbia University Medical Center and Pulitzer Prize–winning author of *The Emperor of All Maladies*.

and providers reading this book—must also keep in mind how the system shapes us. As we begin this next fifty years of the "War on Cancer," we have begun to quantify risks for patients—even *before* they get cancer. The borders of "Cancerland" have begun to feel all-encompassing. In the past, entry into Cancerland was reserved for those with the diagnosis of cancer. But as we move to a risk mitigation and risk assessment model of cancer, we are all becoming citizens with permanent passports.

The shifting borders of this new land hinge on this language of risk: minimizing it, identifying it, managing it. Everyone, in one way or another, slowly becomes a citizen. Yet as we all become cancer patients, how do we exist in a world defined by surveillance, identification of risk, and early detection?

Charting these frontiers leads to an old insight supported by new research. A wealth of data gathered over the past twenty years points to the fact that there are multiple levels of cancer control. One of the major problems we confront is determining how to harmonize them in a way that is more coordinated and integrated than what we know today. Identifying the levels of cancer control also allows us to create a funneled assessment of and response to cancer. This involves lessening harmful exposures and extends to the identification of those at risk. It includes our ability to detect cancer as early as possible while minimizing overdiagnosis. A funneled approach would then consider whether someone's cancer is more likely to progress based on an understanding of host characteristics and the interaction between the host and the tumor. Lastly, where treatment is needed, the aim becomes finding the least toxic therapies. By this point, funneling would hopefully have allowed us to conserve resources best used for those who require the most effective and least toxic treatments.

As we enter this experiment, as we try to create road maps and models for ourselves and for our patients, we must remember the cultural impact of welcoming ourselves and others into Cancerland will outlast and outlive us.

Cancer, Our Genes, and the Anxiety
of Risk-Based Medicine

In the summer of 2005, I met a woman, Laura M., whose life had been overturned by cancer. But she was disease-free: it was the anxiety of cancer in the future that haunted her.

Laura had been diagnosed with a primary tumor in her breast that was small and localized. She had had surgery, radiation, and chemotherapy—a standard treatment protocol—and had then come to see me, an oncologist, to help manage her future care. I suggested doing nothing. Everything about her case suggested a good prognosis; we all agreed that she had likely been cured. But in the wake of her treatment, she became obsessed by the possibility of a relapse. She scoured her family history and discovered a distant aunt who had died of breast cancer at age seventy. Her own mother had died at a young age from a car accident, but Laura became convinced that had her mother lived, she would have been diagnosed with breast cancer.

Laura's visits to the clinic were punctuated by her sense of doom. She often came in with sheaves of papers that she had printed from the internet about "occult metastasis," which had been found in patients who, like her, were thought to be at low risk. She repeatedly asked me to confirm that she "had been given the most aggressive chemo regimen that could be given." (She had, in fact, been treated with the appropriate regimen recommended for her case.) We checked her for genetic susceptibilities, such as inherited mutations in the BRCA1 and BRCA2 genes that increase cancer risk, but found none. Nonetheless, she asked if she and her daughter could undergo "the most intensive form of cancer surveillance" to detect early cancers in her body.

Laura's story highlights a new anxiety about illness that is permeating our culture. It is the anxiety of being under constant diagnostic surveillance, of inhabiting a state of vigilant watchfulness for illnesses before they can take root in one's body. It is the state, as one patient described it, of "feeling under siege from the future." Emblematic of this anxiety is the concept of a "previvor"—a strange new term invented to describe a person who is a survivor of an illness that she is predisposed toward, but has yet to have. For Laura, these states were contiguous. Her survivorship from one breast cancer had turned overnight, it seemed, into "previvorship" for another breast cancer.

As I write this, two kinds of technologies are radically altering the landscape of cancer risk and screening. The first involves what we might call genetic surveillance—an attempt to quantify an individual's inherited predisposition for cancer (that is, you should be surveyed for the disease because of the higher risk conferred by your genes). The second, in contrast, involves chemical surveillance—an attempt to detect chemical markers of incipient cancers in blood (i.e., you should be surveyed because there is a sign of early cancer circulating in your blood). The two technologies converge to increase the supply of those who are forced to enter the domain of surveillance and screening. Both, in short, encourage people without current cancer, but with the prospect of future cancer, to become citizens or permanent residents of what Susan Sontag once described as "the kingdom of the ill."[3]

Cancer Screening and Cancer Risk

For decades, perhaps centuries, we have known of families where some form of cancer (usually the same type: breast or pancreatic) is manifest in multiple individuals across multiple generations. Not every family member is affected, but the risk of cancer in such a family clearly lies beyond the average risk of cancer in the population.

Until recently, our capacity to identify the culprit genes in such families—or, more actionably, to identify the members of the family who carried the heightened risk—was limited to inherited single-gene mutations. These included mutations in such genes as BRCA1, BRCA2, and MLH1 that, if inherited from parents, increase the likelihood of breast, colon, and other cancers by severalfold over normal individuals. But many human traits, including cancer risk, might not track with single-gene mutations. Take human height as an example. Height is highly heritable—we know that tall parents tend to produce tall children, and shorter parents bear shorter children—yet early attempts to pin down the variation in human height to single-gene variations or mutations revealed only a smattering of candidate genes. (For this chapter, I use the terms *variation* and *mutation* interchangeably, although there are subtle differences.) Geneticists described this conundrum, famously, as the "missing heritability" of height. We could infer from the pattern of inheritance that height-determining genes must exist in the human genome, but their precise identity and number remained unknown.

By similar logic, the inherited risk of cancer might be carried by mutations or variations not in one but in multiple genes, each of which acts together to increase an individual's risk of the disease. In the 1990s, some breast cancer patients began to refer to the next, as-yet-unidentified conglomerate of genes for breast cancer as "BRCA3." That name carried both a sardonic and a hopeful edge. Unlike patients with definite BRCA1 and BRCA2 mutations, patients with potential "BRCA3" mutations remained suspended in an anxious limbo. We could not diagnose a woman with this genetic syndrome yet because we had no idea what these genes might be (a few additional single-gene mutations that increased breast cancer risk were identified in the 2000s, but most patients with breast cancer continued to lack a single-gene explanation). A "BRCA3" patient's experience of her terrifying family history and dread of future disease were just as acute as those of a patient with known cancer-risk mutations, but the genes that precipitated the former patient's fate were hidden from our view. As doctors, we would acknowledge the risk that these patients carried—with their family histories scarred by breast cancer—but we were unable to offer a more tangible description of their susceptibility to the disease.

This state of suspension for polygenic (a.k.a. multigene) diseases is finally being relieved: the combinations of gene mutations responsible for such genetically complex diseases are now being identified by powerful computational technologies. Deep-learning algorithms, in particular, have been unleashed on human genomes. By scanning millions of fully sequenced genomes, these algorithms "learn" to dissect how variations in thousands of genes, each exerting a small effect, might ultimately add up to the heightened risk of an illness—a problem of such mind-boggling permutational complexity that ordinary algorithms had failed to capture it. One machine-learning algorithm has learned to predict human height as the consequence of variations in a thousand-odd genes. (Take a moment to digest this startling fact: such an algorithm might soon predict your actual height, or the future height of your unborn child, based on your genetic sequence alone.) Another deep-learning program is learning to predict the risk of cardiovascular disease—again, likely the consequence of hundreds of gene mutations or variations. With such advances, it is likely that an algorithm might identify those of us at highest genetic risk for future cancers. Of course, for many cancers, even ones that run in families, there is still a powerful influence of chance and the environment. A woman with a BRCA1 mutation might increase her risk for breast cancer through certain exposures, by virtue of inheriting other "modifier" genes or by chance alone. These additional variables are not yet part of the deep-learning landscape but could become incorporated into computational algorithms in the future. This technology, then, could serve as a portal of entry into the world of cancer for potentially millions of men and women who seek to be annotated for future cancer risk and potentially surveyed for cancer.

Advancements in Cancer Detection

While computers seek out patients who have an inherited susceptibility to cancer, other machines are seeking to identify chemicals that might currently be in our blood or other organs that signal cancer risk. Termed *liquid biopsy*, or *liquid surveillance*, these methods attempt to discover minuscule amounts of the products shed or spilled by cancer cells—DNA, proteins, and other substances—into the blood or other circulating tissues. Once such trace signs of an incipient cancer are found, the logic runs, cancer will be detected in its earliest stages and can be attacked with more effective therapies. We will scour the body to find ovarian, lung, and prostate cancers, for instance, before these become clinically manifest, thereby enabling better treatments.

These liquid biopsies run the risk of overdiagnosing patients, however. What if someone is found to carry a liquid marker for ovarian cancer, say, but that ovarian cancer never takes root in her body? Cancer cells, we now know, can exist in a body, or a site within the body, without becoming manifest as clinical disease or a detectable metastasis. (Most likely, this is because the "soil" of a particular organ does not allow the "seed" of a cancer to sprout.) Or what if some of the markers turn out to overlap with benign diseases (as was the case with earlier liquid surveillance markers, such as the prostate-specific antigen test for prostate cancer), thereby increasing the risk of false positive results?

Nonetheless, enthusiasm for the liquid surveillance of cancer seems to grow exponentially each day; one private company that hopes to advance this technology goes by the name Grail, emblematic of the near-religious fervor with which some advocates describe the power of liquid biopsies. Many patients in my cancer clinic now come to their appointments armed with brochures about liquid biopsies, wondering whether their tumors might have been detected earlier had such biopsies been performed. These technologies represent a second portal of entry into the world of cancer. By identifying men and women who might be bearing the first markers of cancer, these methods increase the pool of those who must be surveyed and further screened for the illness.

Identifying Whether Cancer Is Likely to Progress

Once a cancer is diagnosed, whether early or not, our capacity to understand which patient is most likely to progress becomes central. Our understanding of how a cancer might progress in a person has evolved in recent years, hinging on host characteristics as well as the interaction between the host and the tumor. Breast cancer provides one example of how recent insights have come to bear. An improved understanding of tumor signatures allowed us to decrease the use of chemotherapy for certain women who we knew were unlikely to have high-risk disease. We also began to better understand the complex collaboration between cancer and its microenvironment. This could more deeply explain why some cancers are likely to progress, whereas others are not. It also leads to a new set of concerns centered on our understanding of the patient's microenvironment. Are there, for instance, aspects of a specific human body's environment that might restrict metastatic spread? An affirmative answer would mean that we would survey an individual's exposures and genetics while also trying to understand what their immune function is like, the nature of their work, and the many elements that define how a host interacts with a tumor. This could allow us to get some sense of whether a person is likely to have progressive disease, local relapse, or metastatic relapse in contrast to someone else who would be better off receiving no intervention beyond a certain point.

A major project initially based at the Wellcome Sanger Institute in Cambridge, England, has been seeking to identify—first in animals and then in humans—the components of an organism's microenvironment that might restrict metastatic spread. One of the early findings to emerge from this project suggests that many of the early genetic determinants happen to be in immune cells, particularly cells of the innate immune system. Approximately thirty genes have been identified by these studies, with only about 15 to 20 percent having been ascribed simple functions. The other approximately 85 percent are of unknown function, manifesting in animal models as well as in certain human data as restrictors of metastatic spread. Better understanding the microenvironment and its relationship to whether and how a tumor might develop— more clearly charting the relationship between "seed" and "soil"— could also impact how cancer is treated.

Finding the Right Treatment

Having followed our road map this far—identifying those at risk of cancer while potentially reducing risk, detecting cancer early, and determining those whose cancer is more likely to progress— how should we think about treatment when it is needed? Finding the least toxic therapies is key. Immunological therapy was not available when I was in training but has subsequently emerged as an effective treatment for several cancers. I once made a personal bet that I did not think that during my lifetime we would ever find an effective treatment for smoking-related lung cancer. The fact that that has happened—at least in some cases of this form of cancer—is a testament to how little we knew back then of other forms of controlling cancer cells as well as of the biology of cancer in general.

There are signs of other intriguing treatment avenues ahead. Take the CANTOS trial as an example. The primary focus of the trial was to try to decrease the risk of cardiovascular disease. The researchers were attempting to test whether there was an inflammatory component to cardiovascular disease caused by inflammatory cells that were ultimately depositing plaque. As a side study, the researchers analyzed data for patients at higher risk for lung cancer. For that cohort, a question was whether a sophisticated anti-inflammatory approach was at play. Results from that study have been used in subsequent research trying to understand whether risk of death from lung cancer or the development of lung cancer can be decreased based on the use of an anti-inflammatory strategy that targets the microenvironment.

There are also new approaches that are much more bespoke—and much more expensive—for certain cancers. Chimeric antigen receptor T cell (CAR-T) therapy, which is a type of human immune engineering, provides one example. Here, T cells are extracted from a patient's body. They are then genetically modified to make them attack her tumor cells before being reinfused back into her body. This is a complex and expensive technology, one that has proven to be successful in a small number of cases by reengineering the immune system to target cancer cells in particular.

Considering these treatments opens onto deeper, as yet unresolved, questions. While we know immune cells contribute to the microenvironment, what other cells play a meaningful part? Widening out even further, what metabolic pathways are Achilles' heels for human cancers? Another insight that has emerged over the past decade addresses microenvironmental failure in cancer—the role of inflammation, immune cell control, and checkpoint deregulation. Could we imagine augmenting immunological strategies with metabolic and other strategies to more effectively treat cancer?

Cancer as a "Total Institution"

What are we to make of these advances, and how will early detection and risk assessment in particular impact the future of cancer as experienced by those who have it and those who fear getting it? My aim is to neither exaggerate nor minimize the transformative potential of these technologies, although it is worth emphasizing this at the outset. The capacity to identify humans with an increased genetic risk for cancer, coupled with the possibility of detecting cancer at its earliest stages using a liquid biopsy, might radically change how we prevent, detect, and treat cancer. But my concern is the effect that such surveillance might have on our bodies and societies.

In the 1950s, the sociologist Erving Goffman wrote a remarkable article about the concept of a "total institution," an idea that he expanded in subsequent work. "A total institution," Goffman explained in his 1961 book *Asylums*, is one "where a great number of similarly situated people, cut off from the wider community for a considerable time, together lead an enclosed, formally administered round of life."[4] Total institutions, such as mental hospitals, prisons, and even boarding schools, have rituals of entry and exit. They inculcate belonging. They invent their own vocabulary and codes of behavior; they have an internal logic, impenetrable to others. They encourage surveillance and create anxiety: members are united by a common sense of purpose, by the feeling of being chosen or marked. Those who are expelled may feel a sense of betrayal, while those who remain can be consumed by the guilt of survivorship.

Cancer, too, runs the risk of becoming a "total institution." A patient, once diagnosed, may be whisked away into a cancer ward, dressed in a patient's smock—"a tragicomically cruel costume, no less blighting than a prisoner's jumpsuit," as I wrote in *The Emperor of All Maladies*—and stripped of his identity.[5] When I once asked a woman with a rare sarcoma about her life outside the hospital, she observed, "I am in the hospital even when I am outside the hospital."

In this new era of cancer treatment, I wonder whether we are unwittingly, but insidiously, intensifying the totality of the "cancer institution" for patients. For people like Laura M., cancer has certainly become a total institution—or a "cancer world." They are in either treatment, remission, surveillance, maintenance, or resurveillance. Mavens of early detection are also working on deep-learning algorithms that will pick up cancerous lesions on patients' imaging results and classify them as malignant, using criteria that seem to defy even the most acute human eye. In an April 2017 article in the *New Yorker*, I wrote about one of the pioneers of this idea, the German computer scientist Sebastian Thrun.[6] Thrun imagines a world in which even the daily instruments of our normal lives are morphed into weapons of diagnostic surveillance—a bathtub that scans your body to detect abnormal masses that might require investigation; a mirror that could check your body for precancerous moles; a computer program that (with your consent) would scour your Instagram or Facebook page while you slept at night, evaluating changes in your photographs that might signal signs of cancer.

Then there's the question of treatment and cost. If an additional tumor—clinically undetectable, but discovered by these novel methods—were detected in Laura M.'s case and the primary lesion removed, what criteria would we use to determine whether we should use some form of adjuvant (extra) medicine, such as cell-killing chemotherapy or targeted therapy, after the initial surgical removal, as is often done for most cancers? The costs of such surveillance and treatment—an astronomical amount if every human had to be genetically annotated, subjected to surveillance, and treated if a tumor was found—would overwhelm current projections of medical costs (although in the most optimistic scenario, the benefits would also be amplified in lives saved via early diagnosis). Thorny issues of overdiagnosis and overtreatment would have to be addressed. We would have to devise careful guidelines about when not to act and whom not to treat.

For Laura M., the answer to each of these questions carries immense consequences. She has entered a strange new world, one of constant diagnostic surveillance; of dealing with the anxiety of relapse and maintenance; of that peculiar desolation of the shuttle from clinical trial to clinical trial, and from hospital to hospital, as she tries to keep one step ahead in this chess game against cancer; and of watching doctors pit their will, wit, and imagination against a formidable enemy that keeps changing its shape. This world has created its own internal vocabulary. A "haircut party" is a celebration thrown in honor of a person about to enter the cancer world as a sign of solidarity, even if the patient is spared hair loss–inducing chemo. "No Exit chemo," as a patient of mine put it, describes the fact that a unique personalized chemo regimen for a patient produces unique toxicities, the phrase "No Exit" borrowed from the Jean-Paul Sartre play in which every human being is assigned his or her own personal hell.

"A world in which cancer is normalized as a manageable chronic condition would be a wonderful thing," medical historian Steven Shapin wrote in a 2010 review of *The Emperor of All Maladies*.[7] "But a risk-factor world in which we all think of ourselves as precancerous would not," he continued. "It might decrease the incidence of some forms of malignancy while hugely increasing the numbers of healthy people under medical treatment. It would be a strange victory in which the price to be paid for checking the spread of cancer through the body is its uncontrolled spread through the culture."

One could argue that Shapin ignores how routine surveillance for other formerly fatal conditions has become woven into our lives to little or no ill consequence: no scientist bemoans the cultural and medical surveillance of, for the sake of argument, cardiac disease. We do not suffer overmuch from automobile safety having dramatically altered our driving habits either. Yet perhaps precisely because cancer encompasses so many different *cancers*, the cultural shift feels totalizing, unstoppable. The very title of this volume hints at the difference: we are in a total war, a century war, with cancer.

The metaphor is telling: total war does not care for its cultural or psychological consequences, but only for vanquishing the enemy. Perhaps the true battle of the next fifty years is to envision ourselves not at war, but at the precipice of a great cultural shift, mediated by cancer, in how Americans collectively conceive of illness and health. The shape of that shift—its borders, to turn back to Cancerland—will depend on how we orient the next fifty years. What shape will the surveillance of cancer take: will it be a great civil project in which all Americans partake, a project of justice? Or will the most vulnerable among us see their health insurance curtailed as we increase genomic surveillance and curtail privacy laws, all while the elites bemoan the inability of "disadvantaged populations" to curtail their smoking or overeating? Will we allow anxiety to dominate our cultural attitude toward risk, or will we find a balance between curative therapies and the condition of being mortal?

To date, Laura M. has not suffered from a relapse of breast cancer. Nor, fortunately, has she had a new cancer anywhere in her body. But the "strange victory" over her body has not spared her mind. She remains haunted by the future prospect of illness. When Sontag wrote of a passport between the kingdom of the well and the kingdom of the ill, she imagined a bidirectional passage: men and women might pass into illness, but some would return to wellness. In inventing cancer's new surveillance culture, I fear that we have closed the borders of the kingdoms. I fear that we now possess one-way passports into the realm of illness. What we will find there in these next fifty years is up to us.

Notes

Portions of this chapter were previously published in *HealthAffairs*: Siddhartha Mukherjee, "Cancer, Our Genes, and the Anxiety of Risk-Based Medicine," *HealthAffairs* 37, no. 5 (2018): 817-820, https://doi.org/10.1377/hlthaff.2018.0344.

1. David Scadden, *Cancerland: A Medical Memoir* (New York: Thomas Dunne Books, 2018).
2. Barbara Ehrenreich, "Welcome to Cancerland," *Harper's Magazine*, November 2001, 43–53.

3. Susan Sontag, "Illness as Metaphor," *New York Review of Books*, January 26, 1978, https://www.nybooks.com/articles/1978/01/26/illness-as-metaphor/.

4. Erving Goffman, *Asylums: Essays on the Social Situation of Mental Patients and Other Inmates* (New York: Anchor Books, 1961), 13.

5. Siddhartha Mukherjee, *The Emperor of All Maladies: A Biography of Cancer* (New York: Simon and Schuster, 2011), 4.

6. Siddhartha Mukherjee, "A.I. versus M.D.: What Happens When Diagnosis Is Automated?" *New Yorker*, March 27, 2017, https://www.newyorker.com/magazine/2017/04/03/ai-versus-md.

7. Steven Shapin, "Cancer World: The Making of a Modern Disease," *New Yorker*, November 8, 2010.

CHAPTER 2

A View from the Ground

The Changing Landscape of Cancer Care

Randall A. Oyer and Erin O. Aakhus

The following are two people: Michael, with a common cancer, and Lisa, with a rare cancer.

Michael is 53 years old, with colon cancer identified during a routine colonoscopy. Michael is able to access surgery followed by preventative chemotherapy in his home community. However, his family history of cancer, as well as pathology findings, indicate the need for cancer genetics counselor services not available locally. Genetics consultation, accessed via telemedicine with an academic medical center, identifies Lynch hereditary cancer syndrome, providing an opportunity to prevent colon cancer in his first-degree relatives, all of whom would be at 50 percent risk of having the same inherited cancer risk gene mutation.

Lisa is 47 years old and notices a lump in her left neck. The patient has a strong family history of cancer, but has not

---

Randall A. Oyer is Medical Director of the Oncology Program at Lancaster General Hospital.

Erin O. Aakhus is Medical Director, Penn Medicine Anne B. Barshinger Cancer Institute.

had prior medical problems. Outpatient biopsy in the local hospital yields unusual results requiring pathology consultation at a distant academic medical center that identifies a rare sarcoma. Lisa then requires multidisciplinary consultation, staging, preoperative chemotherapy, proton radiation, and complex multiorgan surgery with reconstruction available only at an academic medical center. Her sarcoma and family history are recognized as Li Fraumeni syndrome, a high-penetrance hereditary cancer predisposition with profound family implications for multiple types of cancer in children and adults, typically cared for in the academic setting.

Where these patients received cancer care ultimately differed based on the type of cancer identified. Michael, having a common cancer, can stay in the community for the majority of cancer care; however, Lisa, having a rare type of cancer, requires academic specialty consultation and complex care. While the type of cancer is not the only factor influencing where someone receives care, Michael and Lisa's different experiences of cancer in the United States provide a jumping-off point for a larger discussion. Here, we—two oncologists working in different settings, one in community and academic practices since 1986, one in academic and government (Veterans Administration [VA]) practices since 2016—parse out the often-indistinct boundaries between academic and community-based oncology services, as well as government providers.[1] As practicing oncologists, we have been present "on the ground" to witness how the entanglement of these four care locations has its roots in the origins of cancer care in the United States.

Cancer care in the US took form during an era of transformation in both scientific advancement and health-care policy. Although federal investment established the National Cancer Institute (NCI) in 1937, chemotherapy did not find success until the 1950s. In subsequent decades, newly discovered cancer drugs remained inaccessible to most Americans. The 1971 National Cancer Act infused $100 million into cancer research, resulting in the establishment of fifteen federally funded research programs (i.e.,

NCI-designated Cancer Centers) across the country. This expansion brought increased capacity to conduct cancer clinical trials and to train cancer specialists providing care from coast to coast.

Staffed by increasing numbers of academically trained cancer specialists, community-based oncology programs took hold in the 1980s. In this early phase of medical oncology, most patients received chemotherapy infusions while admitted to a hospital. However, medical advancement and changes in health-care reimbursement policy would soon facilitate a transition of chemotherapy to the outpatient setting.

In the early 1980s, revisions to Medicare allowed cancer centers to receive reimbursement for outpatient visits, which, along with cancer care improvements, such as infusion pumps and effective antinausea medications, largely shifted chemotherapy administration from the hospital to an outpatient setting. Declining revenue for inpatient stays led hospital-based oncology units to consolidate or close. Similarly, as outpatient reimbursement has declined, more than 50 percent of oncology practices that were independent in 2007 were integrated with hospitals by 2017.[2]

The workforce of oncology has also changed dramatically since the 1990s. In US cancer care, it comprises medical oncologists, surgeons, pathologists, radiologists, allied health professionals, clinical nurse specialists, and multidisciplinary team coordinators. From the 1990s to 2017, the number of cancer specialists per capita in the US more than doubled, increasing from 1.8 to 4.8 medical oncologists per 100,000 Americans.[3] However, while oncology practices are decreasing, the number of oncologists working per practice grows. In 2017, more than 80 percent of US oncology practices were supported by advanced practitioners, including physician assistants (PAs) and nurse practitioners (NPs).[4] This is notable, as it demonstrates major shifts in where cancer treatment is provided (from small to large practices) and who provides it (from physicians to advanced practitioners).

Whereas most cancer care provided in the community setting is not experimental, community-based oncologists maintain strong connections with academic centers and ongoing clinical research through national societies and research networks. To support these

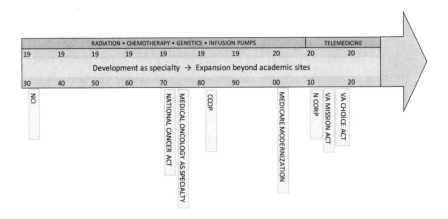

FIGURE 2.1 Trajectory of Cancer Care over Time

alliances and to increase participation in clinical research outside the academic setting, the NCI launched a series of initiatives: the Community Clinical Oncology Program (1983), the NCI Community Cancer Centers Program (NCCCP) (2007), and the NCI Community Oncology Research Program (2014). Today, integration of academic and community oncology care continues to enhance patient access to specialized providers and technologies.

Figure 2.1 depicts a timeline of medical advances in parallel with legislation and national programs that provided structural support for the expansion of cancer care from academia to the community.

Relationship Between Cancer Care and Geography

Where cancer centers are located throughout the United States is driven largely by supply and demand. For example, the southern US, which has the largest proportion (38%) of newly diagnosed cancer patients, likewise has the largest concentration of cancer practices (33%) (Figure 2.2).[5] Despite this grossly proportional regional distribution of oncologists, many cancer patients reside in geographic areas that remain underserved. In 2017, only 7 percent of oncologists worked in rural areas, where 19.3 percent of US citizens reside. The majority of oncology specialists are located in major cities or close suburbs.[6] The geographic distribution of

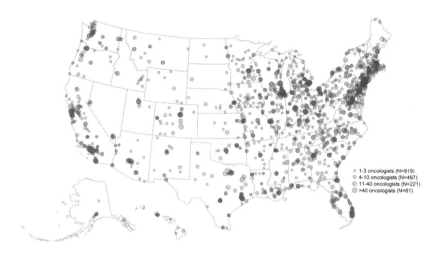

1-3 oncologists (N=919)
4-10 oncologists (N=497)
11-40 oncologists (N=221)
>40 oncologists (N=61)

FIGURE 2.2 Geographic Distribution of Oncologists

the oncology workforce is influenced largely by both professional aspirations (research versus patient care) and salary.[7] This distribution likely contributes to disparities in access to cancer care. Although the percentage of oncologists in rural areas rose from 5.5 percent in 2014 to 7.4 percent in 2019, rural locations are still less likely to have even a single oncologist, rural hospitals have closed at a greater rate than have metropolitan hospitals, and the oncologist-per-population ratio has fallen still lower: 20 percent of rural Americans live more than sixty minutes from an oncologist.

Electronic Health Records

Technology also plays a significant role in cancer care administration. Regardless of where cancer care is provided, the electronic health record (EHR) serves as a billing tool and as a record of care. However, due to lack of integration across institutions, the EHR is underutilized as a tool for care delivery or care improvement. Important information remains trapped in unstructured data because point-of-care natural language processing tools are not readily available. Learning across sites of care is limited to the current status of bioinformatics and health-care delivery research.

This chapter reviews the unique features, capabilities, and challenges characteristic of these four settings: academic research centers, community practices, small private oncology practices, and government providers. Through this careful comparison, we are able to recommend policy measures for the next fifty years of equitable, comprehensive, coordinated cancer care.

Academic Research Centers

The three-part mission of academic research centers, driven by the National Cancer Act of 1971, includes research, education, and patient care.[8] In 1971, fifteen NCI-designated cancer centers across the country received federal funding to establish state-of-the art centers for research, clinical care, and cancer control. Today, fifty-one NCI-designated centers, most of which exist within an academic institution, support clinical and translational research, transdisciplinary disease expertise, and a spectrum of specialty training programs in cancer care. Modern oncology care began in academic medical centers, which continue to yield discoveries that inform the cancer care provided across all other settings. Academic medical centers provide care services unavailable in other settings, develop and lead trials of new therapeutics, and communicate new best practices and guidelines.

Scope of Services

Academic medical centers provide a range of services often unavailable in other settings, including access to subspecialty care. Subspecialties in cancer care include, but are not limited to, medical, surgical, radiation, gynecologic, and pediatric oncology. While subspecialists in these areas may practice in the community, academic cancer centers are set up to support narrowly disease-focused multidisciplinary teams that provide patients with complex, coordinated, and high-quality treatment plans. Academic centers provide high-risk treatments, such as stem cell transplantation, which require expertise in execution as well as complex care coordination for survivors. Also, academic research centers are distinguished from community providers in their ability to devote resources to the study and treatment of rare diseases and disease subtypes (e.g., sarcomas or cancers caused by rare genetic syndromes). For instance, Lisa, with a rare sarcoma, benefits from the expertise and experience of an academic team of medical, radiation, and surgical oncologists who focus entirely on this rare disease.

Research

A central mission of academic research centers is to bring scientific discoveries from the laboratory into practice through clinical trials. Whereas community practices are increasingly involved in clinical research, many early-phase trials require close collaboration between practicing academic oncologists who have framed clinical questions that need to be solved in the laboratory. To safely execute investigations, academic centers employ integrated research teams that include laboratory-based and clinical physician-scientists, regulatory experts, statisticians, trial coordinators, and bioethicists. Academic centers receive substantial financial support from government institutions, industry sponsors, and charitable foundations to conduct such research.

Accessibility and Economic Challenges

Cancer care networks are one solution to extend accessibility of the specialized cancer care provided at academic centers. Increasingly, academic cancer centers form alliances with community oncology practices though acquisition or affiliation agreements. Ideally, these networks facilitate cancer patients receiving benefits of both academic and community care on an as-needed basis, decreasing inequalities in certain areas. For example, Michael, discussed earlier, could receive coordinated follow-up with a cancer geneticist based at a distant academic center while receiving routine surgery and chemotherapy in his community. Through this hub-and-spoke model of cancer care, community-based professionals benefit from the expertise of academic institutions while providing patient-centered care in diverse geographic areas.

In turn, academic institutions benefit through catchment expansion. Academic research centers provide high-level consultations at the request of patients, families, and community oncologists despite the time and resources necessary for records review and the consultation itself, which are not economically supported unless the consultations lead to treatment (surgery, radiation, chemotherapy). This may put academic physicians and their practices in competition with referring physicians and their practices. Such competition can directly affect a patient such as Lisa, who may be encouraged to receive all future cancer evaluation and care that exceeds the scope of the request posed or needed by the referring community oncologist in the academic medical center, rather than in the community.

Community Practices

About 63 percent of US cancer patients are treated in the community setting every year through care delivery, cancer screening, treatment, and clinical research.[9]

Scope of Services

Community oncologists range from generalists who see all cancers and blood disorders to those (mostly in larger group settings) who subspecialize in one or several cancer types. Owing to a strong mission to provide evidence-based and high-quality cancer care across all cancer types, community oncologists maintain broad competency in various cancer types via self-directed continuing education, multidisciplinary prospective treatment planning meetings, and through regular use of electronically available evidence-based guidelines.

For select complex and recurrent cancers, community-based practitioners often collaborate with academic institutions that provide advanced treatments or services. As illustrated earlier, the community hospital where Michael received treatment is not unusual in its practice to refer to an academic medical center for genetic counseling and testing. Many community hospitals would not be able to provide the subspecialization and multidisciplinary teams required for Lisa and her family.

Research

Research in this setting is relevant but challenging due to financial barriers for the majority of community-based cancer programs. Recognizing the need to share research benefits with patients receiving care in the community, the NCI has promoted clinical research in the community setting through the Community Clinical Oncology Program (CCOP) and its successor, the NCI Community Oncology Research Program (NCORP). In past years, CCOP contributed one-third of NCI clinical treatment enrollment and nearly all cancer prevention and control enrollment.[10] However, the cost of doing research through NCI cooperative groups can be prohibitive for community practices. The case reimbursement rate for cooperative group trials is approximately $2,000, compared to the actual case cost of approximately $6,000. Inadequate funding has been cited by practices as a factor that limits their participation in cooperative group trials.[11] Other community-based research groups, including private-practice US Oncology, the Sarah Cannon Research Institute, and the nonprofit Hoosier Cancer Research Network, conduct innovative cancer research in a combination of community and academic sites. Community-based cancer research programs typically have a mixed trials portfolio that includes not only cooperative group trials, but also innovative industry-sponsored trials that have a more sustainable funding model.

Accessibility and Economic Challenges

Across the US, a community oncology practice is within an hour's drive for 90 percent of cancer patients, providing crucial accessibility and convenience. By comparison, nearly 30 percent would have to drive more than one hour to reach an academic research center.[12] Additionally, time to treatment initiation, defined as the number of days from diagnosis to first treatment, is shorter in the community center compared to academic centers.[13] This may be due to a number of factors including limited capacity as well as the actual time involved in planning and coordinating complex care for the types of cancers requiring care in the academic compared to the community setting.

In addition to higher accessibility, cancer care in the community setting is typically less expensive than in the academic setting. The mean monthly cost to the patient for cancer care in the community outpatient clinic setting has been reported at $12,548, compared with $20,060 in a hospital-owned practice.[14] Perhaps due to a lack of transparency, it is unclear whether patient preferences are influenced by these differences in costs.

Practices that provide cancer care in the community face economic challenges that include increasing operational costs, rising costs of drug procurement, unreimbursed investments in the EHR, and time and expense due to insurance prior-authorization and denials. The American Society of Clinical Oncology (ASCO) has reported annual decreases in the total number of active practices as well as increase in practice size, noting that hospital acquisition of oncology practices is more prevalent and increasing at a faster rate in oncology than in other medical specialties.[15] In 2018, the Community Oncology Alliance reported closure of 423 oncology clinics and acquisition of 658 practices over a two-year period.[16]

Medical oncology practices of all types are challenged by costly, complex, and unreimbursed holistic services required under alternative payment models, such as the patient-centered medical home (PCMH) model and the Oncology Care Model (OCM). Due to extra services and time provided, the PCMH can successfully reduce emergency room (ER) visits by 15 to 50 percent and inpatient admissions by 10 to 40 percent.[17] Savings to the payer in such models may not translate to an economic benefit equal to additional care coordination expenses incurred by the community practice, however, calling into question the economic sustainability of this approach in all settings.

Small Private Oncology Practices

The success of small private oncology practices (fewer than six providers) is dependent upon accessibility and strong physician-patient relationships. In 2017, most oncology practices were small and employed somewhere between one and five oncologists.[18] However, in recent years, mergers, acquisitions, and closures have prompted fewer oncologists to open or maintain these types of practices.

Scope of Services

In contrast to academic medical centers or larger community practices, small private oncology practices comprise general hematologist-oncologists providing broad expertise in all types of cancer and blood disorders. Providers in small oncology practices are limited in the type of multidisciplinary care they may have in-house to treat and support complex cases. For example, the majority of services other than chemotherapy (e.g., surgical and radiation oncology) received by both Michael and Lisa would not be available within a small medical oncology office and would require referral to other practices.

Research

Although small private oncology practices are not financially structured to support clinical trials, the medical oncologists that work there strive to provide innovative care. Despite financial strain on the practice, small practice providers often join cooperative groups, such as CCOPs, or contract with industry for late-stage testing of drugs or devices as part of outpatient care. Indeed, one of us (Dr. Oyer) joined such a group in 1986, so as to bring new drugs and trials to patients.

Economic Challenges

The rise and fall of small private oncology practices has been powerfully driven by cancer drug reimbursement. In 2004, drug reimbursement was based on the average sales price (ASP) plus 22 percent to cover overhead costs. However, after Medicare reform in 2003, a new payment system was instituted that decreased reimbursement to ASP + 6 percent.[19] In 2012, a federal budget sequestration, which continues even now, further cut reimbursement to ASP + 4.3 percent. This narrowing of the drug margin for cancer drugs created competitive disadvantage for small oncology practices as compared to larger ones that benefit from volume- or hospital-based discounts. Due to these changes, the percentage of oncologists in small practices fell from 45.8 to 18.7 percent, as private practices have been driven to consolidate into larger groups or to join hospital-based groups.[20]

Government Providers

Government institutions provide access to cancer care for select populations. The following sections examine the characteristics of the government providers of sufficient scale to treat large numbers of cancer patients, to illustrate how they contribute to cancer care in the United States.

Federally Qualified Health Centers (FQHC)

Federally Qualified Health Centers (FQHCs) are a key component of the health-care safety net in the US and provide primary care, as well as cancer prevention and control, annually for twenty million people who are underserved, uninsured, or underrepresented. Despite a lack of resources and their struggle to maintain a sufficient workforce, FQHCs are recognized for cancer prevention services, particularly screening efficiency. FQHCs perform cancer screening and facilitate referrals to cancer specialists but do not provide cancer treatment.[21]

The Indian Health Service (IHS)

The IHS, with urban Indian health programs, provides care to over 2.56 million Americans who are members of 556 federally recognized tribes of American Indians and Alaska Natives (AI/AN); they have the poorest rate of cancer survival. Currently, cancer is the leading cause of death for women in the AI/AN population and the second-leading cause of death for AI/AN men. Despite the impact of cancer on the AI/AN population, the IHS has been significantly underfunded overall.[22] In addition to chronic co-morbidities, lack of access to services is known to be a contributing factor to the prevalence of cancer for the AI/AN populations.[23] Finally, one of the many challenges of the IHS can be the distance beneficiaries must travel for care.

Veterans Health Administration (VHA)

The VHA, a component of the executive branch of the federal government, is the nation's largest health system and makes about 3 percent of all cancer diagnoses every year. The VHA often partners with academic institutions to provide health care with the support of academic faculty and medical trainees. As a result, the majority (70%) of all practicing physicians in the United States trained, at least in part, in VHA hospitals through affiliations with 90 percent of US medical schools. Cancer care in the VHA system varies in nature based on the availability of subspecialty resources accessible through these academic partnerships.[24]

VHA Scope of Services

VHA hospitals with strong academic affiliations may have access to advanced cancer therapies, technologies, clinical trials, and disease-focused specialists. However, many rural VHA hospitals operate similarly to community-based oncology programs. Despite reports of long wait times for veterans seeking care, research suggests that as a population, veterans receive better cancer screening and more evidence-based cancer treatment than do nonveterans.[25] Guideline-concordant care in the veteran system is mandated by a national formulary program, which restricts cancer drug use to evidence-based indications. The VHA also has a National Oncology Program Office that provides centralized quality improvement leadership and research support to oncologists across the country.[26]

The VHA supports developing models of cancer care delivery. The VHA was among the first to provide chemotherapy to remote populations using telehealth.[27] Also unique to the VHA is a "concurrent care" model of palliative and end-of-life care. Whereas nonveterans receive home hospice support only when foregoing all life-sustaining care, veterans with advanced cancer can enroll in hospice care while continuing to receive cancer-directed therapies.[28]

VHA Research

VHA research, developed in alliance with academic medical centers, focuses on population health management and health services (e.g., lung cancer screening), as well as basic and clinical research. In 2018, the NCI and the VHA collaborated to increase veterans' access to therapeutic cancer clinical trials by strengthening clinical research infrastructure. Federal entities including the NCI, Department of Defense, and the VHA often collaborate in cancer research efforts.[29]

VHA Access and Economics

As noted earlier, veteran access to comprehensive cancer care depends on the resources available to a particular VA hospital, which vary greatly. Two major laws increased veterans' access to cancer care services. In response to reports of long wait times, The Veterans' Choice Act of 2014 and the VA MISSION Act of 2018 created pathways for veterans to receive care outside the VA network, expanding cancer care access to veterans who were geographically underserved.[30]

The VHA system benefits economically from being a single-payer national health service. Additionally, the VA is able to buy drugs at discounted prices by statutory mandate, which it can further negotiate due to its national formulary. Out-of-pocket costs for veterans with cancer are modest: veterans incur no out-of-pocket cost for cancer drug infusions. All prescriptions for veterans, including cancer drugs, have the same co-pay: $8. They do pay per-visit co-pays, but that fee operates on a sliding scale. The economies of scale the VA is able to accomplish are used as a benchmark for other government purchasers.

Future Directions

The 1971 War on Cancer Act (P.L. 92-218) strengthened the research mission of the NCI by establishing a National Cancer Program (NCP) that was intended to interact enough with the established cancer care delivery system through planning and coordination to improve the delivery of patient care. But the goals of the 1971 Act could not be met. When the War on Cancer Act was recodified, the scope of the program was redefined to include only the NCI.

Fifty years later, we believe that Congress and the NCI should recommit to the sweeping vision of 1971. To do so, the nation must establish a national cancer program that divides the country into a number of hub-and-spoke delivery regions. Established Comprehensive Cancer Centers (CCCs) would act as regional hubs charged with disseminating knowledge, providing complex cancer care, and continuing all phases of cancer research. Each regional CCC hub would seamlessly connect with a variety of care locations, including community cancer centers, government providers, and private practice oncology locations. Establishing a hub-and-spoke national cancer program would require substantial resources and rigorous national and state policy. Moreover, to function effectively, such a system would require a common EHR system across all care locations. Such an EHR would need to contain critical data elements, including social determinants of health, point-of-care pathways, and telemedicine platforms.

This expansive a hub-and-spoke system is reflective of the recommendations of national organizations, such as the Association of Community Cancer Centers, which recommend that access, equity, precision medicine, holistic care, and clinical trials be available to all cancer patients and families, no matter where, nor what type of institution provides their care. It is imperative that complex cancer care can be delivered across multiple care settings, as growing demand at NCI and academic medical centers may exceed their capacity to provide timely treatment.[31] Many patients, such as Michael, are well cared for across all settings, highlighting the value of a setting that provides the most efficient and accessible care. Other patients, such as Lisa, need a higher level of care, demonstrating the need for academic medical centers. The concrete policy suggestions we make below lay out plans for enacting a hub-and-spoke regional model, reflecting the need for all cancer care locations to communicate effectively and clearly across care settings.

Managed Care and Consolidations

Until the past few decades, physicians controlled both the medical marketplace and medical knowledge, allowing them the freedom to care for and refer patients wherever they chose. In response to rising health-care costs in the early 1990s, a mixture of market and regulatory solutions—notably managed-care plans—were implemented. Combined with an oversupply of hospital beds and some medical specialists, this led to a shift of power away from physicians toward insurers. Physicians' autonomy was sharply curtailed, and insurers could now dictate where patients received care.[32]

The passage of the Affordable Care Act in 2010 expanded the number of Americans covered by health insurance but led to a decrease in the quality of existing coverage through narrowed networks, and an increase in low-quality, high-deductible plans on the market. Superimposed consolidation trends resulted in a decline in small private practices, increased employment of physicians by hospitals, the creation of large physician groups, and vertical integration. Large scale, non-physician-owned practices remain free to dictate referral patterns and exploit a pricing system that rewards market power. For example, hospital-based physicians make referrals at twice the rate of office-based physicians.[33]

Consolidation (both vertical and horizontal) has increased inequities in payment and resources at the community level. Top-tier hospitals with the most market power negotiate significantly higher reimbursement rates than smaller hospitals, especially those caring for poorer populations.[34] Additionally, health-care prices vary from one geographic region to another, further exacerbating disparities in access and quality of cancer care and other health-care services.[35]

The Future of the Oncology Workforce

Along with expansion, the capacity of the oncology workforce presents its own challenges. ASCO predicted that from 2012 to 2025, the demand for cancer care would increase by 40 percent, but that the supply of oncologists would not be able to rise to meet it.[36] This is due to a growing demographic of individuals aged sixty-five and older who are at an increased risk of developing cancer, a growing number of oncologists in the same age range who are retiring, and the complexity of oncology care with individual patients needing more services. These challenges in the labor supply, coupled with the need for oncologists in rural and underserved communities, will undoubtedly shape where cancer care is provided in the near- and long-term future. Underrepresentation of minority groups in the oncology physician workforce is also striking and may exacerbate geographic and racial inequities in access to cancer care. While at least 33.2 percent of the US population identifies as Black, Hispanic/Latinx, or AI/AN, only 7.8 percent of practicing US oncologists are from these groups.[37] With the increasing volume of care both available and needed, as well as improved rates of survival, every patient will require more care over longer periods of time. Improving cancer care equity in the future will require significant expansion and diversification of the oncology workforce with investment in pipeline programs and training in the care of underserved populations.

The Promise of Telemedicine

Changes during the COVID-19 pandemic include trends toward patient-centered care, with patients expecting safety and personalized care, as well as increased home infusions.[38] With this decentralization of care away from medical centers, the entire health-care system has become interested in telemedicine as an effective way to address geographic barriers to access. However, 22 percent of US citizens do not own a desktop computer or laptop and 25 percent do not own a smartphone or other type of wireless handheld computer.[39] It is uncertain whether increasing use of telemedicine will ameliorate or exacerbate disparities in cancer care driven by geographic and sociodemographic factors. A recent study in primary care reported that older patients and non-English-speaking patients had lower rates of telemedicine use generally, and that older patients and Black, Latinx, and poorer patients had less video use.

Technology Toward a Unified Future: Use of EHRs

To ensure cancer care equity, quality, and value across care settings, transformative use of EHRs can and must be implemented to collect relevant clinical data sets, including characteristics that affect both treatment and outcome. We suggest that Congress mandate EHR interoperability using minimum common oncology data elements (mCODE) developed by ASCO and collaborators. Regardless of where care is received, every cancer patient's data can and must be subjected to analytics informed by rigorous methods to furnish real-time, evidence-based, individualized decision support for clinicians in all care settings. Such computational support will enable clinicians with variable expertise and resources to provide state-of-the art cancer care regardless of their practice setting.

As new cancer treatments and technologies become widely available across the US, the boundaries between types of cancer care delivery institutions can and must be broken down. As a specialty, oncology's commitment to cancer care and health equity requires cancer experts to continue researching and advancing not only the scientific understanding of cancer, but also the distribution, economics, and politics of cancer.

Notes

1. A 2020 review of the ten top cancers, representing over four million cases in the National Cancer Database, looked at a narrow subset of these categories. The review showed that between 2007 and 2016, the case distribution across hospital type was 49% community, 23% academic, 14% NCI, and 14% integrated network hospitals (Zachary A. K. Frosch et al., "Association of Hospital Type and Patient Volume Growth with Timely Cancer Treatment," *Journal of Clinical Oncology* 38, no. 15 [2020]: s2022, https://doi.org/10.1200/jco.2020.38.15 _suppl.2022). ASCO reports that 21% of cancer practices are academic practices,

37% health system owned (Megan Kirkwood et al., "The State of Oncology Practice in America, 2018: Results of the ASCO Practice Census Survey," *Journal of Oncology Practice* 14, no. 7 [2018]: e412–e419, https://doi.org/10.1200/JOP.18.00149).

2. Sayeh S. Nikpay, Michael R. Richards, and David Penson, "Hospital-Physician Consolidation Accelerated in the Past Decade in Cardiology, Oncology," *Health Affairs* 37, no. 7 (2018): 1123–1127, https://doi.org/10.1377/hlthaff.2017.1520.

3. American Society of Clinical Oncology, "The State of Cancer Care in America, 2017: A Report by the American Society of Clinical Oncology," *Journal of Oncology Practice* 13, no. 4 (2017): e353–e394, https://doi.org/10.1200/JOP.2016.020743; "Status of the Medical Oncology Workforce," *Journal of Clinical Oncology* 14, no. 9 (1996): 2612–2621, https://doi.org/10.1200/JCO.1996.14.9.2612.

4. Suanna S. Bruinooge et al., "Understanding the Role of Advanced Practice Providers in Oncology in the United States," *Journal of Oncology Practice* 14, no. 9 (2018): e518–e532, https://doi.org/10.1200/JOP.18.00181.

5. Kirkwood et al., "The State of Oncology Practice."

6. Physician Compare National Downloadable File, HealthData.gov, https://data.cms.gov/provider-data/.

7. Christopher E. Desch and Douglas W. Blayney, "Making the Choice Between Academic Oncology and Community Practice: The Big Picture and Details About Each Career," *Journal of Oncology Practice* 2, no. 3 (2006): 132–136, https://doi.org/10.1200/JOP.2006.2.3.132.

8. Nancy J. O. Birkmeyer et al., "Do Cancer Centers Designated by the National Cancer Institute Have Better Surgical Outcomes?" *Cancer* 103, no. 3 (2005): 435–441, https://doi.org/10.1002/cncr.20785; Brian Park et al., "Health Equity and the Tripartite Mission: Moving from Academic Health Centers to Academic-Community Health Systems," *Academic Medicine* 94, no. 9 (2019): 1276–82, https://doi.org/10.1097/ACM.0000000000002833.

9. Frosch et al., "Association of Hospital Type and Patient Volume Growth."

10. Lori M. Minasian et al., "Translating Research into Evidence-Based Practice: The National Cancer Institute Community Clinical Oncology Program," *Cancer* 116, no. 19 (2010): 4440–4449, https://doi.org/10.1002/cncr.25248.

11. Allison R. Baer et al., "Challenges to National Cancer Institute-Supported Cooperative Group Clinical Trial Participation: An ASCO Survey of Cooperative Group Sites," *Journal of Oncology Practice* 6, no. 3 (2010): 114–117, https://doi.org/10.1200/JOP.200028.

12. Gabrielle B. Rocque et al., "Impact of Travel Time on Health Care Costs and Resource Use by Phase of Care for Older Patients with Cancer," *Journal of Clinical Oncology* 37, no. 22 (2019): 1935–1945, https://doi.org/10.1200/JCO.19.00175.

13. Alok A. Khorana et al., "Time to Initial Cancer Treatment in the United States and Association with Survival over Time: An Observational Study," *PLoS One* 14, no. 3 (2019): e0213209, https://doi.org/10.1371/journal.pone.0213209.

14. Lucio Gordan, "The Value of Community Oncology: Site of Care Cost Analysis," Community Oncology Alliance, September 25, 2017, https://

communityoncology.org/the-value-of-community-oncology-site-of-care-cost
-analysis/.

15. Jeffrey D. Clough, Michaela A. Dinan, and Kevin A. Schulman, "Trends in Hospital-Physician Integration in Medical Oncology," *American Journal of Managed Care* 23, no. 10 (2017): 624–627, https://europepmc.org/article/med /29087634.

16. "Practice Impact Reports," Community Oncology Alliance, accessed March 28, 2021, https://communityoncology.org/category/practice-impact -reports/.

17. Mark W. Friedberg et al., "Association Between Participation in a Multipayer Medical Home Intervention and Changes in Quality, Utilization, and Costs of Care," *JAMA* 311, no. 8 (2014): 815–825, https://doi.org/10.1001 /jama.2014.353.

18. Physician Compare National Downloadable File, HealthData.gov . https://data.cms.gov/provider-data/.

19. Wayne Kuznar, "ASP Plus 6% Will Fall by the Wayside, but What Are the Alternatives?" *American Health & Drug Benefits* 8, no. special issue (2015): 31, https://www.ncbi.nlm.nih.gov/pmc/articles/PMC4570048/.

20. Mireille Jacobson et al., "How Medicare's Payment Cuts for Cancer Chemotherapy Drugs Changed Patterns of Treatment," *Health Affairs* 29, no. 7 (2010): 1391–1399, https://doi.org/10.1377/hlthaff.2009.0563.

21. Ronald E. Myers, "Low Rates of Diagnostic Colonoscopy in Federally Qualified Health Centers: A Persistent Problem That Must Be Addressed to Achieve the Promise of Colorectal Cancer Screening," *Cancer* 125, no. 23 (2019): 4134–4135, https://doi.org/10.1002/cncr.32438; US Health Resources & Services Administration, accessed March 28, 2021, https://www.hrsa.gov/.

22. B. Ashleigh Guadagnolo, Daniel G. Petereit, and C. Norman Coleman, "Cancer Care Access and Outcomes for American Indian Populations in the United States: Challenges and Models for Progress," *Seminars in Radiation Oncology* 27, no. 2 (2017): 143–149, https://doi.org/10.1016/j.semradonc.2016.11.006; Jenn Lukens, "Reducing Cancer among Native Populations: Models for Research, Prevention, and Treatment," *Rural Monitor*, May 1, 2019, https://www .ruralhealthinfo.org/rural-monitor/cancer-among-ai-an/.

23. Lukens, "Reducing Cancer Among Native Populations."

24. Folasade P. May, Christine Yu, and Jonathan Kaunitz, "High Quality of Cancer Care in the Department of Veterans Affairs (VA)," *American Journal of Cancer Research* 8, no. 4 (2018): 761–762, https://pubmed.ncbi.nlm.nih.gov /29736320/.

25. Folasade et al., "High Quality of Cancer Care."

26. "National Oncology Program Office," US Department of Veterans Affairs, accessed March 28, 2021, https://www.cancer.va.gov/.

27. Vida Almario Passero et al., "Creation of a Virtual Cancer Care Network for Remote Oncology Treatment," *Journal of Clinical Oncology* 37, no. 15 (2019): s6546, https://doi.org/10.1200/JCO.2019.37.15_suppl.6546.

28. Leah M. Haverhals et al., "The Experience of Providing Hospice Care Concurrent with Cancer Treatment in the VA," *Supportive Care in Cancer* 27, no. 4 (2019): 1263–1270, https://doi.org/10.1007/s00520-018-4552-z.

29. "NCI and VA Collaborate to Boost Veterans' Access to Cancer Clinical Trials," National Cancer Institute, July 10, 2018, https://www.cancer.gov/news -events/press-releases/2018/navigate-va-clinical-trials.

30. Anthony P. Albanese et al., "The VA MISSION Act of 2018: A Potential Game Changer for Rural GME Expansion and Veteran Health Care," *Journal of Rural Health* 36, no. 1 (2020): 133–136, https://doi.org/10.1111/jrh.12360.

31. Frosch et al., "Association of Hospital Type and Patient Volume Growth."

32. P. Starr, *The Social Transformation of American Medicine* (New York: Basic Books, 1982), 450–493.

33. Ann S. O'Malley, Amelia M. Bond, and Robert A. Berenson, "Rising Hospital Employment of Physicians: Better Quality, Higher Costs?" *Center for Studying Health System Change Issue Brief*, no. 136 (2011): 1–4, https://pubmed .ncbi.nlm.nih.gov/21853632/.

34. Paul B. Ginsburg, "Wide Variation in Hospital and Physician Payment Rates Evidence of Provider Market Power," Research Brief no. 16 (2010): 1–11, https://pubmed.ncbi.nlm.nih.gov/21117341/.

35. O'Malley, Bond, and Berenson, "Rising Hospital Employment of Physicians."

36. Kirkwood et al., "The State of Oncology Practice."

37. Curtiland Deville et al., "Diversity by Race, Hispanic Ethnicity, and Sex of the United States Medical Oncology Physician Workforce over the Past Quarter Century," *Journal of Oncology Practice* 10, no. 5 (2014): e328–e334, https:// doi.org/10.1200/JOP.2014.001464.

38. Amy I. Laughlin et al., "Accelerating the Delivery of Cancer Care at Home During the Covid-19 Pandemic," *Catalyst* (commentary), July 7, 2020, https://catalyst.nejm.org/doi/full/10.1056/cat.20.0258.

39. Camille Ryan, "Computer and Internet Use in the United States: 2016: American Community Survey Reports," Census.gov, August 2018, https://www .census.gov/content/dam/Census/library/publications/2018/acs/ACS-39.pdf, 14.

CHAPTER 3

The Health Insurance Landscape and Cancer Care

K. Robin Yabroff

Among high-income countries, health care in the United States is unique, in ways that affect cancer care and outcomes. Americans do not have universal access to health insurance or affordable care. At the same time, the US adopts innovative new cancer therapies at a rapid pace relative to the rest of the world, offering state-of-the-art care to those who can afford it. Novel therapies, such as chimeric antigen receptor T cell (CAR-T) therapy or immunotherapy, can transform cancer outcomes. But such innovations are expensive. Even more routine parts of cancer care, including lengthy inpatient hospitalizations, advanced imaging, and supportive care, contribute to cancer's being one of the most expensive medical conditions to treat. Overall, per capita health-care spending is nearly twice as high in the US compared to other high-income countries.[1] Cancer care is overrepresented in that spending.

National spending on cancer-related care is projected to increase from $183 billion in 2015 to $246 billion by 2030, based only on population aging and growth. Much of this spending occurs in cancer survivors. Survivors experience a higher prevalence of chronic conditions and subsequent cancers due to underlying risk factors (e.g., tobacco use, obesity), as well as late and lasting effects of treatment, than do their counterparts without a cancer history,

---

K. Robin Yabroff is Scientific Vice President, Health Services Research, American Cancer Society.

even many years after a cancer diagnosis. Spending projections incorporating expensive innovations in cancer treatment following
diagnosis and at the end of life suggest even greater growth.[2]

Yet many health outcomes, including cancer outcomes, are not
substantially better in the US. For example, life expectancy is worse
in the US than in other countries with lower health-care expenditures.[3] Further, health outcomes and life expectancy in the US
vary substantially between populations defined by race/ethnicity,
socioeconomic position, and geographic area of residence.[4] Overall, disparities between the most advantaged and least advantaged
populations in the US are among the greatest in the world. Cancers that have effective screening modalities and/or treatments
show the greatest disparity in outcomes across populations. Such
marked inequity in outcomes highlights the central importance of
affordable and adequate health insurance coverage.

Health insurance coverage is one of the strongest predictors of
access to care and health outcomes; lack of coverage plays a central
role in disparities in cancer care and outcomes for historically disadvantaged populations, with large variation in incidence, survival,
and mortality by state.[5] Cancer mortality rates have been and continue to be higher among uninsured populations,[6] with some evidence for widening disparities. Socioeconomically disadvantaged
populations are the most likely to be uninsured, but uninsurance
is associated with worse outcomes regardless of socioeconomic
status.[7] This chapter summarizes evidence for the association between health insurance coverage and access to and receipt of a
broad spectrum of cancer-related care, discusses models of cancer
care delivery, and highlights key issues in the evolving landscape
of health insurance coverage that affect cancer care and outcomes.

Overview of Health-Care Delivery and
Health Insurance Coverage in the United States

Health-care delivery in the United States is deeply fragmented,
with multiple private insurance companies operating independently

of one another as well as from public programs at the federal and state levels. In 2020, there were hundreds of health insurance companies. Some of those companies offer multiple types of health plans, with varying benefits, premiums, and cost-sharing structures. Health care is not explicitly coordinated across multiple insurers, plans, hospitals, and practices. Worse, patient medical records reside in multiple places in different formats without linkage, integration, or interoperability, which limits research and comparisons of care delivery and health outcomes, including cancer outcomes, across insurance types and models of care.

The federal Medicare program provides insurance coverage for more than 96 percent of Americans aged sixty-five years and older and for some adults younger than sixty-five with certain conditions (e.g., end-stage renal disease) or disabilities. It is the largest payer for cancer care in the US, largely because the majority of cancer patients and survivors are aged sixty-five years and older. The state and federal Medicaid programs provide coverage for low-income populations, including about 10 percent of adults aged sixty-five years and older and 24 percent of adults younger than sixty-five years. About two-thirds of working-age adults (aged 18–64 years) have some form of private health insurance coverage, which is mainly employer-based. Adults without employer-based health insurance coverage options can purchase private policies individually. Prior to implementation of the Affordable Care Act (ACA), individual policies could restrict coverage for treatment of preexisting conditions, such as cancer, or deny coverage altogether. In 2010, prior to the ACA, 17.8 percent of people in the US—46.5 million people—did not have health insurance coverage.

Health Insurance Coverage and Access to Cancer Care

Effective interventions across the cancer control continuum (see Figure 3.1), including cancer prevention, screening, treatment, and survivorship care, can reduce cancer mortality. Cancer prevention, such as ending tobacco use, increasing healthy eating, and increasing exercise, can reduce the risk of developing many types of cancers. Moreover, asymptomatic cancer screening and timely

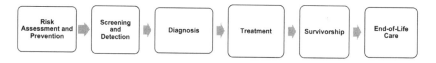

FIGURE 3.1 Healthcare Delivery Across the Cancer Control Continuum

follow-up of abnormal test results can lead to early detection for some cancer, when treatment is more effective. Timely access to effective cancer treatment and palliative care is associated with improved survival and better outcomes, including health-related quality of life. However, uninsured people are less likely to receive high-quality care across the cancer control continuum (see Figure 3.2) than are their counterparts with health insurance coverage.[8]

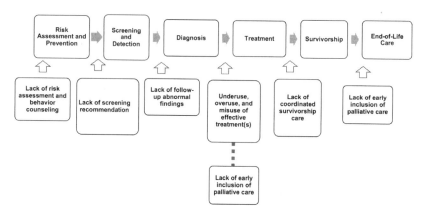

FIGURE 3.2 Lack of Health Insurance Coverage and Potential Breakdowns in Care Across the Cancer Control Continuum

Lack of Health Insurance Coverage and Limitations in Access to and Receipt of Cancer Care

Uninsured people are less likely to have a usual source of health care, and are less likely to receive preventative cancer care, such as cancer risk assessment or help with smoking cessation, diet, weight, or physical activity, than are their counterparts with insurance coverage. These cancer prevention activities typically take place within the primary care setting. Lack of insurance coverage is associated with lack of a usual source of primary care. Both are associated with disparities in age-appropriate breast, cervical, colorectal, and lung cancer screening. Among those who do receive cancer screenings and have abnormal test findings, uninsured people are less likely to receive timely, if any, follow-up diagnostic testing. Having health insurance and a usual source of primary care is strongly associated with receipt of risk assessment, prevention, screening, and evaluation of early signs and symptoms of cancer. Due to these disparities in screening, the uninsured are less likely to be diagnosed with early-stage disease,[9] where treatment can be more effective.

Cancer patients without health insurance are also less likely to receive high-quality, guideline-consistent treatment, including surgery, radiation therapy, and chemotherapy, as well as newer immunotherapies and targeted agents.[10] During and following treatment completion, uninsured cancer survivors are less likely to receive recommended survivorship care, such as surveillance for recurrence and other provider recommendations for reducing risk of other conditions and subsequent cancers. Innovations in cancer prevention, screening, and treatment, including genomic therapies, may also be less available to uninsured populations, potentially widening existing disparities in cancer outcomes. Indeed, recent studies have documented growing cancer survival disparities over the past decades between the uninsured and those with private insurance coverage.[11]

Some uninsured people may receive charity care, but this cannot alleviate the challenges of equitable access to high-quality cancer care. Adults without health insurance coverage are frequently responsible for the entirety of their health-care costs. Not surprisingly, uninsured adults are more likely than their insured counterparts to report medical financial hardship, including trouble paying medical bills, high out-of-pocket cost burden, distress and worry about their financial situation, and delaying or forgoing recommended care because of cost.[12]

Limitations in Access to and Receipt of Cancer Care
Among People with Health Insurance Coverage
Even among adults with current insurance coverage, prior disruptions in coverage are associated with less cancer screening, a later

stage at cancer diagnosis, less recommended cancer treatment, and poorer cancer survival.[13] Most older research addressed coverage disruptions among Medicaid enrollees with regard to cancer care and outcomes; a more recent study found that prior coverage disruptions were associated with problems with access and affordability of care among cancer survivors who reported either current public or private (mostly employer-based) coverage.[14] These findings likely reflect the serious consequences of being uninsured, even for a brief period.

In addition to continuity of coverage, other aspects of coverage affect access to cancer care and outcomes. Even adults with health insurance coverage may experience barriers to care due to deductibles that must be paid out-of-pocket before insurance coverage begins and cost-sharing from co-payments and coinsurance rates that are required after the annual health insurance plan deductible is met. Patient out-of-pocket burden has risen markedly over the past decade. "Underinsurance," where patients have health insurance coverage but are unable to access or afford care, has also risen dramatically. The rising cost of cancer care has exacerbated systemic challenges with affordability while simultaneously increasing the absolute and relative cost borne by patients.[15]

The prevalence of employer-based, private, high-deductible health plans (HDHPs) has increased dramatically in the US, from 15 percent in 2007 to 43 percent in 2017.[16] While deductible thresholds vary across plans, in 2021, maximum HDHP deductibles will be $7,000 for individuals and $14,000 for families. All medical expenses must be paid out-of-pocket before the annual plan deductible threshold, which resets at the beginning of each calendar year. Meanwhile, most Americans report not being able to afford an unexpected expense of $400. Cancer survivors with HDHPs are more likely to delay or forgo care because of cost[17] and experience delays in cancer diagnosis and treatment initiation[18] than their counterparts with low deductibles.

Medicare beneficiaries without supplemental private or public coverage have historically faced coinsurance of 20 percent without an annual out-of-pocket cap for procedures or infusion medications covered under Part B. Oral cancer drugs covered under

Medicare Part D are typically classified as specialty drugs on most formularies. Such drugs have the highest coinsurance rate, as much as 33 percent of the list price, without an annual out-of-pocket cap. Many private insurance plans have structures similar to the Medicare program, with the potential for greater patient cost-sharing for oral cancer drugs on the pharmacy benefit (Part D) than infusion cancer drugs on the medical (Part B) benefit. Most states have passed laws to provide parity between pharmacy and medical benefits, but these laws do not have an impact on adherence to oral treatments, and any benefits in terms of reduced out-of-pocket costs for patients receiving cancer treatment are quite modest.[19] Regardless of which benefit covers prescription drugs, insured patients with greater cost-sharing are more likely to delay or forgo care,[20] including necessary care. Among cancer patients and survivors, medical financial hardship is associated with worse health-related quality of life and even worse survival.[21]

The Affordable Care Act

The landscape of US health insurance coverage continues to evolve within the earlier-described constraints, particularly with the introduction of the ACA. Enacted in 2010, the ACA affects cancer-related care and outcomes through three main mechanisms: expansion of health insurance options, coverage reform, and payment and delivery system reform, accelerating existing efforts in models of care delivery.[22] The coverage expansion provisions of the ACA include dependent coverage expansion (DCE), which allows young adults to remain on their parents' private coverage until age twenty-six; the state-level option to expand Medicaid eligibility to individuals with income up to 138 percent of the federal poverty level; and the establishment of the insurance Marketplace for individuals, families, and small businesses with premium subsidies for purchase.

Following implementation of the ACA, uninsurance dropped to a historic low.[23] The expansion of Medicaid eligibility and the DCE under the ACA are associated with improved access to cancer screening. For cancer patients, these ACA coverage expansions are associated with greater coverage, earlier stage of disease at diagnosis, improved and timelier receipt of cancer treatment, and better survival following diagnosis.[24] Additionally, income, race/ethnicity, and rural/urban residence coverage and financial hardship disparities among cancer patients and survivors have been reduced in states that chose to expand Medicaid, with little changes in disparities in nonexpansion states.[25]

Coverage reform provisions in the ACA include the elimination of cost-sharing for effective preventive services that receive an A or B rating by the US Preventive Services Task Force, including cancer screening tests. Eliminating cost-sharing for preventive services reduces financial barriers to care and is generally associated with increases in cancer screening, especially among low-income populations,[26] and reductions in disparities in receipt of care. ACA coverage reform provisions eliminated preexisting condition exclusions or refusals and coverage limits, which previously allowed insurers to deny or limit coverage for cancer patients and survivors because cancer was considered a preexisting condition.

The ACA also mandated that private insurers provide coverage of routine care for clinical trial participants and the gradual closing of the Medicare Part D donut hole, an annual period where Medicare beneficiaries pay the entirety of the cost of their oral prescription drugs. Further, the ACA introduced annual out-of-pocket spending caps in both the Marketplace and private plans. All of these interventions potentially limit the exposure of insured cancer survivors to high out-of-pocket costs; yet, at present, little work has evaluated these coverage reform provisions.

The highly charged political environment around the passage of the ACA in 2010 led to multiple challenges in state and federal courts. The decision to expand Medicaid was left to each state, and many state governments decided not to expand Medicaid for their residents in 2014. As of 2020, states with some of the highest cancer mortality rates in the country have still not expanded Medicaid. Other actions at the federal level, starting in 2017, undermined the ACA, including limiting enrollment support for Marketplace plans. After historic reductions in the number of uninsured adult cancer patients and survivors in 2014, numbers of uninsured began increasing again in 2017.[27] By 2019, almost 11 percent of people in the United States were uninsured, representing about twenty-nine million people. The data for how many of these twenty-nine million are cancer survivors is not yet available.

Payment and Care Delivery Models

Historically, health care in the United States has been based on a fee-for-service (FFS) model, which reimburses providers for all services delivered to patients. The FFS model results in provider incentives for recommending and delivering a greater volume of health-care services, without consideration of quality of care, patient outcomes, or cost. FFS has played a central role in rising costs of health care in the US and is also thought to be associated with high levels of service intensity at the end of life, which is especially relevant for cancer care. Health-care service intensity and spending is highest at the end of life for most cancers. Further, the use of intensive care at the end of life is higher in the US than in other developed countries.

A fee-for-service structure incentivizes providers to prescribe not only a greater volume of services, but also more expensive infusion prescription drugs. Oncologists purchase infusion chemotherapy, biologics (including immunotherapy), and other drugs that are later administered to patients in their offices, as part of a process known as "buy and bill." Infusion drugs are generally reimbursed under medical benefits by the Medicare program (Part B) and other insurers. Under Medicare Part B, providers are then reimbursed for infusion drugs based on the average sales price of the drug plus an add-on percentage of average sales price for each drug. The add-on percentage is intended to compensate providers for overhead and the administrative complexity of storing and delivering infusion drugs. Because the add-on is proportional to the underlying average sales price for each drug, the add-on reimbursement is more for more expensive drugs, providing incentives for selecting more expensive drugs. The reimbursement approach for infusion drugs is also used by many private insurers. As the list price for new oncology prescription drugs is routinely greater than $100,000 annually, incentives for selecting expensive drugs have become ever stronger. This reimbursement structure for infusion drugs within FFS has been shown to be associated with increased use of higher-cost chemotherapies for newly diagnosed cancer patients.[28] Alternatives to FFS, then, may be needed to optimize cancer care and outcomes.

Managed care, another model of care delivery, organizes, finances, and structures health care differently than FFS. Managed care providers assume responsibility for all the health care for a defined population of patients for a specified time period and are paid a capitated rate for each patient in their defined population. This financial structure does not reward for service volume, but instead incentivizes coordination of care, eliminating duplication of services, and reducing hospitalizations. This structure can result in narrow provider networks. Managed care has grown rapidly in the US, and more than one-third of Medicare beneficiaries and more than two-thirds with Medicaid are enrolled in managed care plans. Historically, enrollment in health maintenance organizations (HMOs), a type of managed care, has been associated with higher rates of cancer screening and earlier stage disease at diagnosis among patients with cancer[29] compared with FFS enrollment. Effects of managed care enrollment on cancer treatment and survival are mixed and few contemporary studies have compared these models of care delivery. Lack of data comparability, patient selection, and underlying differences in patient health status in FFS and managed care limit these comparisons.

Evolving models of care delivery feature greater provider accountability for higher quality of care. That interaction between accountability and quality is based on a specific set of metrics, including pay-for-performance, episodes or bundled payments, and care pathways. These models are sometimes referred to as value-based payment models and can affect receipt of cancer screening and diagnosis, treatment, survivorship, and end-of-life care, even if the models are not designed to be specific to cancer care. Accountable Care Organizations (ACOs) are one type of model that features pay-for-performance. ACOs consist of groups of primary care clinicians, with or without specialty clinicians, usually in partnership with a hospital system. These clinicians organize and are accountable for services provided to a defined population of Medicare FFS beneficiaries. In the few evaluations focused on cancer patients receiving treatment or end-of-life care under this model, however, studies found no effect on hospitalizations, emergency department visits, or chemotherapy use.[30] One study of a pay-for-performance model reported increased use of evidence-based cancer drugs,[31] but to date, none have reported that ACOs or pay-for-performance models reduced cancer care spending in relationship to comparison practices.[32]

The ACA authorized the creation of the Center for Medicare and Medicaid Innovation (CMMI) to develop and test models of health-care delivery. The Oncology Care Model (OCM) is one of the few cancer treatment specific models developed by the CMMI. It was developed within the FFS setting to incentivize care coordination of Medicare beneficiaries undergoing chemotherapy. The expectation was that savings would result from decreases in preventable emergency department visits and hospitalizations, better supportive care, and improved coordination of end-of-life care. Yet while preliminary evaluation of volunteer practices and comparison practices suggests small declines in intensive care use and emergency department visits, research has found no changes in hospitalizations or total payments.[33]

A central challenge is that many of these delivery and payment models have been implemented within the FFS setting, and it may not be possible to alter underlying incentives in FFS for volume, rather than value. Importantly, there are significant methodologic limitations with many evaluations of payment and delivery models. Physician practices that implement these new models typically volunteer to participate, whereas the comparison physician practices do not. Volunteer physician practices can be inherently different from other, nonvolunteer practices in ways that are related to patient care and outcomes, such as the number and types of patients seen each year, the proportion of patients with private or Medicaid insurance, and investment in electronic medical record software. Even with sophisticated statistical modeling, evaluation design is subject to bias. In the future, a more rigorous evaluation design could randomize volunteer practices to the new model of care or standard practice.

Continued Evolution of the Health Insurance Coverage Landscape and Cancer Care in the United States

The health insurance coverage landscape in the United States continually changes in ways that will affect cancer care and outcomes for the next fifty years. Going forward, the profound and growing disparities in cancer care and outcomes must be a central focus of evidence-based health-care policy.

The COVID-19 pandemic exposed multiple fault lines within the organization and delivery of health care in the US. Foremost among these are the continued politicization of public health and health care, the increasing prevalence of medical financial hardship, and the limitations in data infrastructure for informing care delivery. These challenges limit care delivery, including cancer prevention, treatment, and survivorship care, as well as evaluation of payment models described earlier. Widespread unemployment and its attendant loss of access to employer-sponsored health insurance during the pandemic has highlighted the urgency of addressing these three primary challenges.

Politics aside, scientific evidence has consistently demonstrated that affordable, high-quality health insurance and access to care are central to better outcomes overall and better cancer outcomes specifically. Medicaid expansion to provide coverage to low-income populations in all states and expanding comprehensive and affordable health insurance coverage options outside of employment for the working-age population, rather than limiting them, are objectives supported by decades of scientific evidence.

In addition, the rising costs of cancer care and increased patient cost-sharing have led to a growing prevalence of medical financial hardship for cancer patients and their families, even among those with private, employer-sponsored health insurance coverage.

Currently, Medicare beneficiaries with FFS coverage do not have out-of-pocket caps for Part B or Part D spending and are responsible for a percentage of their health-care costs. Paying for health care can be especially challenging for elderly cancer survivors living on a fixed income. Addressing these challenges of affordability will require attention to health insurance benefit design, including the structure of premiums, deductibles, co-payments, and coinsurance.

As noted earlier, higher patient cost-sharing reduces use of health care, regardless of its effectiveness. Realigning benefit design to reduce cost-sharing for highly effective care associated with substantial survival benefits can incentivize its use as recommended and minimize cost-related nonadherence. For example, the introduction of tyrosine kinase inhibitors (TKIs) for treatment of chronic myeloid leukemia led to dramatic improvements in survival. These highly effective treatments are taken for long periods of time and can have substantial patient cost-sharing. Several studies have shown that even small differences in cost-sharing amounts for TKIs are associated with lower treatment initiation and greater discontinuation of potentially life-saving therapies among patients with chronic myeloid leukemia. Realigning benefit design to focus on value would decrease or eliminate cost-sharing for TKIs for patients with chronic myeloid leukemia.

Rigorous health services research and better data infrastructure can inform the optimal structure of health insurance coverage of the future. To date, evaluations of ACOs, pay-for-performance, and episode-based models, such as the OCM, have found only modest effects in terms of reducing hospitalizations and emergency room visits and increasing evidence-based treatment, with little change in spending. Consideration of model development and implementation outside of the FFS setting may alter underlying incentives for volume, rather than value.

Inadequacies in health-care data infrastructure in the US also limit the health services research that could be used to inform cancer care delivery, including the evaluation of different plan benefit design and value-based payment models. Currently, longitudinal data for evaluating care receipt and outcomes in the US are mainly from health insurance claims data, but with so many plan types, frequency of coverage plan changes within and across states, lack of interoperability, and absence of key clinical measures (e.g., stage, tumor markers, recurrence, performance status), comprehensive information about cancer care trajectories and outcomes is not available. Comprehensive information is especially limited for adults with periods of uninsurance. Use of all-payer claims data (APCD), in states where they are available, can help to mitigate these challenges in future research addressing health insurance coverage benefit design, receipt of cancer care, spending, and patient outcomes.

Health insurance coverage is intimately related to the overall picture of cancer prevention, care, and outcomes in the US. Despite spending more on health care per capita than any other high-income nation, the United States continues to experience disparities in cancer outcomes, many of which can be tied to the fractured insurance landscape discussed over the course of this chapter. The next fifty years of the War on Cancer will need to close these gaps. The multifactorial interventions in the health insurance landscape discussed here would help ensure that *all* Americans are able to benefit from innovations in cancer prevention, early detection, treatment, and survivorship care.

Notes

1. Irene Papanicolas, Liana R. Woskie, and Ashish K. Jha, "Healthcare Spending in the United States and Other High-Income Countries," *JAMA* 319, no. 10 (2018): 1024–1039, https://doi.org/10.1001/jama.2018.1150.

2. Angela B. Mariotto et al., "Projections of the Cost of Cancer Care in the United States: 2010–2020," *Journal of the National Cancer Institute* 103, no. 2 (2011): 117–128, https://doi.org/10.1093/jnci/djg495.

3. Papanicolas, Woskie, and Jha, "Healthcare Spending."

4. Robin Osborn et al., "In New Survey of Eleven Countries, U.S. Adults Still Struggle with Access to and Affordability of Healthcare," *Health Affairs* 35, no. 12 (2016): 2327–2336, https://doi.org/10.1377/hlthaff.2016.1088.

5. Rebecca L. Siegel, Kimberly D. Miller, and Ahmedin Jemal, "Cancer Statistics, 2020," *CA: A Cancer Journal for Clinicians* 70, no. 1 (2020): 7–30, https://doi.org/10.3322/caac.21590.

6. Libby Ellis et al., "Trends in Cancer Survival by Health Insurance Status in California from 1997 to 2014," *JAMA Oncology* 4, no. 3 (2018): 317–323, https://doi.org/10.1001/jamaoncol.2017.3846.

7. Ellis et al., "Trends in Cancer Survival."

8. *Delivering Affordable Cancer Care in the 21st Century: Workshop Summary* (Washington, DC: National Academies Press, 2013).

9. Michael T. Halpern et al., "Association of Insurance Status and Ethnicity with Cancer Stage at Diagnosis for 12 Cancer Sites: A Retrospective Analysis," *Lancet Oncology* 9, no. 3 (2008): 222–231, https://doi.org/10.1016/S1470-2045(08)70032-9.

10. *Delivering Affordable Cancer Care.*

11. Ellis et al., "Trends in Cancer Survival."

12. K. Robin Yabroff et al., "Prevalence and Correlates of Medical Financial Hardship in the USA," *Journal of General Internal Medicine* 34, no. 8 (2019): 1494–1502.

13. K. Robin Yabroff et al., "Health Insurance Coverage Disruptions and Cancer Care and Outcomes: Systematic Review of Published Research," *Journal of the National Cancer Institute* 112, no. 7 (2020): 671–687, https://doi.org/10.1093/jnci/djaa048.

14. Jingxuan Zhao et al., "Health Insurance Coverage Disruptions and Access to Care and Affordability among Cancer Survivors in the United States," *Cancer Epidemiology, Biomarkers & Prevention* 29, no. 11 (2020): 2134–2140, https://doi.org/10.1158/1055-9965.EPI-20-0518.

15. Stacie B. Dusetzina, Haiden A. Huskamp, and Nancy L. Keating, "Specialty Drug Pricing and Out-of-Pocket Spending on Orally Administered Anticancer Drugs in Medicare Part D, 2010 to 2019," *JAMA* 321, no. 20 (2019): 2025–2027, https://doi.org/10.1001/jama.2019.4492.

16. Robin A. Cohen and Emily P. Zammitti, "High-Deductible Health Plan Enrollment Among Adults Aged 18–64 with Employment-Based Insurance Coverage," *NCHS Data Brief* no. 317 (2018): 1–8, https://www.cdc.gov/nchs/products/databriefs/db317.htm.

17. Zhiyuan Zheng et al., "High-Deductible Health Plans and Cancer Survivorship: What Is the Association with Access to Care and Hospital Emergency Department Use?" *Journal of Oncology Practice* 15, no. 11 (2019): e957–e968, https://doi.org/10.1200/JOP.18.00699.

18. J. Frank Wharam et al., "Breast Cancer Diagnosis and Treatment After High-Deductible Insurance Enrollment," *Journal of Clinical Oncology* 36, no. 11 (2018): 1121–1127, https://doi.org/10.1200/JCO.2017.75.2501.

19. Stacie B. Dusetzina et al., "Oral Oncology Parity Laws, Medication Use, and Out-of-Pocket Spending for Patients with Blood Cancers," *Journal of the National Cancer Institute* 112, no. 10 (2020): 1055–62, https://doi.org/10.1093/jnci/djz243.

20. Wharam et al., "Breast Cancer Diagnosis and Treatment"; Stacie B. Dusetzina et al., "Cost Sharing and Adherence to Tyrosine Kinase Inhibitors for Patients with Chronic Myeloid Leukemia," *Journal of Clinical Oncology* 32, no. 4 (2014): 306–311, https://doi.org/10.1200/JCO.2013.52.9123.

21. Scott D. Ramsey et al., "Financial Insolvency as a Risk Factor for Early Mortality Among Patients with Cancer," *Journal of Clinical Oncology* 34, no. 9 (2016): 980–986, https://doi.org/10.1200/JCO.2015.64.6620.

22. Jingxuan Zhao et al., "The Affordable Care Act and Access to Care Across the Cancer Control Continuum: A Review at 10 Years," *CA: A Cancer Journal for Clinicians* 70, no. 3 (2020): 165–181, https://doi.org/10.3322/caac.21604.

23. Rachel Garfield, Kendal Orgera, and Anthony Damico, "The Uninsured and the ACA: A Primer—Key Facts About Health Insurance and the Uninsured Amidst Changes to the Affordable Care Act," KFF.org, January 25, 2019, https://www.kff.org/uninsured/report/the-uninsured-and-the-aca-a-primer -key-facts-about-health-insurance-and-the-uninsured-amidst-changes-to-the -affordable-care-act/.

24. Zhao et al., "The Affordable Care Act."

25. Xuesong Han et al., "Changes in Noninsurance and Care Unaffordability Among Cancer Survivors Following the Affordable Care Act," *Journal of the National Cancer Institute* 112, no. 7 (2019): 688–97, https://doi.org/10.1093/jnci .djz218; Xuesong Han et al., "Comparison of Insurance Status and Diagnosis Stage Among Patients with Newly Diagnosed Cancer Before vs After Implementation of the Patient Protection and Affordable Care Act," *JAMA Oncology* 4, no. 12 (2018): 1713–1720, https://doi.org/10.1001/jamaoncol.2018.3467.

26. Han et al., "Comparison of Insurance Status and Diagnosis Stage Among Patients with Newly Diagnosed Cancer."

27. Haley A. Moss et al., "Declines in Health Insurance Among Cancer Survivors Since the 2016 US Elections," *Lancet Oncology* 21, no. 11 (2020): e517, https://doi.org/10.1016/S1470-2045(20)30623-9.

28. Mireille Jacobson et al., "How Medicare's Payment Cuts for Cancer Chemotherapy Drugs Changed Patterns of Treatment," *Health Affairs* 29, no. 7 (2010): 1391–1399, https://doi.org/10.1377/hlthaff.2009.0563.

29. Gerald F. Riley et al., "Stage at Diagnosis and Treatment Patterns Among Older Women with Breast Cancer: An HMO and Fee-for-Service Comparison," *JAMA* 281, no. 8 (1999): 720–726, https://doi.org/10.1001/jama.281.8.720.

30. Miranda B. Lam et al., "Early Accountable Care Organization Results in End-of-Life Spending Among Cancer Patients," *Journal of the National Cancer Institute* 111, no. 12 (2019): 1307–1313, https://doi.org/10.1093/jnci/djz033; Lam et at, "Spending Among Patients with Cancer in the First 2 Years of Accountable Care Organization Participation," *Journal of Clinical Oncology* 36, no. 29 (2018): 2955–2960, https://doi.org/10.1200/JCO.18.00270.

31. Justin E. Bekelman et al., "Association Between a National Insurer's Pay-for-Performance Program for Oncology and Changes in Prescribing of Evidence-Based Cancer Drugs and Spending," *Journal of Clinical Oncology* 38, no. 34 (2020): 4055–4063, https://doi.org/10.1200/JCO.20.00890.

32. Lam et al., "Early Accountable Care Organization Results"; Lam et al., "Spending Among Patients with Cancer"; Bekelman et al., "Association."

33. Gabriel A. Brooks et al., "Early Findings from the Oncology Care Model Evaluation," *Journal of Oncology Practice* 15, no. 10 (2019): e888–e896, https://doi .org/10.1200/JOP.19.00265.

CHAPTER 4

Reductions in Cancer Drug Prices Must Account for the Cross-Subsidies They Provide for Essential Underreimbursed Services

Edward J. Benz Jr.

The fear of getting cancer, enduring cancer treatment, or dying of cancer maintains a grip on our national psyche that exceeds even the magnitude of cancer's public health impact as the second-leading cause of death in the United States. Taken together, the many forms of human cancer are also among the most common illnesses encountered in Western society. One-quarter to one-third of women and one-third to one-half of men will receive a cancer diagnosis in their lifetime.[1] It is thus not surprising that cancer care is a major driver of the overwhelming costs of health care. Indeed, the cost of cancer care has been growing considerably faster than the overall cost of health care. By some estimates, national expenditures for cancer care could climb from about $100 billion to nearly $150 billion in the next eighteen months. Any approaches taken to control overall health-care costs must address the best ways to contain cancer care costs while ensuring access to

Edward J. Benz Jr. is President and CEO Emeritus of Dana-Farber Cancer Institute, and the Richard and Susan Smith Distinguished Professor of Medicine, Professor of Pediatrics and Professor of Genetics at Harvard Medical School.

high-quality care at the cutting edge of rapidly evolving treatment options for all.

Several factors drive the accelerating costs of cancer care. Cancer has transitioned from an acute disease lasting a few months to a few years after diagnosis to a chronic disease, whereby a definitive cure is not often attained but life can be prolonged for many years or even decades. This has been a salutary accomplishment, but it comes with the continuing costs of ongoing monitoring and treatment. High-cost technologies, such as proton beam therapy, intensity-modulated radiation therapy (IMRT), and other contemporary precision radiation therapy techniques; complex imaging modalities, such as positron emission tomography-computed tomography (PET-CT) scanning; and the increasing indications for and use of stem cell transplantation, among others, have become the standard of care essential for both curative and palliative management. During the past twenty-five years, biotechnology has also enabled development of an array of more effective and less toxic but highly expensive drugs. These have become mainstays of treatment for many of the more common cancers. In addition, some providers, patients, and families feel the need to exhaust every means to "fight to the very end" even when the cancer has progressed to an untreatable state. This constellation of factors, complicated by perverse financial incentives and disincentives, tends to promote use of expensive drugs and procedures even when they are likely to be futile. In a very real sense, the partial successes of high technology–driven cancer care in prolonging survival without eliminating the cancer have created multiple structural drivers of rising cancer costs. The challenge for policy makers is finding the opportunities within this rapidly evolving ecosystem for true cost savings without compromising the best outcomes presently achievable or slowing progress toward better outcomes in the future.

While there is general agreement that the pace of growth in the costs of cancer care cannot be sustained, there is little consensus about what costs to target and how, or what strategies to pursue, to maximize quality and enhance positive outcomes at a sustainable cost. Among the most frequently mentioned and targeted objects for reduced costs are the high-priced cancer drugs and the overuse of high-technology surgery, radiation therapy, imaging, and diagnostic testing. Many view slashing these costs as a key component of reducing the overall cost of cancer care. If we are to sustain high-quality cancer care for all who need it, we must develop effective strategies and policies that will slow or even reverse the rising costs of these expensive technologies and therapies to the system, the nation, and the patients.

The premise of this chapter is that cost- and price-reduction strategies and policies must be developed holistically, accompanied by reimbursement reform that recognizes that many high-value and essential services for cancer patients are underreimbursed. The ability to sustain these services, as well as other essential contributions to the national ecosystem of health care, such as workforce development, public health outreach measures focused on prevention and early detection, and research, currently depends heavily on the phenomenon of "cross-subsidization," whereby positive operating margins derived from highly reimbursed goods and services offset operating losses incurred by the delivery of underreimbursed goods and services. Unless policy makers consider the impact of targeted price reductions on this ability to cross-subsidize, critical services could be cut. Price cuts must thus be mitigated by compensatory increases in payment for these critical underreimbursed and thus cross-subsidized services. This correction would necessarily reduce the projected savings in the overall costs of cancer care compared to current projections that count only the reduced expenditures for drugs. This consideration does not relieve our collective obligation to achieve cost reductions for drugs, tests, and procedures. Rather, it delineates the need to achieve that goal in the context of what the current arrangement pays for in the actual settings where care is delivered.

The remainder of this discussion contextualizes cancer care in the United States in light of our overall health-care costs and outcomes. In particular, we explore how the changes we outline above might affect the ability of comprehensive cancer centers to contribute to the national cancer effort and suggest how their current contributions could be preserved.

The Nation's Cancer Care in the Context of the Nation's Health-Care Dilemma

Medical care expenses in the United States far outpace those in other countries in the developed world. Yet, major health outcomes are generally worse despite the higher cost borne by American society.[2] The role of cancer care in this cost escalation is complex. On the one hand, as noted earlier, the rate of rise in cancer care costs outpaces the overall trends; on the other hand, outcomes for cancer care in the US actually compare favorably with other developed countries.[3] This stands in contrast to many other areas of medicine. Cancer care in the US needs a cost-reduction strategy that preserves performance in areas that contribute to our relatively good outcomes and recognizes the resources needed for improvements in access and performance in other areas, while fostering a sustainable investment in the nation's efforts to eradicate the fear and suffering caused by cancer.

Many remedies have been proposed to decelerate or even reverse the worrisome growth of overall health-care costs, both absolutely and as a percentage of the annual gross national product. These remedies include replacing the traditional fee-for-service forms of reimbursement with "value-based" algorithms that tie reimbursements to certain pre-agreed outcomes deemed to improve the quality of the care delivered. Within health policy, *value* is often defined in terms of the degree to which the processes and outcomes are favorable to patients, society, and payers; innovations that improve cost efficiency while maintaining quality are rewarded as well. Alternatively, some health-care stakeholders recommend massive shifts in the reimbursement formulae away from current algorithms that favor procedures, high-cost diagnostics, and pharmacy charges, and toward important underreimbursed services, such as "evaluation and management" (that is, the charge for a visit with a provider and the provider's time), preventive health measures, palliative and end-of-life care, hospice care, and mental health services. Finally, still other stakeholders propose blanket, prepaid health-care formulae whereby the providers and provider institutions receive flat monthly or annual fees per patient for the management of certain populations, for example, hypertension or diabetes patients. Various pilot programs sponsored by the government, health insurance companies, and the Veterans Administration have been tried with varying, but usually limited, degrees of success. An imperative to move the financial risk of care onto providers, be they institutions or individual practitioners, underlies many of these proposals, while supplying safeguards intended to prevent compromises in the quality or quantity of services delivered for financial reasons.

The challenge for many of these "population medicine" strategies with regard to cancer care is that cancer is a not a single disease within which one can organize the very large populations needed to define the cost and services calculations that yield predetermined per-patient or per-episode reimbursements. Cancers are highly heterogeneous, comprising over five hundred distinct types,[4] with diverse physician, nursing, hospital, and outpatient needs for optimal care. Moreover, recent advances in dissecting the molecular roots of cancers in individual patients have revealed even greater heterogeneity. For example, molecular analysis has uncovered over a dozen forms of breast cancer and several forms of non-small-cell lung cancer (NSCLC),[5] each dictating the use of distinct therapeutic modalities and agents. This "precision oncology" paradigm is spreading rapidly to many other forms of cancer. It has created an impediment to establishing population-based reimbursement paradigms that must balance the rapid shift toward highly individualized treatment regimens with the desire to define coherent populations upon which to calculate appropriate reimbursements and allocation of risk. The costs of individual goods and services in a fee-for-service setting may thus continue to be targeted in the cancer domain, even as shifts to population medicine take hold in the overall system.

The Issue of Drug Costs and Drug Prices

There is no question that the reimbursement system in the United States is broken or that it creates perverse incentives for overutilization by both patients and providers. It is heavily skewed toward procedures (e.g., surgery or interventional radiology) and testing (e.g., magnetic resonance imaging [MRI] or PET imaging), and away from some of the key parts of medical intervention, such as evaluation and management of the patient's condition and supportive care of patients and their loved ones.[6] Within the health-care industry, among patient advocacy groups, and in the political arena, attention has focused on the rising prices of highly reimbursed pharmaceuticals. Both policy makers and public opinion prominently implicated high drug prices as a major cause of the American health-care cost disaster and a prime target for correction of the overall problem. Drug costs for general health care make up 17 percent of the total health-care "bill" and are rapidly rising.[7] For cancer care, the percentage is somewhat higher and rising faster.[8]

There are several reasons the prices of new drugs are rising at the alarming rate that has attracted the attention and ire of the public and policy makers. One is that the search for more effective drugs now depends heavily on applying complex scientific experimentation and technology to identify more precisely targeted, efficacious, and safe agents. A consequence of this is that the "market size" for any single drug is much smaller, useful only for those in whom the target drives the disease. For example, non-small-cell lung cancer, an extremely common cancer, and the major cause of cancer deaths, can no longer be regarded as a single diagnosis. Rather, the availability of molecular technologies to characterize the tumors in individual patients has revealed that there are many subtypes of NSCLC driven by myriad genomic alterations.[9] These create a variety of targets for therapy, but each treatment is useful only in those patients having that target. This population can comprise as little as 1 to 2 percent of the general lung cancer population.[10] Thus, these drugs are useful only to much smaller groups of patients and development costs must be amortized over these smaller groups. A second driver is the methodology for financing new drug development. A potential drug candidate often starts with a discovery in an academic laboratory that is then patented. Start-up companies are founded on the basis of this intellectual property and the promise that the candidate will ultimately achieve sufficient utilization in clinical practice to generate a return on investment. These start-ups are supported at the earliest high-risk stages by multiple rounds of financing from angel investors, venture funds, etc. Often, such start-ups enter the public market, sometimes long before a single agent has received FDA approval. The total private and public market investments in this process frequently amount to hundreds of millions or even billions of dollars before the product reaches patients and generates revenue.[11] Those investing in these endeavors demand extremely high rates of return, on the order of six- to tenfold, on individual drug successes, so as to offset the failure rate for new drug development, which can be close to 90 percent of all drugs entering Phase 1 clinical trials.[12] Drug development is also a prolonged process. Patents issued at the time of the discovery of a target, compound, or application sometimes have a limited postapproval life span.[13] Investment costs must, in these cases, be recouped over a shorter time frame.

Despite these acknowledged drivers of the high cost of drugs, public outrage over the perception that pharmaceutical companies charge overinflated prices for these agents persists, driven in part by the companies' annual profit margins and stock performance. Moreover, the price of drugs in the United States is aggravated by the fact that many other countries regulate drug prices or permit government-run health systems to negotiate drug prices with the industry. Public and political opinion holds that both drugs and drug development are provided to the public much less expensively outside the US. Regardless of the reasons for the rapidly rising costs of drugs, there is an unquestionably strong public and political momentum for reducing the costs of pharmaceuticals, as an at least partial solution to the overall excessive costs of American health care. While a few practical approaches have been proposed (for example, permitting Medicare and Medicaid to negotiate directly with drugmakers, allowing importation of drugs from Canada at their price points, etc.), it seems increasingly likely that concrete proposals will come either in the form of legislation or Medicare/Medicaid policy and regulations.

Drug Costs, Drug Reimbursements, and
Comprehensive Cancer Centers

Cancer centers, particularly the National Cancer Institute's fifty-one designated Comprehensive Cancer Centers (CCCs), remain wary of a sudden reduction in drug prices.[14] These centers are the nation's hubs for highly specialized and subspecialized cancer care; education and training of the national cancer care workforce; basic, translational, clinical, and population-based research; and community outreach for prevention and early detection. For these single-specialty hospitals, the margins on cancer drugs are high, particularly for some of the newer agents that are based on precision medicine and therefore given to select smaller groups of patients. The margins (i.e., net revenues) for drug charges are among the highest that CCCs receive for any of their activities, because of purchase-price markups that are permitted under existing formulae. This is especially important to the sustainability of the CCCs, even those with robust inpatient and surgical activity, because cancer care has shifted significantly to the ambulatory setting, where reimbursements for most health-care services tend to be lower.[15] The arc of cancer care is now associated, fortunately, with longer survival, but often in the setting of continued presence of the cancers, making cancer more of a chronic disease akin to diabetes or hypertension, requiring intensive but less well reimbursed ambulatory care.[16] The responsibility for palliative care and end-of-life care falls disproportionately on CCCs, even in general health-care systems.[17] While imaging, surgery, and certain testing do provide positive reimbursement margins, cancer care drugs have become an important component of net revenues available to cross-subsidize these and other critical activities of the CCCs.[18]

The true costs and value of cancer care are thus mismatched with the reimbursements for services, tests, and procedures in such a way that slashing reimbursements for drugs, procedures, and infusions might reduce expenditures, but only at the expense of the provision of a broad array of high-value, moderate-cost services. The latter are currently cross-subsidized because they are underreimbursed or nonreimbursed. Abrupt reductions in drug prices without compensating improvements in reimbursement for money-losing services could have a substantial negative impact on CCCs and the national cancer care effort. These mismatches have profound effects on the operations and sustainability strategies of both large cancer centers with substantial investments in research and training, and smaller cancer centers that are often embedded in communities with lesser access to economies of scale and other opportunities for cross-subsidization. These challenges inevitably influence the utilization of services, the competition for privately insured patients, and the outcomes of cancer care in the United States.

The foregoing concerns are amplified by the fact that, in addition to delivery of highly sophisticated subspecialized care for all cancers, including rare and particularly complex cancers, the CCCs are the nation's primary generator of the cancer care workforce, including oncology-trained physicians, nurses, pharmacists, social workers, research scientists, and so on.[19] They are the major national hubs for the performance of clinical research, particularly the critical and highly complex early-stage "first in human" clinical studies that determine the viability of potential new drug candidates.[20] They engage, frequently with little or no reimbursement, in major community outreach activities that are critical to improving national cancer health outcomes, such as mammography screening, human papillomavirus (HPV) vaccination, colorectal cancer screening, and malignant melanoma cancer prevention efforts, among others. Finally, CCCs comprise by far the largest and most robust hubs for basic, early, and late-stage translational, applied clinical, and population research in the nation. Efforts to recoup the costs of these essential services are necessarily fragmented, expensive, and invariably incomplete: in other words, the financial resources sufficient to offset the structural fixed costs of these highly expensive activities at CCCs are already precarious.

The Need to Cross-Subsidize Might Limit Savings
from Reduced Drug Costs

It is widely accepted throughout the American health-care system that provider institutions must cross-subsidize to survive under the current reimbursement formulae.[21] For example, emergency services, mental health services, primary care clinics, addiction medicine services, and so on are reimbursed at or below actual cost and sustained by cross-subsidization from highly reimbursed services such as pharmaceuticals, surgery, and imaging.[22] Reliable statistics on the extent and intensity of cross-subsidization as a survival mechanism are hard to come by, but at least one study shows the negative impact that loss of highly reimbursed activity can have on the provision of less-reimbursed services by an institution.[23] In this study, a hospital providing a comprehensive array of services was operating in a health-care market into which an entity focusing solely on highly reimbursed cardiovascular services entered. This entry resulted in the loss of this activity by the generalist institution. In response, the institution was forced to reduce its provision of underreimbursed services, such as mental health services, that had been made possible by the margins from cardiovascular medicine.[24] The complexities of cross-subsidization are also at work in CCCs.

Second opinion consultations are a vital service performed by CCCs. One major cancer center, MD Anderson Breast Center, felt that it could no longer meet the growing need for these consultations and temporarily curtailed them. MD Anderson stated, among other reasons, that the cost of providing second opinions was too high, compared to the reimbursement recovered.[25] This policy was later rescinded, but not because second opinions became more lucrative; rather, the CCC simply accepted higher operating losses from this service line. In CCCs, pharmaceutical prices provide significant amounts of the margin available for this form of cross-subsidization.

The preceding discussion makes apparent one aspect of the discussions around pharmaceutical reimbursement that extant conversations often do not recognize. That is, what patients and society are paying for when reimbursing a CCC for a cancer drug is not simply the all-in costs of the cancer drug itself and the indirect costs associated with storing, handling, and dispensing the drug, and so on, but also a significant contribution to the broad array of comprehensive clinical services, public health activities, education, training, and research that make CCCs important national resources. It follows that abrupt reductions in the reimbursements for cancer drugs will need to be balanced by recognition, either by reimbursement reform or subsidies, of the essential services that could be negatively impacted by a sudden loss of substantial revenue from pharmaceuticals. The need to account for those no longer cross-subsidized costs implies that the savings anticipated by reduced drug prices might thus be lower than anticipated. The alternative could otherwise be a reduction in vital services.

Reducing Drug Prices Must Be Accompanied by Other Payment Reforms

There is no doubt that drug prices are escalating far too rapidly. The trend needs to be significantly slowed and reversed. This chapter argues that the reduction in drug prices needs to be accomplished holistically, with anticipation of unintended consequences. At least in the case of cancer drugs, one should not expect to recoup the total reduction in drug costs in the form of health-care savings, unless one is prepared to forgo in part or completely the availability of other critical services both to patients and to society that CCCs perform. The goal of any solution should be to rationalize the reimbursement system so that the prices charged for drugs are reduced to levels appropriate for the costs of their development, production, utilization, and monitoring. The portion that results in net revenue loss to provider institutions should be mitigated by implementing appropriate levels of reimbursement for services that now operate at a loss. In other words, the price of goods and services should directly reflect their cost and value, both to patients and society.

Another approach to reducing the cost of cancer drugs to consumers and society is to reduce the cost of development. The chances of an early drug candidate that is matched to a promising physiologic target, such as a particular cancer mutation, progressing through the long and complex process of drug development, testing, and approval are about 5 to 10 percent.[26] Much of the expense associated with that high failure rate occurs because the knowledge and technology are not always available to advance those agents with a higher chance of success or eliminate those unlikely to succeed at earlier stages of development.

Given that situation, a national priority should be to de-risk some of the earliest stages of pharmaceutical research, thus reducing a portion of the enormous but necessary early-stage investments in companies or development programs. This would involve creating funding mechanisms, whether governmental or private, that would pool funds and drug development candidates, subsidizing rigorous interrogation of many therapeutic targets and many approaches to manipulating promising targets at the earliest, least expensive stages of drug development. In that manner, drug candidates destined for failure would be eliminated early. Only the most promising candidates would need to be supported by investment in the later, more expensive stages.[27] The return on agents that do succeed would offset the costs and risks of evaluating the broader array of early candidates. Mechanisms to achieve this, such as those proposed by Dr. Andrew Lo and colleagues, are under investigation.[28]

CANCER CARE AND research in the United States continue to improve both the quality of care and the quantity of positive outcomes. At least some of these gains are due to services that are underreimbursed but supported by cross-subsidization from more highly reimbursed goods and services, including cancer drugs. However, the rate of rise of overall cancer care costs is unsustainable. Innovative mechanisms to reduce costs are essential if cancer care is to remain anything close to affordable for patients, the government, insurers, and employers. Managing the rate of rise of cancer drug prices must constitute a significant part of policy discussions involving such mechanisms. Such discussions must take into consideration the consequences, intended and un-intended, of abrupt changes in drug-related reimbursements to providers. Indeed, the savings from reducing drug prices will ul-timately be less than one might predict if one takes into account the indispensable services delivered by cancer care centers that pharmacy revenues cross-subsidize. Compensatory increases in cost recovery for currently underreimbursed services and under-funded activities must accompany reduced drug prices. In taking such a holistic approach, the United States can still anticipate a salutary reduction in overall health-care costs, as providers will be able to increase the availability of services, such as preventive cancer medicine and palliative care, which are known to improve patient outcomes and satisfaction, reduce the cost of care, and prolong high-quality survival.

Notes

1. American Cancer Society, "Lifetime Risk of Developing or Dying from Cancer," Cancer.org, last modified January 13, 2020, https://www.cancer.org /cancer/cancer-basics/lifetime-probability-of-developing-or-dying-from -cancer.html.

2. Roosa Tikkanen and Melinda K. Abrams, "U.S. Healthcare from a Global Perspective, 2019: Higher Spending, Worse Outcomes?" Commonwealth Fund, January 30, 2020, https://doi.org/10.26099/7avy-fc29.

3. Claudia Allemani et al., "Global Surveillance of Trends in Cancer Survival 2000-14 (CONCORD-3): Analysis of Individual Records for 37,513,025 Patients Diagnosed with One of 18 Cancers from 322 Population-Based Registries in 71 Countries," Lancet 391, no. 10125 (2018): 1023–1075, https://doi.org/10.1016 /S0140-6736(17)33326-3.

4. National Cancer Institute, "What Is Cancer?" Cancer.gov, last modified February 9, 2015, https://www.cancer.gov/about-cancer/understanding/what-is -cancer.

5. International Agency for Research on Cancer, World Cancer Report 2014, ed. Bernard W. Stewart and Christopher P. Wild (Geneva: World Health Or-ganization, 2014).

6. "Chapter 13: Radiology Services and Other Diagnostic Procedures," in Medicare Claims Processing Manual (Baltimore, MD: US Centers for Medicare

& Medicaid Services, last revised March 27, 2019), https://www.cms.gov/Reg ulations-and-Guidance/Guidance/Manuals/downloads/clm104c13.pdf.

7. "Observations on Trends in Prescription Drug Spending," Office of the Assistant Secretary for Planning and Evaluation, US Department of Health and Human Services, Washington, DC, March 2016, https://aspe.hhs.gov/system /files/pdf/187586/Drugspending.pdf.

8. Roland Turck, "Oncology Drug Costs—the Imaginary Crisis?" *Annals of Oncology* 28, no. 2 (2017): 427–431, https://doi.org/10.1093/annonc/mdw548.

9. Larissa A. Pikor et al., "Genetic Alterations Defining NSCLC Subtypes and Their Therapeutic Implications," *Lung Cancer* 82, no. 2 (2013): 179–189, https://doi.org/10.1016/j.lungcan.2013.07.025.

10. Lucian R. Chirieac and Sanja Dacic, "Targeted Therapies in Lung Cancer," *Surgical Pathology Clinics* 3, no. 1 (2010): 71–82, https://doi.org/10.1016/j .path.2010.04.001.

11. Olivier J. Wouters, Martin McKee, and Jeroen Luyten, "Estimated Research and Development Investment Needed to Bring a New Medicine to Market, 2009–2018," *JAMA* 323, no. 9 (2020): 844–853, https://doi.org/10.1001/jama .2020.1166.

12. Chi Heem Wong, Kien Wei Siah, and Andrew W. Lo, "Estimation of Clinical Trial Success Rates and Related Parameters," *Biostatistics* 20, no. 2 (2019): 273–286, https://doi.org/10.1093/biostatistics/kxx069.

13. Eric Budish, Benjamin N. Roin, and Heidi Williams, "Do Firms Underinvest in Long-Term Research? Evidence from Cancer Clinical Trials," NBER Working Paper No. 19430, National Bureau of Economic Research, Cambridge, MA, last revised February 2015, https://doi.org/10.3386/w19430.

14. "NCI-Designated Cancer Centers," National Cancer Institute, Cancer .gov, last modified June 24, 2019, https://www.cancer.gov/research/infrastructure /cancer-centers.

15. Tamela Sterrett Williamson, "The Shift of Oncology Inpatient Care to Outpatient Care: The Challenge of Retaining Expert Oncology Nurses," *Clinical Journal of Oncology Nursing* 12, no. 2 (2008): 186–189, https://doi.org/10.1188 /08.CJON.186-189.

16. Joanna Lion et al., "Case Mix and Charges for Inpatient and Outpatient Chemotherapy," *Healthcare Finance Review* 8, no. 4 (1987): 65–71, https://www .ncbi.nlm.nih.gov/pmc/articles/PMC4192853/.

17. David Hui et al., "Availability and Integration of Palliative Care at US Cancer Centers," *JAMA* 303, no. 11 (2010): 1054–1061, https://doi.org/10.1001 /jama.2010.258.

18. Edward J. Benz, "The Jeremiah Metzger Lecture. Cancer in the 21st Century: An Inside View from an Outsider," *Transactions of the American Clinical and Climatological Association* 128 (2017): 275–297, https://www.ncbi.nlm.nih.gov /pmc/articles/PMC5525421/.

19. Lawrence N. Shulman, Lisa Kennedy Sheldon, and Edward J. Benz, "The Future of Cancer Care in the United States—Overcoming Workforce Capacity Limitations," *JAMA Oncology* 6, no. 3 (2020): 327–328, https://doi.org/10.1001 /jamaoncol.2019.5358.

20. Benz, "The Jeremiah Metzger Lecture."

21. Guy David et al., "Do Hospitals Cross-Subsidize?" *Journal of Health Economics* 37, no. 1 (2018), https://doi.org/10.1016/j.jhealeco.2014.06.007.

22. David et al., "Do Hospitals Cross-Subsidize?"

23. David et al., "Do Hospitals Cross-Subsidize?"

24. David et al., "Do Hospitals Cross-Subsidize?"

25. Todd Ackerman, "M.D. Anderson Breast Center Halts 2nd Opinions," *Houston Chronicle*, last modified July 20, 2011, chron.com/news/health/article /M-D-Anderson-breast-center-halts-2nd-opinions-1486242.php.

26. Wong, Siah, and Lo, "Estimation of Clinical Trial Success Rates and Related Parameters."

27. Andrew W. Lo, "Can Financial Engineering Cure Cancer?" Tangerine Lecture in Finance, November 3, 2016, https://www.ivey.uwo.ca/cmsmedia/377 4733/20161103_tangerine_hardcopy.pdf.

28. Lo, "Can Financial Engineering Cure Cancer?"

CHAPTER 5

Save Physician-Owned Practices to Save Money in Health Care

Barbara McAneny

Cancer care is the canary in the coal mine for any discussion of the costs of health care. On top of a devastating medical diagnosis, cancer patients face bankruptcy at the most vulnerable time in their lives. High out-of-pocket costs and the prospect of losing employer-based health insurance are exacerbated by the ever-increasing costs for cancer care. Community oncology practices evolved as the lower-cost option when antinausea drugs made outpatient chemotherapy possible. Patients then had an option for care close to home, with a practice that could provide a friendlier, less institutional atmosphere, as well as lower costs. Over time, however, the payments independent practices received under the physician fee schedule were significantly outpaced by the payments to hospital systems with greater negotiating power and the benefits of a fee schedule that was increased every year.

The allure of cancer drug reimbursement for hospitals with a profit margin greater than that of independent practices made acquisition of oncology practices highly profitable for hospitals. Oncology practice consolidation has increased 21 percent in the last two years, resulting in higher prices and less choice for patients. Cancer patients are mostly unaware of the difference in

---

Barbara McAneny is a former President of the American Medical Association and Founder and CEO of the New Mexico Cancer Center.

price and out-of-pocket costs between hospital and physician office care.

The COVID-19 pandemic has created unprecedented challenges, including for smaller practices that may not be able to weather the financial shock or may be overwhelmed by needing to provide traditional public health services to their patients. Rather than further entrenching a system that deprives society's most vulnerable, we should take charge of this opportunity to control cancer care costs by better understanding the true costs of oncology care, increasing transparency at all levels, facilitating competition and preventing health-care concentration, and restructuring the health-care insurance system to serve patients more effectively. Solving problems with cancer care requires addressing problems within the entire health-care system—the two are inseparable.

This chapter will begin by diving into some of the issues that make cancer care so expensive for patients, such as opaque drug pricing and the holes in the insurance safety net. Then, the chapter will explore the forces driving consolidation and their impact on community oncology practices and patients. The chapter concludes with suggestions for meaningful reform.

A Cancer Diagnosis Is a Medical and Financial Catastrophe for Patients

For cancer patients, costs can be overwhelming. Cancer patients are 2.65 times more likely to go bankrupt than people without cancer. Two-thirds of bankruptcies are triggered by a health-care event, and two-thirds of the people declaring bankruptcy have health insurance. Younger cancer patients have two to five times higher rates of bankruptcy than cancer patients aged sixty-five or older, indicating that Medicare and Social Security might ease some of the bankruptcy risk. The high financial burden stems in part from astronomical oncology drug prices, made worse by opaque middlemen driving up costs, paired with health insurance companies that shift the cost to cancer patients by co-pays and deductibles.

Cancer Patients Face Losing Employer-Based Health Insurance with Inadequate Fallback Options

Employer-based insurance can be problematic for cancer patients. Inability to work can cause them to lose their insurance. The Family Medical Leave Act allows unpaid time off and job retention if a worker can return in time, but it does not pay the insurance premiums. The Consolidated Omnibus Budget Reconciliation Act of 1985 permits patients to retain their insurance for eighteen months, if they pay both the employer's and the employee's parts of the full payment. Without a salary, that is often impossible. If the insurance lapses, the patient incurs the full cost of treatment, and if they return to work, there is usually an additional month before their coverage resumes.

Clearly, employer-based insurance is designed for people with short-term, limited illnesses or for managing chronic diseases that do not interfere with the ability to work. It is not designed for the people who need insurance the most: people with an illness so severe they cannot work.

As employers attempt to control insurance costs, narrow networks and patient cost-shifting through defined benefit plans have gained popularity. The cost-shifting to patients has resulted in a decrease both in necessary valuable care as well as unnecessary care. Cancer patients need to know that their portion of the cost of care can be significantly lower at independent physician fee schedule (PFS) practices than at hospital-owned practices.

Social Security Disability Insurance and Medicare take two years to obtain, so that is not an option for cancer patients either. The average American family has under $50,000 for retirement and an emergency fund of less than $500. A diagnosis of cancer, especially in a family where two employed adults are needed to make ends meet, can plunge an entire family into poverty.

Our safety net has large holes, and cancer patients fall right through them.

Insurance Gaps Also Plague Medicare-Eligible Cancer Patients

Medicare-eligible cancer patients enrolled in Medicare Fee-for-Service (FFS) still need to purchase a Medigap plan, which covers the 20 percent of the Medicare allowable price not covered under Medicare. They must also purchase Part B coverage and a Part D prescription drug plan. The cost of cancer drugs for a Medicare patient without the Medigap, Part B, and Part D coverage would make care unaffordable.

Medicare Advantage (MA) plans are another attempt by the Centers for Medicare and Medicaid Services (CMS) to decrease the cost of care. MA plans are paid a capitated rate, usually 14 to 19 percent more than the per capita cost of FFS Medicare. The hope was that the commercial payers' negotiating power would lower overall costs. The plans try to control costs by narrowing the network of physicians and hospitals, and by utilization management tools, such as prior authorization, co-pays, coinsurance, and narrow formularies. This does not work well for cancer patients, however, who need to see specialists who may not be in network and need drugs that may not be on the formulary. Patients who get seriously ill tend to switch back to Medicare FFS with a Medigap plan.

Astronomical Drug Costs

The gaps in insurance coverage make it difficult for cancer patients to afford ever-rising oncology therapy prices. For example, innovative therapies, such as chimeric antigen receptor T cell (CAR-T) drugs, can carry price tags close to half a million dollars for a single dose.[1] The effectiveness of these drugs is irrelevant if patients cannot afford them.

Drug costs are everyone's favorite target for the high cost of care. The manufacturers deserve some of the blame for creating consolidated markets that maximize profits. Often, the original research that leads to a new drug is federally funded by the National Institutes of Health (NIH) and is acquired by the pharmaceutical company. The FDA process is particularly expensive to navigate, encouraging further consolidation of manufacturers. Manufacturers also regularly extend patent profits by paying companies to delay bringing a generic or biosimilar drug to market, or by developing minor variations to restart the patent clock. For example, the seven-month delay in the generic entry of the leukemia therapy Gleevec is estimated to have cost the health-care system at least half a billion dollars.[2]

Pharmacy Benefit Managers Hike Up Chemotherapy Costs
Manufacturers are not entirely to blame, however, for high drug prices. The American Medical Association has estimated that 42 percent of the cost to the patient is added once the drug leaves the manufacturer. Pharmacy benefit managers (PBMs) are companies created by the insurance industry to negotiate discounts with pharmaceutical manufactures. However, PBMs have evolved to be extremely profitable, have acquired commercial pharmacies and distributors and created specialty pharmacies, and are now large enough that they are buying the insurance companies.

PBMs negotiate discounts as a percentage of the list price, keep some of the discount and pass some to the parent insurance company. The higher the price, the more money the PBM makes. Sometimes the markup is so high that the co-pay charged to the patient is higher than the price of the drug, and the contracts with pharmacies forbid the pharmacist from letting the patient know! Because a percentage-based discount on chemotherapy is profitable, PBMs have persuaded insurance companies to mandate that all purchases must go through their specialty pharmacy. They can add a dispensing fee and lower the amount paid to independent pharmacies until the latter cannot afford to stay in business. The PBMs then "invite" the pharmacy to join their network, adding more profit to their bottom line. Data sales, both to the manufacturers and to the insurers, add another revenue stream to the PBMs. And PBMs claw back direct and indirect remuneration fees from the pharmacy, often months after the drug was purchased.

We need to demand transparency from PBMs so that they cannot generate large profits without adding value for cancer patients.

The Origins and Impact of Consolidation in Oncology

Cancer care costs are predicted to reach $230 billion by 2023, putting cancer care on center stage because of the high cost of drugs, concerns about unnecessary care, and worries about rationing. Without the control of costs, we could see poor people or people of color having even worse access to care than they receive now.

The acquisition of community oncology practices is driving increases in cancer costs. Since 2008, nearly 1,750 independent community oncology clinics and practices have either been closed, acquired by hospitals, or merged due to financial hardship.[3] The rate of consolidation has increased 21 percent in the last two years. Taking an extraordinary toll on small businesses, the COVID-19 pandemic will likely exacerbate this issue, resulting in diminished patient choice and higher costs.

The American health-care system is stacked against community practices in many ways, including outdated Medicare reimbursement models that favor large hospitals and cancer centers both for services and drug reimbursement, as well as newer insurance models that force practices to take on substantial financial risk, requiring data resulting in further consolidation. Ultimately, insurers and cancer patients overpaying for services in hospital settings are subsidizing the acquisition of independent oncology practices, leading to decreased choice of site of care and causing their own expenses to rise.

Outdated Reimbursement Practices Prioritize Large Hospital Systems, Pushing Community Practices to Consolidate

In 1965, when President Lyndon Johnson created Medicare, cancer care was largely surgical, if it happened at all, and chemotherapy and radiation were still in the future. Medicare Part B, for outpatient services, was an afterthought. Everything that a physician could do in 1965 could be carried into people's homes in a little black bag, so the cost was minimal.

Originally, Medicare fees for services were set based on a doctor's usual and customary charges, which varied significantly by location. Even today, prices are adjusted by geography, with the assumption that a physician practice's overhead will reflect the costs of living in the region. For cancer care though, the equipment cost does not vary by location, and recruiting is done through a national market, so the geographic price adjustments harm oncology practices serving rural or less-affluent populations.

Oncologists built infusion centers in their offices and stopped admitting patients to the hospital for chemotherapy once nausea was no longer uncontrollable. Stemming from outdated distinctions between hospital and outpatient delivery of care, CMS continues to pay community health providers pursuant to the Physician Fee Schedule (PFS) and hospitals according to the Hospital Outpatient Prospective Patient System (HOPPS). However, these two payment schedules have not evolved at the same pace.

Managing cancer patients outside the hospital is better for patients and their families, and improves the patient's and the health-care system's finances, just not the bottom line of the hospital. As care shifts to outpatient settings and the revenue from inpatient services drop, hospitals have responded by hiring entire oncology practices. Because hospitals bill under HOPPS, they can charge higher fees and add on a facility fee, even for outpatient services, such as chemotherapy. In those areas where no independent community practices exist, nothing acts as a brake on the prices charged by hospitals. The facility fees paid by the cancer patient are used to pay for the emergency department, the operating room, the intensive care unit, and other high-priced items the community needs to have available, with enough left over for a profit margin.

Despite the burden of quality measures and data submission, electronic medical records, and other requirements, CMS estimates that practice expense has only increased by 30 percent. The proportion of people eligible for Medicare increased, and the costs of delivering care in the PFS practices have increased, but Medicare payments have not kept up, as the last survey of practice expense occurred in 2010. However, because hospital outpatient services are paid through HOPPS, they continue to receive a "market basket" increase every year. The average increase for the HOPPS is 2 to 3.5 percent yearly, whereas the PFS has changed very little over the last twenty years. HOPPS has increased by almost 50 percent and the PFS by 6 percent between 2002 and 2015, when the law changed. For 2021, the hospital fees were increased by over 2 percent, while the physician fee schedule decreased by 10.4 percent.

In addition, when the diagnosis-related group (DRG) system was implemented in 1983, eleven cancer hospitals were exempted and paid based on their costs plus a margin. The rationale was that cancer length of stay was much longer than for other diseases. Those eleven hospitals, now hospital systems with multiple satellite facilities, are still exempt, making them highly profitable and very expensive. Today, almost all hospitals admit cancer patients, and most of cancer care is done on an outpatient basis, so the need to compensate these hospitals more generously has diminished, but this carefully guarded anachronism is protected by an army of lobbyists.

These reimbursement disparities created the site of service differential: practices being paid below cost for Medicare patients, and hospitals being paid at almost twice the rate for exactly the same services. Hospitals justify the higher payment because of the cost of uninsured patients requiring care, even though the physicians delivering care who are not employed by the hospitals are billing at the PFS rate. Practices are relying on the better payments from commercial plans to cover the shortfall in payment from governmental payers or are limiting the number of governmental patients they accept.

Furthermore, as hospitals merge into hospital systems, their ability to negotiate higher price increases, and the gap between the charges from a self-employed PFS physician and a hospital-employed physician increased for both Medicare and for commercial health plans. The result of the widening payment gap has been that many physician practices have found no alternative to being acquired by hospitals when they could not cover expenses. Empirical research has shown that prices tend to increase with consolidation, without an increase in the quality of care. Over the last twelve years, nearly two thousand community oncology practices have closed or merged with hospitals as a result of these disparities. The remaining independent practices have had to become very lean to survive.

Independent Cancer Providers Cannot Bear
the Financial Risks Required

In 2015, the Medicare and CHIP Reauthorization Act discouraged fee-for-service (FFS) payments in favor of Accountable Care Organizations (ACOs). ACOs pay groups of clinicians a predetermined fee for a particular type of care, regardless of the ultimate cost of care. Groups with more patients can accept more risk. Smaller practices are disadvantaged by the actuarial risk of managing fewer patients and inadequate financial reserves to offset the risk. If they go out of business or are acquired by a hospital, costs increase and choice for patients goes down. Furthermore, the differential between payments for the services of hospital-employed and independent physicians was carried forward. The PFS still lags 30 percent lower, and the HOPPS reimbursement is significantly higher than cost as estimated by the Medicare Economic Index, disadvantaging small, independent cancer providers.

Financial risk may also prevent smaller practices from benefiting from alternative care models. The Community Oncology Medical Home (COME HOME), a team-based care innovation that aggressively managed cancer patients' side effects to avoid the need for hospitalization, saved over $600 per patient on average. However, when it was adopted by the CMS ACO Oncology Care Model, the target price was developed from national averages, leaving smaller practices at risk if more patients with expensive needs than predicted obtained care from the practice. Two-thirds of the practices have since abandoned the model. Although it focused practices on the value of keeping patients out of the hospital, it did not decrease the spending on drugs as CMS had hoped.

CMS Chemotherapy Drug Reimbursement Practices and 340B Subsidies Drive Consolidation

CMS designs alternative payment models that expect oncologists to either control the drug cost or pay for the increased costs over their target price. The assumption is that oncologists select the more expensive drugs for the add-on of 6 percent over average sales price (ASP). The number of drugs with medically equivalent options is relatively small, and newer, more expensive immunotherapies are remarkably effective with much less toxicity. Selecting older, cheaper, more toxic regimens would be unethical. In addition, in the current risk-based models for value-based care, accepting a cancer patient requiring an expensive biologic drug for a benign condition means that the target of total cost of care is not attainable. Physicians are finding that if the best regimen for a patient includes an expensive new drug, their practice misses the target price.

Further, the requirements of an infusion center that conforms with United States Pharmacopeia (USP) regulations, Occupational Safety and Health Act (OSHA) regulations, and specialty society requirements have outpaced the CMS payments for infusion. The National Cancer Care Alliance (NCCA) did a time and motion study on the costs of the first hour of an infusion, and found the costs to be $200 more than CMS paid, and that the drug margin did not make up the difference.[4]

CMS pays within a few weeks, but commercial insurers often delay four to six weeks. In the interim, the ASP may have dipped below their purchase price. Because ASP is an average, large practices or systems that buy in large quantities or pay the same day get a significant discount, so the average is sometimes below the price paid by a smaller practice. Without a significant markup on the chemotherapy payments of commercial payers, smaller independent practices would not be able to stay in business.

For practices with increasing numbers of Medicare and Medicaid patients—that is, those treating the poor and the elderly—the prospect of being acquired by a hospital is often irresistible. The facility fee paid to hospitals for chemotherapy makes even Medicare profitable. Underpaying the PFS practices therefore increases costs for the entire health system over time.

Another contributing factor to drug prices, particularly important for cancer patients, is the 340B program. This program was designed so that tax-exempt designated hospitals and entities, such as Federally Qualified Health Centers, can receive significant discounts from pharmaceutical manufacturers when they purchase drugs to be given in the outpatient setting. The money received from the discount is supposed to cover the costs of unreimbursed care. When a hospital-employed physician writes a prescription for a drug, and the hospital fills that prescription for a commercially insured patient, they can bill the insurance company the full contracted price and then obtain an additional rebate of 30 to 50 percent of the drug cost from the manufacturer. Manufacturers are required to participate in the 340B program if they wish to sell their medicines to patients with governmental payers.

As chemotherapy became more expensive in the early to mid-2000s, that discounted amount started to make a significant contribution to the bottom line of hospitals. A busy oncologist prescribes $2 million to $3 million of drugs every year. A 340B hospital that acquired an oncologist found that the 340B program delivered $1 million to $1.5 million of rebate profit to their bottom line. When that amount is added to the significantly higher prices hospitals negotiate with all payers, the amount of imaging needed by oncologists, and the volume of referrals for surgery or other services needed by cancer patients, it becomes obvious why hospitals targeted oncology practices for acquisition. As independent oncologists lose the drug margin in their practices and have trouble making their overhead, 340B hospitals can entice them with a nice salary increase and still add millions to their own bottom line.

The number of 340B hospitals when the program began was under four hundred, and now it is above four thousand, with over 80 percent of community oncology mergers occurring with hospitals with existing 340B programs.[5] When manufacturers are forced to give this rebate to an ever-increasing number of hospitals, they raise the prices for everyone else to cover their loss. The price of drugs goes up again. The cancer patients do not get the 340B discount, the hospitals do. You can tell a 340B hospital by the opulence of its lobby, although the hospital CEO will claim it needs the 340B money to cover its overhead.

Our system seems designed to maximize the profit of the insurance companies, the consolidated hospital systems, and the pharmaceutical companies. They are all doing well, while patients go bankrupt. We must decide whether the for-profit insurance companies provide value, if the value of a hospital system is greater than the value of a community hospital, and whether the consolidation of the various parts of the industry is contributing to efficiency, or just raising prices.

COVID-19 Presents New Challenges for Providers and Cancer Patients

The COVID-19 pandemic has unmasked the flaws of how we deliver health care. The social determinants of health have an enormous impact on health outcomes. With COVID-19, disadvantaged populations have been disproportionately represented in ICU admissions and in deaths.

Take the population of the Navajo Nation in Arizona and New Mexico. One-third of the Navajo do not have running water. Few have internet or cellular network access, and many live in small, multigenerational houses. Social distancing is not possible when you must haul water to wash your hands. The Navajo nation has a very high per capita infection rate. Years of neglect in providing electricity and running water, compounded by government underfunding of the Indian Health Service (IHS), has led to a public health disaster. The courage and dedication of the medical staff is inspiring, but the lack of resources is devastating. Oncology care in IHS hospitals was placed out of reach by the limited budgets approved by Congress.

My practice has had a cancer center serving the Navajo Nation since 2007. We are used to having the IHS run out of money every July and be unable to pay us until the new fiscal year every October. However, providing cancer care during the COVID-19 pandemic has been a new experience. Patients, relieved that we were providing treatment, are afraid to go home to a possibly infectious family. We have had to provide food support, help with transportation, masks, rent, and utilities out of the practice and our foundation. Telemedicine requires an internet connection or a smartphone, and often our patients have neither. The health-care system cannot provide all the needed infrastructure to keep a population healthy, and the additional burden certainly cannot fall on community practices operating on ever slimmer margins and smaller reserves.

The fragility of the health-care system is exposed as small rural hospitals close, small and medium-size practices shuttered during the pandemic may not be able to reopen, and people delay care for fear of contamination. Larger hospitals have furloughed employees, yet some of the richest hospitals, often with billions in reserves, have received generous handouts from the federal government response. Further entrenching provider disparities, $50 billion of the Coronavirus Aid, Relief, and Economic Security Act (CARES) funding for provider relief was distributed through Medicare, using a formula that gave more money to providers that tend to have higher margins.[6] For example, Baylor University was given $454 million, even though it eventually made a surplus of $815 million.[7]

An Opportunity for Reform

After this pandemic, the worst scenario would be that the remaining large, profitable hospitals acquire even more of the health-care infrastructure, consolidating their control and eliminating the competition that currently puts restraint on prices. More consolidation will lead to increased prices and decreased choice.

If small practices and hospitals in rural areas, small towns, or inner cities do not recover, a significant number of Americans will be left without access to cancer care. If a small town loses its health-care infrastructure, the town will die as surely as if it lost running water and power. Patients will be forced to travel to the increasingly expensive, highly consolidated hospital systems and their monopolistic control of both inpatient and outpatient care. As prices rise, fewer people will be able to afford care, and health disparities will increase.

The system, our medical industrial complex, is clearly not sustainable.

Fixing the System

1. Transparency is key. For every cost-shifting process, and every proprietary price structure, money is funneled off into profits for corporate entities, consultants, and administrative bloat. The actual costs of *care*, NOT charges, must be tabulated by universally accepted accounting parameters, and made publicly available. Rational approaches to fixing every aspect of the system will never be possible without access to accurate and updated cost data. The "Site of Service Differential" could be eliminated if processes were accurate and the need for cost-shifting eliminated.

2. If the price of care is altered by characteristics of the patient or the cancer, then the compensation should match that price. If two systems charge very different amounts for equivalent treatment, payers should only pay the lower amount. To control costs, we must first adopt tools to determine the adequate price for optimal care. Making Accountable Sustainable Oncology Networks (MASON) is a proposal to CMMI that would combine the clinical data of NCCA practices with claims data to create accurate pricing using data science techniques. Here is how it works:

   MASON uses cost accounting techniques to determine the infrastructure costs of delivering care, such as for infusion centers. NCCA practices have agreed to accept invoice price for the drugs, thus removing any concern that drugs are selected for profit. Target prices determined by data science give the practices the opportunity to manage patients even more efficiently to share in additional savings. Practices would thrive while still providing cost-effective care.

   Quality of care is determined by adherence to evidence-based pathways and by patient satisfaction. Oncology is fortunate to have reputable guidelines developed by the National Comprehensive Cancer Network, a group of academic centers. However, once we show that the MASON process works for cancer care, it can be applied to accurately price other types of care.

3. The pharmacy benefit manager system must be made transparent and accountable, if indeed it needs to exist at all. Knowing what the insurer was charged for the drug and not allowing the markup of the PBM would be a good start to manageable drug prices. Eliminating direct-to-consumer advertising would save the manufacturers a lot of money, which could then be used to reduce prices.

4. Emergency departments should not be paid for by people using the other parts of the health-care system, but by the tax structure of local, state, and federal governments. We pay for police, fire fighters, and ambulance services by tax base, regardless of whether or not we use them as individuals. Cancer patients would benefit because the facility fee and the markup of services to cover unreimbursed care would be unnecessary if the emergency services costs were covered separately.

5. The tax-exempt status and the role of hospitals should be reexamined. Hospitals are needed in every community to provide emergency services, treat people whose chronic diseases are out of control, provide recovery space for people with severe acute illnesses or surgeries, and provide a setting for the local infrastructure of care, such as imaging. Accountability for the amount of charity care provided could lead to payment for that care, which would decrease if everyone had insurance. We could eliminate the need for tax-exempt hospitals to possess wholly owned for-profit subsidiaries or have huge endowments that they invest in competition with those who pay taxes. Localities would do better if hospitals paid their share of taxes.

6. Hospital systems that do not show value should be broken up by antitrust actions. Hospitals should be based on community need and logical provision of services, not

pricing advantages. Data show that hospital systems increase price but not quality. Actions that return hospitals to the control of the communities they serve should be encouraged.

7. The DRG-exempt cancer hospital financial structure should be eliminated. The eleven DRG-exempt cancer centers have used profits not available to other hospitals to consolidate ownership and stifle competition, further increasing the overall costs of cancer care to everyone. Clinical oncology research and outpatient services can be provided in ways that better match community needs, so we should eliminate this historical relic.

8. The 340B system should be entirely redesigned. Money paid by the federal government should follow the patient for whom the support is designed, NOT be given to hospitals to advance their bottom line. At a minimum, the discount for Medicare patients should accrue to Medicare similarly to how the discount goes to Medicaid.

9. Insurance must be redesigned. The employer-based system works only for employees, not for people too sick to work. Commercial payers have a very lucrative system, collecting premiums throughout the healthy years, then dumping patients onto Medicare when they age into infirmity. The pandemic has taught us that leaving anyone out of care endangers all of us. Everyone must have true access, not just an insurance card that does not cover the costs of delivering care. If people could have health insurance that covered the costs of care, without cost-shifting, we would not need special programs like Medicaid and Medicare. Insurance companies would not be nearly as profitable, but would charge enough to cover the costs of determining actuarial rates, collecting premiums, and paying claims.

We must first decide whether we want insurance as a profitable industry or as a utility that provides service for nominal costs. The Affordable Care Act took a major step toward insurance as a utility, even though the transformation was deliberately slow. The call for "Medicare for All" is focused on providing Medicare as a not-for-profit insurance. By moving towards an insurance safety net that catches all Americans and adequately covers the legitimate costs of care, cancer patients can fully focus on their recovery.

THE CURRENT MONOPOLIES of hospitals, health plans, and pharmaceutical manufacturers should be broken up so that hospitals can be restructured to fit the needs of the communities they serve, with a transparent funding process. We must preserve the low-cost, high-quality option of independent physician practices.

As we examine our system and the flaws uncovered by the pandemic, we can either use the opportunity to create a rational system, or we can return to our current, highly profitable medical industrial complex without change. We can develop a system that treats all patients, or we can have a system that can only be accessed by the very wealthy. We are the richest nation on the planet; surely we can afford to invest in our own population.

Notes

1. Gillian Mohney, "Concern Rises over $475,000 Price Tag for Breakthrough Cancer Treatment," *Healthline*, last modified October 16, 2019, https://www.healthline.com/health-news/concern-rises-over-price-tag-for-breakthrough-cancer-treatment.

2. Hagop Kantarjian and S. Vincent Rajkumar, "Why Are Cancer Drugs So Expensive in the United States, and What Are the Solutions?" *Mayo Clinic Proceedings* 90, no. 4 (2015): 500–504, https://www.mayoclinicproceedings.org/article/S0025-6196(15)00101-9/fulltext.

3. Rebecca Pifer, "Community Oncology Practices Turn to Mergers, Private Equity to Avoid Hospital Acquisition," Healthcare Dive, April 24, 2020, https://www.healthcaredive.com/news/community-oncology-practices-turn-to-mergers-private-equity-to-avoid-hospi/576722/.

4. These data have not been published.

5. Pifer, "Community Oncology Practices."

6. Karyn Schwartz et al., "What We Know About Provider Consolidation," KFF.org, September 2, 2020, n72, https://www.kff.org/report-section/what-we -know-about-provider-consolidation-issue-brief/#endnote_link_481999-72.

7. Jordan Rau and Christine Spolar, "Some of America's Wealthiest Hospital Systems Ended Up Even Richer, Thanks to Federal Bailouts," *Washington Post*, April 1, 2021, https://www.washingtonpost.com/us-policy/2021/04/01 /hospital-systems-cares-act-bailout/.

PART TWO

CANCER AND THE COMMUNITY

CHAPTER 6

Racial Disparities and Cancer Injustice

Matt K. Nguyen and Otis W. Brawley

The murder of George Floyd, a Black man, in May 2020, and many others at the hand of American law enforcement touched off nationwide protests with millions taking to the streets to decry state-sanctioned racial injustice. At the same time, the COVID-19 pandemic engulfed America—and the world—and a mountain of empirical evidence has shown that communities of color have disproportionately borne the brunt of its harmful effects. While COVID-19 laid bare the pervasiveness of racial inequality in American medicine, it is by no means the first example.

Racial injustice pervades the US health-care system—especially the field of cancer medicine. For the past half century, Black Americans have suffered from the highest cancer death rates of any US racial or ethnic group for most cancers. But members of the Black community are not innately more susceptible to cancer. Rather, profound racial inequities in our health-care system and across American society compound to produce this unjust result. Even more, the unjust realities of contemporary medicine are particularly evident because the capacity to achieve cancer equity is already within our reach.

Matt K. Nguyen a racial justice attorney, policy advocate, and educator whose racial justice advocacy includes voting rights, immigrants' rights, school discipline reform, equitable jury selection, K-12 funding parity, and school desegregation.

Otis W. Brawley is Bloomberg Distinguished Professor of Oncology and Epidemiology at Johns Hopkins University and former Chief Medical and Scientific Officer for the American Cancer Society.

Our chapter proceeds as follows. We begin by rejecting the flawed view that biological factors constitute a key driver of racial disparities in cancer. In doing so, we clarify that the social realities of race in America largely define disparate cancer outcomes. We then delve into how ethnicity, geographic origin, systemic racism, and socioeconomic status all exacerbate racial disparities in cancer screening, treatment, and ultimately outcomes. We close with a brief survey of policies that broaden health-care access and utilization, underscoring their invaluable role in the fight against cancer injustice.

Defining Cancer Populations: The Myth of Biologic Race

The field of minority health gained prominence during the civil rights movement to highlight the unique health challenges identified in the Black community and other populations of color. More recently, the field has centered on health disparities to highlight the fact that fellow Americans suffer unnecessarily. There is now a movement toward achieving health equity.[1] Implicit in this conversation is a recognition that health justice is not only feasible, but also long overdue.

When assessing health disparity measures, it is important to define meaningful populations. Populations can be defined by race, ethnicity and culture, socioeconomic status, geographic origin, ancestry, or area of residence (e.g., north/south or urban/rural). There are disparities when using all of these categories. Across all these dimensions, however, the central question is *why* the disparity exists. For example, differences in cancer outcomes arise from socioeconomic status because income deprivation presents obstacles to health insurance, preventative care, timely diagnosis, and quality treatment.

With respect to race, the correlation is much more complicated. Historical research into health disparities has centered predominantly on race, especially Black-white differences. Black Americans, who make up 12 percent of the US population, have higher

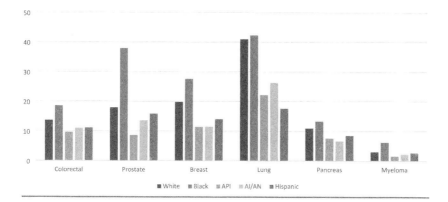

Age-Adjusted Mortality Rates (per 100,000 population) by Race and Ethnicity

	Colorectal	Prostate	Breast	Lung	Pancreas	Myeloma
White	13.6	17.9	19.8	41	10.9	3
Black	18.5	37.9	27.6	42.3	13.3	6.2
API*	9.6	8.6	11.4	22.2	7.6	1.6
AI/AN*	11	13.6	11.5	26.3	6.6	2.2
Hispanic	11.1	15.8	14	17.6	8.5	2.7

*API—Asian Pacific Islander, AI/AN—American Indian or Alaskan Native. Rates are age-adjusted to the 2000 standard.

FIGURE 6.1 US Cancer Mortality Rates by Age and Race/Ethnicity, Annualized 2013–2017

death rates for a number of diseases, including most cancers (see Figure 6.1). It is a systemic feature of American society that income deprivation correlates with racial minority status. Other social determinants of health often correlate with race as well. Thus, disentangling interwoven racial, socioeconomic, and geographic factors is central to any attempt to rectify cancer injustice.

A long-standing assumption, dotted across the scientific and lay literature, is that these disparities are due to inherent genetic differences among racial groups. Inherent biological differences resulting in differential health outcomes are clearly correlated with sex. For instance, men and women naturally have different rates of breast cancer.

But in America, racial categories are constructed almost entirely on visible traits associated with skin color, facial features, and presumed geographic origin. Consequently, the medical anthropology community has soundly rejected race as a biologic categorization, concluding race is at most a sociopolitical demographic.[2] Self-declared race correlates more with shared experiences and outward identification than with common genetics. So, while illuminating in narrow circumstances (i.e., ethnicity and genetic isolation), biological justifications tend to have weak explanatory power for the prevalence of racial disparities in cancer.[3]

Despite this, the fields of policy and medicine have historically encouraged physicians and society writ large to presume race-based biology.[4] Part of this long-standing misconception is predicated on federal data collection. The US Office of Management and Budget (OMB) defines race to collect health data[5] and publishes its definitions about two years before each decennial census. Importantly, the preamble to the OMB's definition of race confirms that these categories are *not* based in biology. Moreover, the OMB's rough definitions are fluid. Only in 1990 did federal law begin to require collecting demographic data beyond Black and white. The most recent definitions appear in Table 6.1. The federal definitions also change over time. People with Indian ancestry were considered Caucasian in 1960, Asian/Pacific Islander in 1980, and finally Asian since 2000.

The OMB's racial definitions are also quite broad. People from more than 840 areas of geographic origin are considered white. There are 109 areas of African geographic origin. Migration histories and interracial marriage further complicate efforts to group by race. Indeed, many view attempts to divide the population into racial groups as akin to trying to slice soup.

One need not look hard to find salient examples of how the error-ridden biologic view of cancer has driven policy making. In 1993, Congress enacted the National Institutes of Health (NIH) Revitalization Act, which mandated inclusion of women and people of color in federally funded research on the premise that, without equitable participation, these groups may not benefit from the fruits of clinical breakthroughs. This requirement was predicated on Congress's concern that "minority groups" would react "differently than other subjects" (i.e., white patients) to treatment.

The NIH revitalization legislation is controversial among clinical trialists because it is scientifically flawed.[6] The law failed to

TABLE 6.1 OMB Race and Ethnicity Categories

Current categories were developed in 1997 by the Office of Management and Budget (OMB). The OMB stresses in the introduction that these categories do not denote scientific definitions of anthropological origins.

Individuals are asked to first designate ethnicity as:

- Hispanic or Latino or
- Not Hispanic or Latino

Second, individuals are asked to indicate one or more races that apply among the following:

- American Indian or Alaska Native
- Asian
- Black or African American
- Native Hawaiian or Other Pacific Islander
- White

- **Hispanic or Latino:** a person of Cuban, Mexican, Puerto Rican, South or Central American, or other Spanish culture or origin, regardless of race.

- **American Indian or Alaska Native:** A person having origins in any of the original peoples of North and South America (including Central America) and who maintains tribal affiliation or community attachment.

- **Asian:** A person having origins in any of the original peoples of the Far East, Southeast Asia, or the Indian subcontinent, including, for example, Cambodia, China, India, Japan, Korea, Malaysia, Pakistan, the Philippine Islands, Thailand, and Vietnam.

- **Black or African American:** A person having origins in any of the Black racial groups of Africa.

- **Native Hawaiian or Other Pacific Islander:** A person having origins in any of the original peoples of Hawaii, Guam, Samoa, or other Pacific Islands.

- **White:** A person having origins in any of the original peoples of Europe, the Middle East, or North Africa.

- The 1997 OMB standards permit the reporting of more than one race. An individual's response to the race question is based upon self-identification.

acknowledge that disparate health outcomes by race arise primarily due to differences in receipt of quality health care.[7] Ironically, the legislation prompted large cancer studies that generally show that equal treatment yields equal outcomes among equal patients. For example, studies show that even though Black patients have a higher incidence of prostate cancer, Blacks of the same stage who receive comparable treatment to their white counterparts have equal mortality outcomes.[8] Yet, most patterns of care studies confirm Black patients are more likely to receive inadequate care compared to white patients.[9]

Thus, the biologic view of cancer disparities rests on a fundamental misunderstanding of cancer medicine. In reality, most racial disparities in cancer arise from socioeconomic deprivation, systemic racism, and limited access to quality care—whether preventive, diagnostic, or therapeutic. In addition, by failing to appreciate the dominant causes of cancer disparities, focus on biologic race as a cause of disparate cancer outcomes obscures the reality that many low-income white Americans also bear an outsized cancer burden. Because timely health-care access and utilization contributes to most lopsided cancer outcomes in the United States, curbing racial disparities in cancer is, at bottom, a question of equalizing health provision across demographic groups. In other words, achieving cancer justice does not require some novel cancer therapy, it simply demands that all Americans have equal access to timely, quality care.

Defining Populations: Ethnicity and Geography

Ethnicity relates to culture and habits. As such it can influence risk of cancer and acceptance to therapy. It relates to what we eat. And among cigarette smokers, people of different ethnicities differ substantially in their smoking preferences—a key cause of lung cancer.

The OMB recognizes only two ethnicities: Hispanic and non-Hispanic. Individuals classified as ethnically "Hispanic"—a subgroup defined not by genetics, but language heritage and Spanish colonization—hail from more than twenty countries and countless cultures. Of note, the Asian American, Latin American, and Native American communities have lower age-adjusted death rates for cancer overall compared to white and Black Americans. Trends in mortality rate by race/ethnicity from 2000 to 2018 are shown in Figure 6.2. Rather than biology, social and cultural factors associated with these groups may contribute to or prevent cancer. Still, there are certain cancers where Asian Americans have higher rates. For example, women of Southeast Asian descent have higher cervical and liver cancer mortality rates than do other Americans.[10]

There are also genetic and biologic differences among populations as defined by area of geographic origin. This classification is very different from race, which remains too broad a category. For example, the gene mutation HLA-B*1502 is found in 20 percent of people living within 150 kilometers (about 90 miles) east or west of the Thai-Burmese border.[11] People with this mutation develop Stevens-Johnson syndrome (a condition with peeling of skin, painful lesions in the mouth and flu-like symptoms) when given the antiseizure drug carbamazepine. The key distinction here is not race, but a narrow area of geographic origin. This is not an allele common to all Asians, the racial category, or Southeast Asians. It is not even common to all people of Thai or Burmese descent.

Likewise, men of West African heritage have higher incidence and mortality from prostate cancer. Researchers are actively looking into the root cause of this disparity. It is not blackness or even African descent; the disparity is seen exclusively in men of West African heritage. As noted earlier, studies do show that Blacks of the same stage who receive comparable treatment to their white counterparts have equal mortality outcomes.[12]

Social segregation on the basis of race, income, culture, area of geographic origin, or other factors can also contribute to the preservation of a specific gene in the segregated population. This is seen with a number of genetic diseases, among them Tay-Sachs, cystic fibrosis, and sickle cell disease.[13] Each disease has a higher prevalence in, but is not exclusive to, a specific group. Perhaps the best example is that of BRCA mutations. Women with certain mutations of the BRCA-1 and BRCA-2 genes are at higher than average risk for the development of breast and ovarian cancer.

Mutations of BRCA-1 and BRCA-2 have been found in women of all races, but three specific mutations are common in about 2 percent of the Ashkenazi Jewish population.[14] These mutations are not exclusive to those with Ashkenazi Jewish ancestry.[15] Population modeling suggests that the 185delAG mutation is linked to a small number of individuals alive about one thousand to twelve hundred years ago.[16] These mutations should be considered ancestral or familial, and they are more common among Jewish families due to historical segregation and intrareligious matching preferences. A growing literature has begun to clarify specific mutations of BRCA and other genes in women of western African heritage—likewise leading to greater breast cancer risk.[17]

Thus, several sociocultural factors and some genetic factors related to geographic origin and population isolation may manifest in differential rates of cancer among certain populations.

Systemic Racism and Cancer Outcomes

Race does not matter biologically; race matters *socially*. Like other facets of American society, systemic racism exists along every dimension of our health-care system, prompting such entities as the Centers for Disease Control and the American Medical Association in recent months to designate systemic and structural racism "a serious public health threat"—and one of the "primary drivers of racial health inequity."[18]

Race, therefore, matters when seeking to illuminate the root causes of cancer disparities—namely structural barriers to high-quality prevention, screening, diagnosis, and treatment among populations of color. Black patients are more likely to experience disruptions in health insurance and provider continuity, leading to untimely screening and later cancer staging. Black patients are also more likely to receive lower quality of care. In other words, quality cancer treatment often does not necessarily result in better

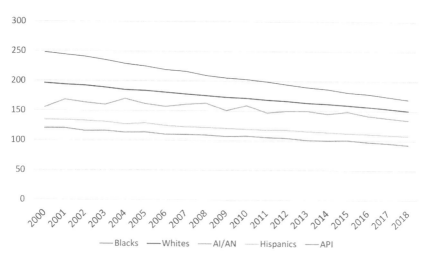

US cancer mortality rates by year, by race and ethnicity. AI/AN—American Indian or Alaskan Native, API—Asian Pacific Islander. Rates are age-adjusted to the 2000 standard.

FIGURE 6.2 US Age-Adjusted Cancer Mortality by Race, 2000–2018

outcomes in the Black community because Black patients are less likely to receive such treatment. Even when these patients receive guideline-adherent treatment, they are still more likely to face other disruptions in their treatment regimen and may even discontinue treatment altogether, often due to the magnified costs associated with later screening and staging. Further, insurance premiums, deductibles, and health-care costs have risen precipitously over the last several decades, leaving quality care beyond the reach of many. Together, these factors contribute to higher cancer mortality rates—especially for low-income patients of color.

Like the policy landscape, the medical literature is also replete with erroneous assumptions that racial subgroups differ biologically. Some of these assumptions are flawed methodologies based on observation of a small number of individuals. Early in the twentieth century, syphilis was believed to affect people of color differently than whites.[19] Ethically abhorrent studies, such as the Tuskegee Syphilis Study, inadvertently demonstrated that this is not true.[20] Medical schools commonly teach that the best initial therapy for Black patients with hypertension is a diuretic, whereas whites should be treated with an angiotensin-converting enzyme inhibitor.[21] Objective analysis of clinical studies shows that this teaching is false. Blacks have meaningful blood pressure response to angiotensin converting enzyme inhibitors and whites have meaningful responses to diuretics.[22]

One recent study demonstrated how race-based biology in medicine has gone to extremes. A survey of medical students showed most believe Black patients do not perceive pain as whites do. There is simply no data to support this view.[23] Such implicit biases held by medical professionals often lead to misdiagnoses, undertreatment, and worse outcomes for Black patients.

Another recent study challenged the long-standing assumption that colorectal cancer is more aggressive in Blacks compared to whites. This common belief was borne out of data showing that Black patients with Stage 2 colorectal cancer disproportionately relapse after surgery. The study found that Black patients with colorectal cancer are more often treated in hospitals with over-worked pathologists, who assess five or six surgical specimens per day.[24] These clinicians do not have time to accurately stage each patient. If adequately staged, these Black patients with Stage 2 disease would be upstaged to Stage 3 or even Stage 4. By contrast, white patients tend to be treated in hospitals where pathologists assess only one or two specimens a day. Accordingly, these physicians have time to perform proper staging assessments.

In other words, imprecise staging exists not *because* of race, but as an interwoven socioeconomic and geographic issue arising from the overcrowded, busy hospitals where Black patients tend to get their care versus the better-resourced hospitals where whites tend to receive theirs. Indeed, studies comparing outcomes by race in NCI cooperative groups and single institutions demonstrate that equal access to high-quality treatment yields equal outcomes.[25] Yet, before these findings came to light, years of quiet injustice contributed to misconceptions about race-based biology as a driver in colorectal cancer disparities.

Systemic racism in health care is best seen in the case of breast and colorectal cancer mortality trends from the 1970s to present (Figures 6.3 and 6.4). In the 1970s, there were few Black-white disparities. The disparities that existed actually showed that white

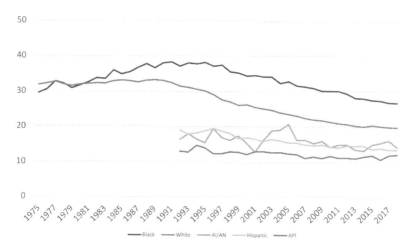

Age-adjusted US breast cancer mortality rates by year, by race and ethnicity for Blacks and Whites. Data for other races and ethnicities were collected beginning in 1990. AI/AN—American Indian or Alaskan Native, API— Asian Pacific Islander. Rates are age-adjusted to the 2000 standard.

FIGURE 6.3 Breast Cancer Death Rate by Age and Race/Ethnicity, 1975–2018

patients had slightly worse death rates. In the late 1970s, screening and treatment for these cancers improved. Yet, patterns of care studies showed that, during this time, income-deprived populations and communities of color were less likely to get adequate care.[26] Accordingly, one perverse consequence of innovations in cancer medicine has been an attendant increase in racial disparities, as underresourced communities are less likely to benefit from these novel screening or treatment interventions.

In the case of breast and colorectal cancer, whites were more likely to access new therapies. As a result, by the early- to mid-1980s, Black breast and colorectal mortality rates surpassed white mortality. Today, even though both Black and white mortality rates have declined since that time, the Black-white breast cancer mortality disparity remains higher than it has ever been. Why? Throughout this time, white Americans—whose cancer mortality rate was already fairly low—captured the lion's share of the cancer mortality decline made possible by technological innovations in cancer screening, diagnosis, and treatment. Moving forward, while *future* therapies will assuredly contribute to further reductions in cancer mortality writ large, it is important to not discount the vital

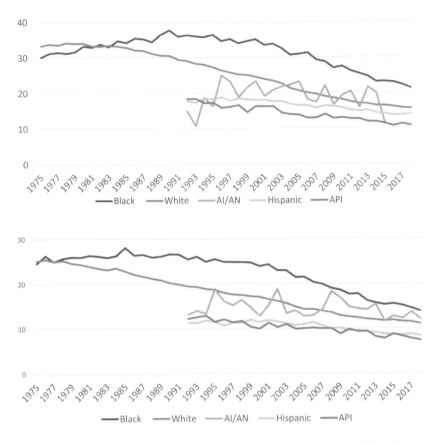

Age-adjusted US colorectal cancer mortality rates by age, race/ethnicity, and sex for Blacks and Whites from 1975 to 2018. Data for other races and ethnicities were collected beginning in 1990. AI/AN—American Indian or Alaskan Native, API—Asian Pacific Islander. Rates are age-adjusted to the 2000 standard.

FIGURE 6.4 Colorectal Death Rates by Age and Race/Ethnicity, 1975–2018; Males (top), Females (bottom)

role that delivering high-quality *existing* treatments to underserved populations of color can play in curbing racial disparities in cancer.

Indeed, there are grave treatment disparities across racial subgroups. For example, Mary Jo Lund and colleagues studied breast cancer patterns of care in Georgia.[27] They found that more than 7 percent of Black women with an early stage, and potentially curable, breast cancer diagnosis received *no treatment* whatsoever in the first two years after their initial diagnosis. Delayed treatment worsened their cancer staging, increased treatment cost and severity, and worsened mortality rates.

More generally, inadequate cancer care can take the form of unavailability or poor quality of screening and diagnostics, surgery, radiotherapy, or chemotherapy.[28] The reasons for inadequate care are many. They range from lack of access to health-care systems or providers that can provide quality care, affordability or convenience issues, or lack of adherence due to the physician-patient relationship or the complexity of the US health-care system. Ultimately, the root cause is systemic racism—encompassing not only racial bias on the individual and structural levels but also socioeconomic, geographic, and other societal factors closely correlated with race.

Defining Populations: Socioeconomic Deprivation

Studies have also shown socioeconomic deprivation exacerbates racial disparities in cancer.[29] Most important, employer-based health insurance is a major obstacle to preventative care, early screening, and long-term treatment for low-income Americans. Because the vast majority of Americans are insured through their employer, unemployed and underemployed Americans are typically underinsured or lack insurance altogether. And even when they have insurance, their insurance status may be unstable and their coverage often less favorable, with high deductibles that make expensive cancer care infeasible.

Socioeconomic status has an even more complex relationship with racial disparities. A higher proportion of Black women with breast cancer have harder-to-treat triple-negative breast cancer compared to whites (approximately 24% to 12%).[30] Patterns of care studies have shown that the racial disparity in breast cancer outcomes is largely a product of disparities in the treatment of estrogen receptor positive (non-triple-negative) disease. Epidemiologic studies suggest white Americans have a higher incidence rate of breast cancer and non-triple-negative breast cancer, because white women often delay childbirth until after the age of thirty or do not have children. These factors are known to increase the risk of not just breast cancer, but estrogen receptor–positive (non-triple-negative) breast cancer.[31]

On the other hand, having a child and not breastfeeding increases the risk of triple-negative breast cancer. This is more common among young Black women who, due to systemic racism, are more likely to have children earlier because of inequitable access to family planning, higher education, and upward career trajectories.[32] Many public hospitals where poor women of color deliver their children send the new mother home with coupons for formula, rather than encouraging breastfeeding. This, alongside other social pressures, such as the need to work extra shifts to make ends meet in physically demanding jobs that are less likely to offer the space and privacy to pump, discourages breastfeeding and may increase the risk of the worse forms of breast cancer in low-income communities of color.

Risk factors associated with low socioeconomic status also increase cancer incidence. Crucially, tobacco use is the cause of a third of all cancers. Low-income communities tend to be the primary targets of tobacco advertisements, and these communities have been a lower priority for robust antitobacco public health campaigns. Low-income Americans are also more likely to smoke to curb hunger or stress. Whereas US smoking rates in 1966 were nearly identical across all socioeconomic groups, the smoking rate in the highest income group declined by approximately 36 percent by 1999. By contrast, the smoking rate in the poorest populations remained unchanged from 1966 to 1998, at 56 percent. Today, huge differences in smoking prevalence remain among poor versus middle-class Americans, and in high school graduates compared to college graduates. Because smoking causes 80 to 90 percent of all lung cancer deaths in America, the racial disparities in lung cancer originated in part from divergent smoking patterns over the last half century.

Similarly, the second-leading cause of cancer (nearly 30% of all cancers) is obesity—the energy imbalance arising from the consumption of too many calories and lack of exercise. Obesity is more common in low-income communities and in certain geographical regions (i.e., inner cities and rural areas). Beyond affordability, low-income Americans commonly live in food deserts lacking equal access to healthy foods, resulting in cheap but unhealthy diets.

The socioeconomically deprived are also more likely to live near industrial polluted areas and suffer the health consequences, including increased cancer risks. Environmental exposure is believed to be the reason for increased Black rates in myeloma. Some of the deleterious effects of environmental exposure may be passed down from one generation to the next, giving rise to the nascent field of epigenetics. As practitioners gravitate toward precision medicine, there is even greater risk of conflating structural racism, geography, and socioeconomics with cancer biology.

Moving Toward Cancer Justice

In 2018, American Cancer Society (ACS) scientists tried to estimate the size of and describe the cancer disparate population in the United States.[33] They made some important observations regarding death rate and area of residence. Breast cancer is perhaps the most studied of all cancers for disparities. Notably, six states have Black populations whose breast cancer death rates are very similar to their white populations. In ten or more states, the breast cancer death rate of white women exceeds the breast cancer mortality rate for Black women in Massachusetts.

Since 1990, there has been a 40 percent decline in the breast cancer death rate in the United States.[34] But these results were lopsided. The reduction was as high as 51 percent in Massachusetts and as low as 20 percent in Mississippi.

What explains this difference? For colorectal cancer, the U.S. death rate has halved since 1980. The decline by state varies from a high of 63 percent to a low of 12 percent. In both breast and colorectal cancer statistics, southern states performed poorly. The data demonstrate the importance of area of residence and the importance of getting the entire population high-quality care.

Public health policy also plays an important role in curbing cancer injustice. Enacted in 2010, the Patient Protection and Affordable Care Act (ACA) gave financial incentives to states to expand the Medicaid income eligibility threshold for adults aged eighteen to sixty-four years. Thirty-four states have implemented this provision of the ACA, but many states in the South rejected Medicaid expansion altogether. Perhaps unsurprisingly, these contrarian states experienced only minor declines in breast and colorectal cancer mortality. Although the ACA's Medicaid expansion took place over the past decade and, as such, has little effect on these data, the variation in state implementation portends increased interstate disparities in cancer outcomes as low-income Americans struggle to access care. Early efficacy studies of the ACA suggest that states that expanded Medicaid coverage—thereby removing access as a persistent barrier to care in low-income populations—will achieve lower cancer death rates compared to states that did not. In short, federal- and state-level policy decisions undoubtedly contribute to disparities in cancer.

In addition, access to quality education is an amazing cancer preventative. For almost every cancer, the 30 percent of Americans with a college education have a lower death rate compared to those without a college education.[35] Education is more influential to health outcomes than race. ACS epidemiologists routinely publish estimates of the number of Americans who will die of cancer. They estimate that about 600,000 Americans die of cancer annually. But if all Americans had the risk of death of college-educated Americans, the death toll would be cut to around 468,000.[36] This means that 132,000 deaths could be averted if all Americans had the quality prevention, screening, diagnosis, and treatment that college-educated Americans receive.

These deaths could be prevented without any new research breakthrough, no new treatment, no new screening test or diagnostic. Educational opportunity enables socioeconomic mobility, geographic flexibility, and—given the deliberate link between employment and insurance access in America—more continuous health coverage and sustained utilization. This includes sustained access to care from prevention to treatment, insurance, and the logistical assistance (including patient navigation, health coaching, and transportation) to navigate our complex health infrastructure.[37] So, fundamentally, broadening educational opportunity involves getting every American the high quality care that already exists for more advantaged populations.

The 132,000 per year who make up the disparate population live in every state, but disproportionately live in the southeastern United States. Of the 132,000, approximately 80,000 are white.[38] It is interesting that when we speak of cancer disparities, we generally think of race and especially Black patients. But cancer disparities and health equity affect all races. The data speak to the importance of social determinants of health.

To make cancer justice a reality, policy makers at every level of government must target the distinct features of our health-care system that proliferate these cancer disparities. At the onset, policy makers must work to provide all Americans equal access to and utilization of long-term, affordable health care, whether through greater ACA/Medicaid expansion, a government-subsidized public option, or Medicare for all. Crucially, to the extent feasible, health insurance must be decoupled from employment status—which is especially unstable for millions of working-class families—as well as immigration status—which, as a practical matter, slams shut the doors of primary and specialty care for millions of undocumented and mixed-status families.

At the same time, policy makers must incentivize health providers to universalize low-cost proven effective cancer screening, especially in disadvantaged communities. Use of unproven late-stage interventions can discourage patients and divert resources from needed proven interventions. Mobilizing resources on the front end to identify and treat cancers in their earliest—and least costly—manifestations will pay important dividends for the patient and society as a whole, including longer life expectancy, continued participation in the workforce, and lower emergency care costs. Buy-in and partnerships with local leaders and organizations serving communities of color will be central to any universal screening program.

Finally, there must be a serious reckoning with systemic racism in our health-care system at the doctor-patient and provider-patient levels, as well as across American society writ large. Such efforts must not fall into the trap of accepting the fundamentally flawed biologic race premise that undergirded past policies. Instead, decision makers serious about cancer justice must ensure that health professionals and health systems identify and disrupt their own implicit biases that increase cancer risk factors, foment patient distrust, and undermine treatment efficacy. For patients of color, guideline-adherent treatment must be the norm, not the exception. And in society more broadly, policy makers must tackle social determinants including, but not limited to, tobacco advertising and consumption, family planning, environmental racism, and urban/rural disparities.

Moving forward, the most important question is: How can we ensure *all Americans* receive high-quality cancer care, including preventative care, timely screening, and quality treatment? Only then can we turn the page on cancer injustice.

Notes

1. Heidi D. Nelson et al., "Achieving Health Equity in Preventive Services: A Systematic Review for a National Institutes of Health Pathways to Prevention Workshop," *Annals of Internal Medicine* 172, no. 4 (2020): 258–271, https://doi.org/10.7326/m19-3199.

2. Edison T. Liu, "The Uncoupling of Race and Cancer Genetics," *Cancer* 83, no. S8 (1998): 1765–1769, https://doi.org/10.1002/(SICI)1097-0142(19981015)83:8+<1765::AID-CNCR19>3.0.CO;2-4.

3. Ralph J. Coates et al., "Anatomic Site Distribution of Colon Cancer by Race and Other Colon Cancer Risk Factors." *Diseases of the Colon & Rectum* 38, no. 1 (1995): 42–50, https://doi.org/10.1007/bf02053856; Tim E. Byers et al., "The Impact of Socioeconomic Status on Survival After Cancer in the United States: Findings from the National Program of Cancer Registries Patterns of Care Study," *Cancer* 113, no. 3 (2008): 582–591, https://doi.org/10.1002/cncr.23567.

4. Deborah A. Bolnick, "Combating Racial Health Disparities Through Medical Education: The Need for Anthropological and Genetic Perspectives in Medical Training," *Human Biology* 87, no. 4 (2015): 361–371, https://doi.org/10.13110/humanbiology.87.4.0361; Ritchie Witzig, "The Medicalization of Race: Scientific Legitimization of a Flawed Social Construct," *Annals of Internal*

Medicine 125, no. 8 (1996): 675–679, https://doi.org/10.7326/0003-4819-125-8 -199610150-00008.

5. Daniel J. Friedman et al., "Race/Ethnicity and OMB Directive 15: Implications for State Public Health Practice," *American Journal of Public Health* 90, no. 11 (2000): 1714–1719, https://doi.org/10.2105/ajph.90.11.1714.

6. L. S. Freedman et al., "Inclusion of Women and Minorities in Clinical Trials and the NIH Revitalization Act of 1993—The Perspective of NIH Clinical Trialists," *Controlled Clinical Trials* 16, no. 5 (1995): 277–285, 286–289, 293–309, https://doi.org/10.1016/0197-2456(95)00048-8.

7. Vickie L. Shavers and Martin L. Brown, "Racial and Ethnic Disparities in the Receipt of Cancer Treatment," *Journal of the National Cancer Institute* 94, no. 5 (2002): 334–357, https://doi.org/10.1093/jnci/94.5.334.

8. Robert T. Dess et al., "Association of Black Race with Prostate Cancer-Specific and Other-Cause Mortality," *JAMA Oncology* 5, no. 7 (2019): 975–983, https://doi.org/10.1001/jamaoncol.2019.0826.

9. Brandon A. Mahal et al., "Getting Back to Equal: The Influence of Insurance Status on Racial Disparities in the Treatment of African American Men with High-Risk Prostate Cancer," *Urologic Oncology: Seminars and Original Investigations* 32, no. 8 (2014): 1285–1291, https://doi.org/10.1016/j.urolonc .2014.04.014.

10. Moon S. Chen Jr., "Cancer Health Disparities Among Asian Americans: What We Do and What We Need to Do," *Cancer* 104, no. S12 (2005): 2895–2902, https://doi.org/10.1002/cncr.21501.

11. Chaichon Locharernkul, Vorasuk Shotelersuk, and Nattiya Hirankarn, "Pharmacogenetic Screening of Carbamazepine-Induced Severe Cutaneous Allergic Reactions," *Journal of Clinical Neuroscience* 18, no. 10 (2011): 1289–1294, https://doi.org/10.1016/j.jocn.2010.12.054.

12. Dess et al., "Association of Black Race."

13. Liu, "The Uncoupling of Race and Cancer Genetics."

14. Yael Laitman et al., "The Spectrum of BRCA1 and BRCA2 Pathogenic Sequence Variants in Middle Eastern, North African, and South European Countries," *Human Mutation* 40, no. 11 (2019): e1–e23, https://doi.org/10.1002 /humu.23842.

15. D. B. Berman et al., "Two Distinct Origins of a Common BRCA1 Mutation in Breast-Ovarian Cancer Families: A Genetic Study of 15 185delAG-Mutation Kindreds," *American Journal of Human Genetics* 58, no. 6 (1996): 1166–1176; K. Offit et al., "Germline BRCA1 185delAG Mutations in Jewish Women with Breast Cancer," *Lancet* 347, no. 9016 (1996): 1643–1645, https://doi .org/10.1016/s0140-6736(96)91484-1.

16. Berman et al., "Two Distinct Origins."

17. Frederick M. Howard and Olufunmilayo I. Olopade, "Epidemiology of Triple-Negative Breast Cancer: A Review," *Cancer Journal* 27, no. 1 (2021): 8–16, https://doi.org/10.1097/ppo.0000000000000500.

18. Media Statement from CDC Director Rochelle P. Walensky, MD, MPH, on Racism and Health, Centers for Disease Control and Prevention (2021), https://www.cdc.gov/media/releases/2021/s0408-racism-health.html.

19. Otis W. Brawley, "The Study of Untreated Syphilis in the Negro Male," *International Journal of Radiation Oncology, Biology, Physics* 40, no. 1 (1998): 5–8, https://doi.org/10.1016/s0360-3016(97)00835-3.

20. Brawley, "The Study of Untreated Syphilis."

21. J. Kahn, "Race in a Bottle," *Scientific American* 297, no. 2 (2007): 40–45.

22. J. M. Flack, G. A. Mensah, and C. M. Ferrario, "Using Angiotensin Converting Enzyme Inhibitors in African-American Hypertensives: A New Approach to Treating Hypertension and Preventing Target-Organ Damage," *Current Medical Research and Opinion* 16, no. 2 (2000): 66–79, https://pubmed.ncbi.nlm.nih.gov/10893650/.

23. Megan M. Miller et al., "Assessment and Treatment Recommendations for Pediatric Pain: The Influence of Patient Race, Patient Gender, and Provider Pain-Related Attitudes," *Journal of Pain* 21, no. 1–2 (2020): 225–237, https://doi.org/10.1016/j.jpain.2019.07.002.

24. K. F. Rhoads et al., "Adequacy of Lymph Node Examination in Colorectal Surgery: Contribution of the Hospital Versus the Surgeon," *Medical Care* 51 no. 12 (2013): 1055–1062. https://doi.org: 10.1097/MLR.0b013e3182a53d72.

25. George Rust et al., "Counties Eliminating Racial Disparities in Colorectal Cancer Mortality," *Cancer* 122, no. 11 (2016): 1735–1748, https://doi.org/10.1002/cncr.29958.

26. Shavers and Brown, "Racial and Ethnic Disparities."

27. Mary Jo Lund et al., "Parity and Disparity in First Course Treatment of Invasive Breast Cancer," *Breast Cancer Research and Treatment* 109, no. 3 (2008): 545–557, https://doi.org/10.1007/s10549-007-9675-8.

28. Shavers and Brown, "Racial and Ethnic Disparities."

29. Byers et al., "The Impact of Socioeconomic Status."

30. Carol E. DeSantis et al., "Cancer Statistics for African Americans, 2019," *CA: A Cancer Journal for Clinicians* 69, no. 3 (2019): 211–233, https://doi.org/10.3322/caac.21555.

31. M. E. Roseland et al., "Influence of Clinical, Societal, and Treatment Variables on Racial Differences in ER-/PR- Breast Cancer Survival," *Breast Cancer Research and Treatment* 165, no. 1 (2017): 163–168, https://doi.org/10.1007/s10549-017-4300-y.

32. Fatma P. Turkoz et al., "Association Between Common Risk Factors and Molecular Subtypes in Breast Cancer Patients," *Breast* 22, no. 3 (2013): 344–350, https://doi.org/10.1016/j.breast.2012.08.005.

33. Rebecca L. Siegel et al., "An Assessment of Progress in Cancer Control," *CA: A Cancer Journal for Clinicians* 68, no. 5 (2018): 329–339, https://doi.org/10.3322/caac.21460.

34. Rebecca L. Siegel, Kimberly D. Miller, and Ahmedin Jemal, "Cancer Statistics, 2020," *CA: A Cancer Journal for Clinicians* 70, no. 1 (2020): 7–30, https://doi.org/10.3322/caac.21590.

35. Rebecca Siegel et al., "Cancer Statistics, 2011: The Impact of Eliminating Socioeconomic and Racial Disparities on Premature Cancer Deaths," *CA: A Cancer Journal for Clinicians* 61, no. 4 (2011): 212–236, https://doi.org/10.3322/caac.20121.

36. Siegel et al., "An Assessment of Progress."

37. Ana Natale-Pereira et al., "The Role of Patient Navigators in Eliminating Health Disparities," *Cancer* 117, no. s15 (2011): 3543–3552, https://doi.org/10.1002/cncr.26264; Uchechukwu K. A. Sampson et al., "Reducing Health Inequities in the U.S.: Recommendations from the NHLBI's Health Inequities Think Tank Meeting," *Journal of the American College of Cardiology* 68, no. 5 (2016): 517–524, https://doi.org/10.1016/j.jacc.2016.04.059.

38. Siegel et al., "An Assessment of Progress."

CHAPTER 7

Cancer and Health Justice

Blase N. Polite and Lindsay F. Wiley

Why are Black patients diagnosed with cancer at a higher rate, why are they more likely to die from cancer than their white counterparts, and how can we reverse these trends?[1] However one defines health disparities, health equity, and health justice, fundamentally it comes down to questions like these. Researchers have devoted growing resources and attention to Black-white disparities in cancer outcomes for at least the last twenty to thirty years. Hundreds, if not thousands, of articles have been written on the subject. Yet we are left with an uncomfortable set of facts that for colorectal and other cancers, Black-white disparities in outcomes are actually getting worse and not better.[2] The same can be said for other subordinated identities, including for people from other racial, ethnic, and cultural backgrounds; women; people living in low-income households and communities; people with disabilities; and lesbian, gay, bisexual, and transgender people. Black-white racial disparities in cancer outcomes are not necessarily the most important or the starkest among a multitude of health injustices in the United States. But disparities caused by other forms of subordination have not been subjected to the same intense, multidecade attention from

Blase N. Polite is Professor of Medicine; Deputy Section Chief for Network and Strategy and Executive Medical Director for Cancer Accountable Care at the University of Chicago.

Lindsay F. Wiley is Professor of Law and Director, Health Law and Policy Program at American University Washington College of Law.

researchers. For other groups and outcomes, the need for more research may forestall calls for immediate action. For Black-white cancer disparities, the research could hardly be clearer. Action is clearly long overdue for all subordinated identities, but we would argue that if the changes we recommend in this chapter are put into place, then it is likely that health equity would be achieved for other marginalized groups as well.

How can so much effort by very bright and well-meaning researchers, public health and public policy experts, and engaged community groups resulted in such a failure? The answer is that we have tried to implement incremental changes within a health-care system that is fundamentally broken and is in many ways designed to achieve this very result.

This reality is not lost on those who live under this system. A recent American Society of Clinical Oncology/Harris research poll of 4,012 adults aged 18-plus and 1,142 adults with cancer found that 71 percent of Black adults believe that Blacks are less likely to have access to the same quality of cancer care as whites and 27 percent believe race has an impact on a person's likelihood of surviving cancer. These same beliefs were shared by 47 and 16 percent of white adults, respectively.

In this chapter, we will describe a health justice approach to eliminating racial disparities in health, discuss how anti-Black racism is foundational to the US health system and functions as a social determinant of cancer disparities, and show concrete proof that when elected leaders prioritize health justice, we can build new systems that eliminate racial disparities while saving costs. Finally, we will propose specific changes to the existing health-care system where health justice can be imbedded as a core principle in the incentive structure as a way to achieve health equity. If our elected leaders choose not to make these changes, they should at least make it clear that the decision not to achieve health justice is a conscious one. We hope that exposing that truth will support public demands for action.

We could elaborate on health inequity and health justice for any number of cancers, such as breast, prostate, lung; hematologic malignancies; or for other health conditions, such as diabetes and cardiovascular disease, and the message from this chapter would not change: Anti-Black racism is embedded in the structural sinews of our health-care system. We instead chose to use colorectal cancer as a test case for the health justice approach. Colorectal cancer inequity has been intensely researched. More significantly, policy changes implemented in targeted geographic areas have narrowed racial disparities in key outcomes. Focusing on colorectal cancer also allows us to examine multiple failures of public health policy and the health-care system. Along the progression from community prevention to screening to diagnosis to treatment to follow-up, there are multiple points at which structural, institutional, and interpersonal racism shape outcomes.[3] Focusing interventions at any one point along this pathway may achieve progress, but will ultimately fall short. In the end, achieving health justice will require fundamental changes to the entire system to dismantle the structural racism embedded in its very foundations. Specifically the system will need to (1) define, with measurable outcome metrics, what is meant by health equity; (2) hold state and local governments and private entities who are receiving trillions of health-care dollars financially accountable, at a level that they would notice, for these outcomes; and (3) adequately fund and empower community-based organizations to assist with this goal.

The Problem

Black individuals are more likely to get colorectal cancer and more likely to die from it than are their white counterparts.[4] The epidemiology is not contested. More concerning is that the inequity has worsened rather than improved over the last decade. Epidemiologists from the American Cancer Society have estimated that from 2008 to 2010, more than twenty-three thousand deaths resulting from colorectal cancer could have been averted if all population groups in all states had had colorectal cancer death rates equal to the five states with the lowest death rates for the most educated whites.[5] If one dismisses such an analysis as a far-fetched thought experiment, then one has to ask, why do we view it as an unattainable future? These are real body counts, not just some statistical fantasy.

The reasons for these excess deaths are multifold, but none of the reasons is without solutions. Let us start with community prevention. For colorectal cancer, there is evidence that a diet high in fat and refined grains, physical inactivity, high glycemic load, and high body mass index (BMI) all play a role in colorectal cancer incidence and, in some studies, survival from colon cancer.[6] In each of these areas, Black people are more exposed to risk factors than their white counterparts.[7] Environmental factors such as a lack of safe and enjoyable opportunities to be physically active; lack of access to affordable and appealing whole grains, low-fat dairy, and fresh produce; psychosocial stress; and lack of leisure time clearly contribute to these risk factors. These factors do not occur at random or as a result of individual choices unconstrained by social and physical realities. Rather, they are a clear result of historical neglect and active harm for areas with Black majority populations.[8] Agricultural subsidies and other policies contribute to fresh foods' being more expensive and more challenging to procure than refined grains and products with added sugars. Zoning, licensing, education, employment, housing, and transportation policies shape the environments in which people live, work, and make decisions about physical activity and diet.

Colorectal cancer screening saves lives. There is little to no debate about this among health-care professionals. In 2015, The American Cancer Society and the National Colorectal Cancer Roundtable set an ambitious goal of achieving 80 percent screening rates by the year 2018. Had we achieved that goal, 277,000 colorectal cancers would have been prevented and 203,000 deaths avoided. The new goal is 80 percent in every community. The longer it takes us to achieve that goal, the more deaths we will see. Black patients are less likely to be screened or to be referred for appropriate follow-up after screening than their white counterparts are, and therefore make up a disproportionate percentage of those preventable deaths. A microsimulation model estimated that differences in screening accounted for 42 percent of the disparity in colorectal cancer incidence and 19 percent of the disparity in colorectal mortality between Black and white patients.[9] Differences in screening may be influenced by lack of access to health care, including lack of insurance coverage, lack of available and racially congruous providers, limited time and transportation, and discrimination against Black patients by health-care providers. Health-care providers may not spend as much time with—or offer the same recommendations to—Black patients and may treat these patients in other ways that make them reluctant to return.[10]

Finally, once diagnosed with cancer, lives are actually only saved by making sure the patient gets treated appropriately and in a timely fashion. Multiple studies over the last two decades have consistently shown that Black patients are less likely to receive treatment for colorectal cancer.[11] At the same time, a nearly equal number of studies have shown that when Black patients are treated equally, such as occurs within a cancer clinical trial or within such settings as the Military Health System, survival outcomes are the same.[12] This bears repeating: if we were to treat Blacks and whites equally, health equity would be achieved and excess deaths for Blacks would be averted. That they are not treated equally goes to the heart of why we have persistent and growing health inequities in this country. Even more gut-wrenching, Black patients may be less likely than their white counterparts to receive appropriate palliative care, including at the end of life.[13]

Health Justice, Racism, and the Social Determinants of Cancer Outcomes

Achieving health justice requires inquiry and action on the full range of social determinants of poor health and premature death. In the health-care industry, the phrase "social determinants" has become something of a buzzword associated with "initiatives that buy food, offer temporary housing, or cover transportation costs for high-risk patients."[14] But these efforts to meet the immediate material needs of individual patients fall far short of meaningful action to improve the underlying social, environmental, and economic conditions that are the root causes of poor health. In the World Health Organization's original vision, the social determinants of health "encompass [...] the full set of social conditions in which people live and work," including "structural determinants" and "intermediary determinants."[15] Structural determinants of health are "social and political mechanisms that generate, configure and maintain social hierarchies."[16] Structural determinants—including racism and other forms of subordination, as well as the laws and policies in which subordination is embedded—shape the intermediary determinants of health. The intermediate determinants include material circumstances (such as housing, employment, and neighborhood factors), psychosocial circumstances, and interactions with the health system.

To put it another way, racism is a social determinant of health. It takes many forms—interpersonal, institutional, and structural. Interpersonal racism is present in interactions in which the explicit and implicit racial bias of one individual (e.g., a physician or nurse) affects other individuals (e.g., the patients they are tasked with serving).[17] Institutional racism operates through the seemingly neutral practices and policies of institutions, such as hospitals and schools. Structural racism encompasses the structuring of health care, public health, education, employment, housing, and law enforcement systems to advantage people in power and subordinate racial minorities. Structural racism typically operates through laws and policies that secure racial subordination.

Anti-Black racism is deeply embedded in the core fixtures that have shaped the US health system: privatization, federalism, fiscal fragmentation, and individualism.[18] One need look no further than the decision of state governments to refuse the Affordable Care Act's expansion of Medicaid eligibility, which the Supreme Court rendered optional for states in 2012.[19] As of this writing, fourteen states have made the conscious choice to reject this heavily subsidized expansion, and half of those states are clustered in the southeast. If we were to overlay a map focusing on almost any health inequity on the Medicaid expansion map, the maps would be carbon copies of each other. Six in ten Black Americans live in states that have not expanded Medicaid. The frequently cited reason is one of financial concern. Putting aside that the state liability for this expansion was limited, even that argument makes it clear that there is no desire to redistribute money from a predominantly white, higher-income majority to a Black minority population. Indeed, the decision in 1965 that, unlike Medicare, Medicaid would be jointly financed and administered by the federal government and the states has racist roots.

Social-Ecological Interventions

Health disparities are often discussed in ways that express and reinforce racist beliefs about individual blameworthiness for behaviors that are constrained by social circumstances and the supposed futility of addressing those social circumstances. Often the argument is that the fault lies with the Black individuals themselves: "If they worked harder or received more education, they would have access to private insurance and would not need the help of the state." "If they changed their lifestyles, they would be at less risk for deadly diseases." In other cases, rhetoric about health disparities seeks to shift blame from the health-care system to social realities that are characterized as too firmly entrenched to be amenable to intervention. "Poverty and the social determinants of health are complex and cannot be solved by elected officials." "Health-care systems should not be penalized for poor outcomes that are attributable to social factors beyond their control."

The notion that it is the health-care system itself, and the broader legal and political systems that are its foundation, that from birth until death ignores the needs of Black people or actively seeks to harm them, is almost never acknowledged. More broadly, we must grapple with the ways in which our health-care system reinforces, rather than confronts, privatization, federalism, fiscal fragmentation, and individualism. Finally, we must expand our focus beyond the health-care system to ensure that Black people are empowered and equipped with the resources, civil and political rights, and other legal protections they need to create health-promoting communities and secure access to healthy living and working conditions.

Empowering Communities

Central to achieving health justice is empowerment of and self-determination for Black communities and individuals. Laws and policies must be reformed to equip Black people with the legal protections and material supports they need to care for themselves, their families, and their communities. Legal protections relevant to the social determinants of health include protections from discrimination in education, employment, housing, law enforcement, and health care, and protections to ensure the safety of working and residential conditions. Financial supports include assistance with housing, food, and other basic needs. Health inequities embody the failures of our social, economic, political, and legal systems to serve all people equally. Or, to put it another way, health injustice is the result of systems of subordination that were designed to achieve it. Health justice is furthered when the tools of civil rights law—voting rights, employment and housing protections, and health-care rights—are supported by legislatures and the courts.[20]

Concrete Solutions

The solution is there, if we want to pursue it. We say this not as an empty statement, but because we have concrete evidence in both New York City and in the state of Delaware that when achieving health equity in colorectal cancer prevention and treatment is the priority, health equity is realized. As one of us has written about elsewhere, in 2003, the New York City Department of Health and Mental Hygiene initiated the Citywide Colon Cancer Control Coalition (C5 program). In addition to increasing colonoscopy screening rates for all New Yorkers, the other stated goal was to eliminate racial and ethnic screening disparities. This was achieved by crafting health messages to physicians and patients about the benefits of colonoscopy for detecting colon cancer, developing an open access colonoscopy system throughout the area allowing patients to be directly scheduled for colonoscopies without having to

see a gastroenterologist for an office visit first, and providing patient navigation to make sure patients understood the colon prep
and had transportation to and from the screening visit. As part
of the public education campaign, the coalition recruited racially
and ethnically diverse celebrity spokespeople for radio and poster
campaigns to be displayed in the subway and bus shelters, created
palm card distribution in check-cashing offices frequented by racial and ethnic minorities, and targeted radio campaigns to select
racial and ethnic radio stations. The result, between 2003 and 2013,
was an increase in colonoscopy rates from 30 to 70 percent, and the
Black-white difference in screening rates was eliminated.[21]

The state of Delaware created a comprehensive, statewide colorectal cancer screening program with the elimination of health-
care disparities between Blacks and whites as the stated, upfront
goal. The program provided coverage for colon cancer screening for
the uninsured, provided patient navigation, and agreed to pay for
twenty-four months of colon cancer treatment for the uninsured.
Like New York, the state of Delaware also placed an emphasis on
public education by partnering with over sixty community-based
organizations to communicate cancer-related information. The results: between 2001 and 2009, colon cancer screening rates for both
Blacks and whites reached 75 percent, colon cancer incidence rates
reached parity, and the mortality rate disparity was significantly
reduced (and, in the most recent data, has actually been eliminated). This was achieved while simultaneously saving money for
the state.[22]

What both Delaware and New York City's programs have
in common is that they began with a primary goal of achieving
health equity and then engaged a diverse set of stakeholders to
help reach this goal. Certainly a key component was a centralized
commitment to coordinate navigation and fund the various initiatives, but equally as important was the very early involvement of
diverse stakeholders with an emphasis on community-based organizations who were empowered to come up with solutions that
made the most sense for the communities they serve. While not
discussed in this chapter, a not-for-profit consortium in Chicago,
the Metropolitan Chicago Breast Care Task Force, was able to

reduce breast cancer disparities with a similar focus. It went a step further and included the lessons learned from the lived experiences of patients who have navigated breast cancer screening to advocate for change at the state level. As a result, the task force was able to secure additional funding for the Illinois Breast and Cervical Cancer Screening Program and helped pass the Breast Cancer Excellence in Survival and Treatment Act (BEST Act, HB3673) in 2015, which put an increased focus not just on mammography access but also on the quality of mammography that women of color received. These are examples of what can be achieved when racial and ethnic minority communities are "empowered" rather than ignored or subverted. Several local governments have used their zoning and licensing authority and shared-use arrangements for public property to promote access to healthier food options and physical activity. In 2014, the Minneapolis City Council strengthened an ordinance to promote equitable access to better dietary choices in low-income neighborhoods. The ordinance requires retail food stores that are licensed as grocers to carry a minimum stock of staple foods, including fruits, vegetables, legumes, whole-grain products, and low-fat dairy products.[23] Cleveland, Ohio, has launched an initiative to convert vacant properties owned by the city into appealing open spaces for physical activity and community gardening. Many cities have updated their zoning and land-use ordinances in recent years to ensure urban agriculture is permitted on public and private property.[24] The Delaware Cancer Consortium has increased its focus on physical activity and nutrition and has created a "Wellness Map" that allows residents to find local farmers' markets, where people can find fresh and local produce, as well local fitness centers, yoga studios, and parks and trails.

Finally, we have the opportunity to redesign the health-care system at the federal and state levels to make health equity a high-stakes quality metric where financial incentives flow to those who can show tangible improvements in health equity. One can start with state Medicaid programs and their contracts with the privately managed care companies that provide the majority of care for Medicaid patients in this country. Reducing if not eliminating health inequity in multiple health outcomes, from hypertension to diabetes to cancer screening and treatment, can easily be a requirement for a portion of the payments to these organizations or to the automatic assignment of patients to these plans. For example, patient assignment and/or substantial payments (enough that organizations would notice their absence) would be tied to the percentage of racial and ethnic minorities who have completed colon, lung, and breast cancer screening. These metrics could be expanded to include timeliness of care (time from diagnosis to definitive treatment) and ultimately to the survival of these underserved populations compared to majority patients in the state registry. Over time, as resources and patients are redistributed to those companies who do it well, this will likely incentivize the other companies to either change their strategies and methods or exit from the system. Risk-rated payments and fraud and abuse controls are critical to prevent gaming through patient selection and to not unfairly punish the organizations caring for patients with the most complex social needs, but if one organization achieves better health equity outcomes for the same group of patients compared to another, they should be rewarded for doing so. In the current system, very few real financial incentives exist to hold payers accountable for the outcomes of the patients they insure, and none that we know of specifically incentivizes health equity as a high-stakes quality outcome. Payments tied to quality are often less than 5 percent of total payments. At that level, they can be ignored as a cost of doing business. Imagine a world where they represented 50 percent of total payments—you can almost guarantee that these health-care companies would figure out how to meet the quality metrics. With our government payments, we can send a strong signal of what we hold to be important. The federal government could choose to likewise hold the states accountable for achieving health equity by tying federal match payments to this goal. While some state elected leaders may not care about the goal, they will surely care about the flow of federal funds. More fundamentally, Medicaid and other social support programs must be adequately funded at the federal level to ensure residents of states with fewer resources are not penalized for the actions of state leaders who may not be committed to serving all of their constituents equally. At the root, empowerment will require attention to the basic mechanisms of our constitutional democracy, including voting rights and other civil rights.[25]

THE ROAD MAP to achieving health equity is clear. First, the federal government and all fifty states should definitively state that achieving health equity is their goal and hold themselves accountable to a date when this will be achieved. This should be a required part of all state Medicaid plans. Second, federal and state policy makers should impose real financial incentives that will reward or penalize stakeholders in the system for their health equity outcomes, such as achieving parity in cancer screening and prevention and eventually achieving equity in cancer survival from diagnosis across a broad range of subordinated groups. Third, they should commit to adequately and equitably funding a health-care system where no individual goes without proper care because they cannot afford it. That is, they must commit to equitable health *outcomes* (not just health-care *access*) as a fundamental human right. We need to move beyond being satisfied that individuals are insured. As we are learning in the COVID-19 vaccine rollout, vaccines do not save patients, vaccinations do. Similarly, health insurance does not save people: getting high-quality, timely prevention and treatment does. This is most likely to be achieved with a national insurance funding model that obviates the need to try and set this goal at every level of our fragmented public-private health-care delivery system. Finally, federal and state leaders should adequately fund, empower, and work closely with community-based organizations to secure the living and working conditions necessary to achieve the health equity goal. These organizations know what the barriers to achieving health equity are, and in many cases they know how to solve them. They have to be given the financial resources and true stakeholder power to help put those solutions into action. To sum this up succinctly, this is how we should structure our health-care system to actually achieve health equity:

1. Define, with measurable outcome metrics, what we mean by *health equity*.
2. Hold state and local governments and private entities who are receiving trillions of health-care dollars financially accountable, at a level that they would notice, for these outcomes.
3. Adequately fund and empower community-based organizations to assist with this goal. Set the incentives right and empower those who are on the front lines of this injustice, and the creative solutions will follow.

It is easy to get bogged down in the nuances of health equity research, and we can be accused of oversimplifying a complex problem. However, it is also easy to use the complexity argument as a cover for a system that has inequity as its implicit, if not explicit, goal. Coming to terms with that difficult reality is the crucial first step to actually achieving health equity. The only real question that remains is, will we?

Notes

1. American Cancer Society (ACS), *Cancer Facts & Figures for African Americans 2016–2018* (Atlanta, GA: American Cancer Society, 2016).

2. Anthony S. Robbins, Rebecca L. Siegel, and Ahmedin Jemal, "Racial Disparities in Stage-Specific Colorectal Cancer Mortality Rates from 1985 to 2008," *Journal of Clinical Oncology* 30, no. 4 (2012): 401–405, https://doi.org/10.120/JCO.2011.37.5527.

3. Ruqaiijah Yearby, "Structural Racism and Health Disparities: Reconfiguring the Social Determinants of Health Framework to Include the Root Cause," *Journal of Law, Medicine & Ethics* 48, no. 3 (2020): 518–526, https://doi.org/10.1177/1073110520958876.

4. ACS, *Cancer Facts & Figures.*

5. Ahmedin Jemal et al., "Inequalities in Premature Death from Colorectal Cancer by State," *Journal of Clinical Oncology* 33, no. 8 (2015): 8298–35, https://doi.org/10.1200/JCO.2014.58.7519.

6. ACS, *Cancer Facts & Figures*; Jeffrey A. Meyerhardt et al., "Influence of Body Mass Index on Outcomes and Treatment-Related Toxicity in Patients with Colon Carcinoma," *Cancer* 98, no. 3 (2003): 484–495, https://doi.org/10.1002/cncr.11544; Meyerhardt et al., "Physical Activity and Survival After Colo-

rectal Cancer Diagnosis," *Journal of Clinical Oncology* 24, no. 22 (2006): 3527–3534, https://doi.org/10.1200/JCO.2006.06.0855; Meyerhardt et al., "Impact of Physical Activity on Cancer Recurrence and Survival in Patients with Stage III Colon Cancer: Findings from CALGB 89803," *Journal of Clinical Oncology* 24, no. 22 (2006): 3535–3541, https://doi.org/10.1200/JCO.2006.06.0863; Meyerhardt et al., "Association of Dietary Patterns with Cancer Recurrence and Survival in Patients with Stage III Colon Cancer," *JAMA* 298, no. 7 (2007): 754–764, https://doi.org/10.1001/jama.298.7.754; Meyerhardt et al., "Dietary Glycemic Load and Cancer Recurrence and Survival in Patients with Stage III Colon Cancer: Findings from CALGB 89803," *Journal of the National Cancer Institute* 104, no. 22 (2012): 1702–1711, https://doi.org/10.1093/jnci/djs399.

7. ACS, *Cancer Facts & Figures*; Robbins, Siegel, and Jemal, "Racial Disparities;" Penny M. Kris-Etherton et al., "Barriers, Opportunities, and Challenges in Addressing Disparities in Diet Related Cardiovascular Disease in the United States," *Journal of the American Heart Association* 9, no. 7 (2020): e014433, https://doi.org/10.1161/JAHA.119.014433.

8. Dayna Bowen Matthew, *Just Medicine: A Cure for Racial Inequality in American Health Care* (New York: New York Press, 2015).

9. Iris Lansdorp-Vogelaar et al., "Contribution of Screening and Survival Differences to Racial Disparities in Colorectal Cancer Rates," *Cancer Epidemiology, Biomarkers, and Prevention* 21, no. 5 (2012): 728–736, https://doi.org/10.1158/1055-9965.EPI-12-0023.

10. Matthew, *Just Medicine.*

11. Laura-Mae Baldwin et al., "Explaining Black-White Differences in Receipt of Recommended Colon Cancer Treatment," *Journal of the National Cancer Institute* 97, no. 16 (2005): 1211–1220, https://doi.org/10.1093/jnci/dji241; Blase N. Polite et al., "Colorectal Cancer Model of Health Disparities: Understanding Mortality Differences in Minority Populations," *Journal of Clinical Oncology* 24, no. 14 (2006): 2179–2187, https://doi.org/10.1200/JCO.2005.05.4775; Daniel R. Simpson et al., "Racial Disparity in Consultation, Treatment, and the Impact on Survival in Metastatic Colorectal Cancer," *Journal of the National Cancer Institute* 105, no. 23 (2013): 1814–1820, https://doi.org/10.1093/jnci/djt318.

12. Polite, Dignam, and Olopade, "Colorectal Cancer Model."

13. Jennifer J. Griggs, "Disparities in Palliative Care in Patients with Cancer," *Journal of Clinical Oncology* 38, no. 9 (2020): 974–979, https://doi.org/10.1200/JCO.19.02108.

14. Brian C. Castrucci and John Auerbach, "Meeting Individual Social Needs Falls Short of Addressing Social Determinants of Health," *Health Affairs* Blog, January 16, 2019, https://www.healthaffairs.org/do/10.1377/hblog20190115.234942/full/; see also Brietta R. Clark, "A Critical Race Perspective on Social Risk Targeting in the Health Care Sector," Bill of Health Blog, October 20, 2020, https://blog.petrieflom.law.harvard.edu/2020/10/20/a-critical-race-perspective-on-social-risk-targeting-in-the-health-care-sector/#more-29370.

15. O. Solar and A. Irwin, *A Conceptual Framework for Action on the Social Determinants of Health Paper 2 (Policy and Practice)* (Geneva: World Health

Organization, 2010), 9, 27, 37, https://www.who.int/sdhconference/resources
/ConceptualframeworkforactiononSDH_eng.pdf?ua=1.

16. Solar and Irwin, *A Conceptual Framework for Action*, 5.

17. Ruqaiijah Yearby et al., "Memo: Racism Is a Public Health Crisis. Here's
How to Respond," Data for Progress, September 3, 2020, https://www.datafor
progress.org/memos/racism-is-a-public-health-crisis.

18. Erin C. Fuse Brown et al., "Social Solidarity in Health Care, American-
Style," *Journal of Law, Medicine & Ethics* 48, no. 3 (2020): 411–428, https://doi
.org/10.1177/1073110520958864.

19. "Status of State Action on the Medicaid Expansion Decision," KFF.org,
accessed March 22, 2021, https://www.kff.org/health-reform/state-indicator
/state-activity-around-expanding-medicaid-under-the-affordable-care-act
/?activeTab=map&currentTimeframe=0&selectedDistributions=status-of
-medicaid-expansion-decision&sortModel=%7B%22colId%22:%22Location
%22,%22sort%22:%22asc%22%7D.

20. Angela P. Harris and Aysha Pamukcu, "The Civil Rights of Health: A
New Approach to Challenging Structural Inequality," *UCLA Law Review* 67,
no. 4 (2020): 758–832.

21. Steven H. Itzkowitz, "New York Citywide Colon Cancer Control Coalition: A Public Health Effort to Increase Colon Cancer Screening and Address
Health Disparities," *Cancer* 122, no. 2 (2016): 269–277, https://doi.org/10.1002
/cncr.29595.

22. Stephen S. Grubbs et al., "Eliminating Racial Disparities in Colorectal
Cancer in the Real World: It Took a Village," *Journal of Clinical Oncology* 31, no.
16 (2013): 1928–30, https://doi.org/10.1200/JCO.2012.47.8412.

23. "Case Studies, Minneapolis, MN," Healthy Food Policy Project, accessed
March 22, 2021, https://healthyfoodpolicyproject.org/case-studies/minneapolis
-mn.

24. Ben Winig and Heather Wooten, *Dig, Eat, and Be Healthy: A Guide
to Growing Food on Public Property* (ChangeLab Solutions, 2013), https://www
.changelabsolutions.org/sites/default/files/Dig_Eat_and_Be_Happy_FINAL
_20130610_0.pdf.

25. Harris and Pamukcu, "Civil Rights of Health."

CHAPTER 8

Cancer and Public Health

Melinda L. Irwin, Abigail S. Friedman,
Nicole C. Deziel, and Linda M. Niccolai

While approximately one-third of all cancer cases are preventable,[1] policies often emphasize diagnosis and treatment of diseases rather than the public health interventions that could reduce onset in the first place. Indeed, the United States directs less than 3 percent of its health expenditures towards prevention and public health.[2] A recent systematic review found the return on investment from public health interventions in high income countries was fourteen to one, suggesting that such measures are highly cost-effective.[3] Concurrently, underinvestment in public health gives a false impression that public health interventions are inexpensive and require fewer resources. Yet, as demonstrated by the COVID-19 pandemic, significant investment in high-quality public health infrastructure is crucial to protecting population health, particularly when facing unexpected or wide-ranging threats.

Melinda L. Irwin is the Susan Dwight Bliss Professor of Epidemiology, Yale School of Public Health and Associate Director (Population Sciences) at Yale Cancer Center.

Abigail S. Friedman is Associate Professor of Public Health (Health Policy), Yale School of Public Health.

Nicole C. Deziel is Associate Professor of Epidemiology (Environmental Health Sciences), Yale School of Public Health.

Linda M. Niccolai is Professor of Epidemiology (Microbial Diseases), Yale School of Public Health; Director, HPV Working Group at Yale.

Prioritizing public health as a national policy goal has the potential to propel us from a reactive paradigm that primarily emphasizes treatment of individuals with disease to a proactive approach of reducing disease onset in the first place, yielding vast improvements in population health and welfare. To that end, this chapter discusses modifiable risk factors that are critical to cancer prevention, including tobacco, obesity, environmental carcinogens, and HPV, with a specific focus on how research can inform evidence-based policies to advance public health.

Tobacco Control and Cancer

For decades, tobacco use has been the leading cause of preventable mortality worldwide. In the United States, conventional cigarette use (smoking) is responsible for more than one in six adult deaths each year. Considering adults aged thirty-five and up, data from 2005 through 2009 indicate that over one-third of US smoking-attributable deaths are due to malignancies, about 80 percent of which are lung cancers.[4]

Over the past twenty years, however, US smoking rates have fallen markedly, from 24.7 percent of adults in 1995 to 13.7 percent in 2018.[5] Tobacco control policies implemented since the landmark 1964 Surgeon General's Report on Smoking are estimated to account for over 50 percent of the reduction in smoking from that point to 2014, driven primarily by tobacco advertising restrictions and antismoking campaigns, increased cigarette taxes, and smoke-free indoor air laws.[6]

More recently, federal enactment of a nationwide minimum tobacco sales age of twenty-one could further reduce tobacco use. Specifically, studies of earlier local and state "tobacco 21" laws found that these policies yielded significant reductions in smoking among eighteen- to twenty-year-olds, with evidence for social multiplier effects; that is, if the policy reduces propensity to smoke for both a given teen and their friends, then peer effects—the relationship between peer- and own-behavior—may amplify the law's impact.[7] If delaying nicotine exposure until youths have gained better impulse control and less exaggerated reward-responsiveness—consistent with the typical course of adolescent brain development—produces lasting effects on smoking uptake, such policies could, in the long run, reduce smoking rates across age groups.[8]

Although policy changes and smoking trends point to substantive reductions in tobacco use over time, these effects have been uneven across the population. Geographically, more lenient tobacco policies in southern states likely contribute to higher smoking rates in that census region. Nationwide, individuals with lower educational attainment remain more likely to become regular smokers and less likely to quit, contributing to ongoing socioeconomic disparities in smoking and smoking-attributable mortality. Moreover, despite marked declines in overall smoking rates, smoking did not fall among individuals with mental illness over the first decade of the twenty-first century.[9]

With almost one-third of US cancer mortality attributable to smoking, the growing gap in smoking rates has substantive consequences for health disparities. In California, tobacco-related conditions accounted for over 50 percent of deaths among adults hospitalized with a primary diagnosis of schizophrenia or depression between 1990 and 2005.[10] Consequences are compounded for low-income individuals, who are more likely to receive late-stage cancer diagnoses and less likely to receive standard care.

Electronic cigarettes complicate this landscape. While e-cigarettes can serve as an effective smoking cessation aid,[11] youth vaping poses concerns: 20.8 percent of high school students reported vaping in the past month in 2018. Yet from 2011 to 2018, there was no significant change in youths' rates of "any tobacco product use" alongside significant declines in use of conventional cigarettes, cigars, smokeless tobacco, and pipe tobacco, suggesting that some would-be-youth-smokers took up e-cigarettes instead.[12] Indeed, the decline in smoking rates steepened as e-cigarettes became popular,[13] consistent with substitution. Still, vaping's potential to stimulate nicotine addiction among youths who would not otherwise smoke remains a concern.

Current evidence on e-cigarettes' health effects suggests that, while not safe per se, these products are likely less harmful than conventional cigarettes.[14] Switching from smoking to vaping is expected to yield a "considerable reduction in risk of lung cancer [. . .] due to lower exposure to tobacco-related carcinogens."[15] Consequently, e-cigarettes' net health impact is likely to hinge on how they affect smoking. This complicates regulation: state minimum legal sales ages for e-cigarettes were associated with relative *increases* in youth smoking,[16] while e-cigarette taxes appeared to increase adult smoking.[17] Thus, policies restricting the price or accessibility of lower-risk options may have unintended consequences.

Tobacco's health toll in the twenty-first century will depend on the direct health effects of new tobacco products and, perhaps especially, how those products impact smoking. Given tobacco control policies' substantive effects on tobacco use to date, as well as consumers' tendencies to move between products when incentives change, a more strategic approach to tobacco control policy is needed going forward, accounting for consumer substitution between different tobacco products as well as their varying risks. Getting these policies right—that is, ensuring that more harmful products are also more expensive, harder to access, and less addictive—could lead to vast reductions in tobacco-related morbidity and mortality, particularly from cancer.

Obesity and Cancer

Although smoking is currently the major cause of preventable cancer cases and deaths, recent reports estimate that obesity could overtake smoking as the primary modifiable cause of cancer.[18] As cancer mortality rates have declined over the last two decades, the prevalence of obesity in the United States and globally has increased significantly. Whether increased obesity rates will negatively affect the decline in cancer mortality rates remains unclear. At present, 40 percent of US adults are obese (defined as a body mass index [BMI] ≥ 30 kg/m^2), which is a sixfold increase in obesity prevalence since the 1970s.[19] Further, the prevalence of obesity in adults with a history of cancer increased from 22 to 32 percent between 1997 and 2014, and the rate of increase in cancer survivors was greater than in the general population.[20] Rates of obesity are also the highest in underrepresented minority groups. With such alarming statistics, the impact of obesity on cancer prevention and control should not be underestimated.

Obesity is associated with an increased incidence of thirteen cancers and increased mortality of fourteen: breast, uterine, ovarian, colorectal, liver, gallbladder, kidney, esophagus, pancreas, multiple myeloma, gastric, thyroid, meningioma (risk only), prostate (mortality only), and non-Hodgkin's lymphoma (mortality only).[21] The mechanisms through which obesity may increase cancer risk and mortality include changes in hormones involved in glucose and energy metabolism (e.g., insulin, leptin, and adiponectin), cellular growth factors (insulin-like growth factors and their binding proteins), steroid hormone metabolism, inflammatory mediators, DNA oxidative damage, and immune function.[22] Further, obesity may be associated with worse adherence to adjuvant treatments as well as reduced cancer treatment efficacy.[23] It is important to understand how obesity affects cancer outcomes so that clinical care can be improved for patients with cancer and obesity.

Obesity is rooted in a web of genetic, physiological, psychosocial, and environmental factors and behaviors that increase caloric intake and reduce physical activity. Numerous lifestyle interventions including exercise, nutrition, and weight management have been conducted in cancer survivors, finding improvements in treatment-related side effects, overall quality of life, body composition, serum inflammatory and metabolic biomarkers, and tumor tissue biomarkers.[24] A handful of large-scale trials of weight loss and/or exercise on disease-free survival are in progress among patients with breast, colon, prostate, and ovarian cancer. These therapeutic trials, as well as the trials of nutrition, exercise, and weight management on biological/surrogate markers and patient-reported outcomes, will provide evidence of the role of modifiable lifestyle behaviors for cancer prevention and control, and how oncology care adapts to ideally include services for lifestyle behavior counseling.

For achieving and maintaining a healthy weight, the American Cancer Society recommends following a dietary pattern that is high in vegetables, fruits, and whole grains, avoiding sugar-sweetened beverages, and limiting the consumption of processed and red meats, as well as alcohol. It also advises an exercise regimen that includes 150 minutes per week of aerobic exercise and at least two sessions of strength training exercise per week for cancer survivors and decreasing sedentary time.[25] Despite these lifestyle recommendations, a majority of cancer survivors are overweight or obese, and fewer than one-third of cancer survivors meet the nutrition and physical activity recommendations.[26]

The reason for low adherence to lifestyle guidelines is likely multifactorial. It is difficult to make lifestyle changes and this may be further complicated by lack of access to and reimbursement for structured weight management and exercise programs. In general, for adults with obesity, the United States Preventive Services Task Force (USPSTF) recommends obesity behavioral interventions that entail twelve to twenty-six visits over the course of a year.[27] However, few providers have been trained in the delivery of behavior change therapies. Currently, few major insurance plans provide reimbursement for the duration of care recommended by the USPSTF. In 2011, the Centers for Medicare and Medicaid Services (CMS) initiated coverage of intensive behavioral therapy (IBT) for obesity in primary care settings, providing beneficiaries twenty-two brief, individual counseling visits in twelve months. However, CMS's requirement of having physicians and other primary care providers (PCPs) provide IBT likely has contributed to the very low (<1%) utilization of this benefit. Thus, a recommendation would be to allow registered dietitians to provide IBT. Additional reasons for lack of utilization may involve limited access to care, the time constraints of primary care physicians, and a lack of training available for learning to deliver effective behavioral counseling. The low priority attributed to obesity is reflected in the failure to fund comprehensive approaches to population-wide obesity prevention and evidence-based treatments.

Several organizations have enacted policies designed to increase the availability of services and develop guidelines, which may become the basis for policy change. As mentioned, the American Cancer Society provides guidelines and resources directed to both patients and clinicians.[28] The American Society of Clinical Oncology offers online resources for patients, including a position statement on obesity and cancer, citing its commitment to reducing the impact of obesity on cancer through a multipronged initiative to increase education and awareness of the evidence linking obesity and cancer.[29] The American Physical Therapy Association (APTA) has established board certification in oncology. Similarly, the Academy of Nutrition and Dietetics offers certification in oncology nutrition. Lastly, the American College of Sports Medicine has been the most active in promoting exercise programming for the primary and secondary prevention of diseases including cancer.[30]

Additional policy approaches to mandating obesity prevention and treatment services include the Commission on Cancer (CoC) certification.[31] The CoC mandates that its certified cancer centers ensure the availability of cancer rehabilitation services, including physical therapy. Expansion of this certification to include weight management counseling may result in prevention of weight gain and improved cancer outcomes among cancer patients overall and among our most vulnerable groups, including Black and Hispanic adults. Other policy approaches towards obesity prevention and treatment include the Oncology Care Model requiring weight management counseling in its bundled payment initiatives to ensure the availability of effective services.[32]

In sum, a new standard of practice in cancer care is warranted because of the improvement in outcomes evident when lifestyle interventions, including nutrition, exercise, and weight management, are integrated into cancer care from diagnosis through treatment. The value proposition of prospective personalized lifestyle behavioral counseling and/or referrals to such programs in oncology is that they promote early detection of adverse changes in body weight and prompt interventions that prevent weight gain and also attenuate or improve many cancer treatment–related side effects, enhance return to work, and positively influence additional health outcomes such as hospitalization rates and reduction of other chronic diseases. Oncologists and primary care physicians should be encouraged to counsel cancer survivors proactively about weight management, nutrition, and physical activity. We envision a future where an accreditation is created for centers that deliver optimal obesity care. However, with no set policy or reimbursement for obesity prevention and treatment services in the oncology care clinic, our advances in lowering cancer mortality rates are in jeopardy.

Environmental Exposures and Cancer

Environmental and occupational exposures have been identified as carcinogens for more than two centuries. In 1775, the British surgeon Percivall Pott observed a higher frequency of scrotal cancer cases in young men employed as chimney sweeps and identified the culprit as soot exposure; later, the combustion by-products polycyclic aromatic hydrocarbons were implicated as the specific etiologic agents. Pott's research helped pass of some of the first legislation protecting child laborers and their working conditions (e.g., the Chimney Sweepers Act) and informed primary prevention strategies of personal protective gear and increased hygiene, ultimately leading to the decline in scrotal cancer. This case illustrates how identification of occupational and environmental carcinogens can pave the way for exposure mitigation and avoidance of new cancer cases.

Countless other notable associations between occupational agents and cancers have been identified, including aromatic amine dyes and bladder cancer, asbestos and mesothelioma, radium and bone sarcomas, ambient tobacco smoke and lung cancer, and pesticides and prostate cancer. In fact, based on an analysis in 2004, 186 individual agents, jobs, or industries were classified as known, probable, or possible human carcinogens by the International Agency for Research on Cancer (IARC).[33] A more recent analysis observed that of the 120 known human carcinogens assessed by IARC from 1971 to 2017, fifty-nine were work-related agents, occupations, industries, or processes.[34] Many of the individual occupational chemicals are also present in the environment at lower levels, posing an additional risk to the general population.

In 1981, Doll and Peto published their famous study on proportions of cancer deaths attributable to extrinsic factors, with "occupation," "pollution," and "industrial products" combined yielding a total of ≤7 percent.[35] Recent analyses estimate that 6 to 10 percent of incident cancer cases are caused by occupational chemical exposures.[36] Incidence of certain pediatric cancers, including leukemia, brain tumors, and thyroid cancer, have been increasing globally, with up to 15 percent attributable to environmental causes. Some experts, including the President's Cancer Panel (established under the National Cancer Act of 1971), have argued that the percentages of cancer attributable to environmental exposures in the general population are grossly underestimated due to the limited testing and research on the thousands of chemicals in commercial use.[37] Indeed, of the universe of eighty thousand commercial chemicals in the United States, only approximately two hundred have been adequately assessed for carcinogenic effects.[38]

Many environmental exposures are outside individual control and thus difficult to avoid, as they are present in the air, drinking water, food, consumer products, building materials, and workplaces. Therefore, we rely on government regulations to protect the public from these environmental carcinogens. Yet the United States' regulatory system generally allows production and use of chemicals until they are demonstrated to cause harm, rather than requiring manufacturers to prove safety. Furthermore, few chemicals have been banned due to their carcinogenicity, as this burden of proof generally requires decades of research and many cases of occupationally and environmentally attributable cancers.

Some of the difficulties in studying occupational and environmental carcinogens in population-based studies lies in the exposure assessment. Cancer has a long latency period, requiring exposures to be assessed over years or decades. The increasing cancer incidence among younger populations may inculpate in utero and early-life exposure to environmental carcinogens, and there is a recognition that even adult cancers may originate from exposures that begin in early life. People are also concurrently exposed to complex combinations of numerous carcinogens, and measuring and disentangling these coexposures is challenging.

The absence of strong public health policies facilitates inequities, as certain racial/ethnic groups and lower socioeconomic status populations experience disproportionately higher exposures to known and suspected carcinogens, and have limited access to crucial services, such as health care and healthy foods. This problem is also pronounced in low- and middle-income countries, where 70 percent of global cancer deaths occur. Patients often do not receive diagnosis or treatment until the cancer is in its late stages. Therefore, mitigation of environmental risk factors would be even more effective in reducing cancer mortality and morbidity.

Overcoming these challenges requires reenvisioning the relationship between environment, lifestyle, economy, and health and embracing environmental policies that prioritize a precautionary approach, exposure monitoring, long-term thinking, and sustainable design.[39] The concept of the "exposome" (i.e., measure of all the exposures of an individual in a lifetime and how those exposures relate to health) articulates the need to attend to the dynamic and modifiable factors experienced by individuals across the course of their lives.[40] Further, we must improve and expand the monitoring infrastructure for chemicals in our environment and harness the tremendous advancements in laboratory- and informatics-based tools and technologies that have been developed to operationalize the concept of the exposome.[41] Additionally, information, interventions, and actions which empower individuals to protect themselves would complement new population-based public policies.[42] Research agendas which advance the evaluation of the complex interrelationships between multiple external environmental exposures with lifestyle factors and internal genetic and epigenetic factors would facilitate progress.[43] Finally, applying transdisciplinary approaches can help address the environmental and social context for cancer disparities.[44]

In summary, occupational and environmental exposures are important risk factors for cancer. More attention is needed in pediatric populations and populations experiencing disproportionate burdens of exposures. Early-life exposures and assessment of multiple exposures across the life course will help improve our ability to understand the contributions of the environment to the burden of cancer.

HPV and Cancer

Vaccination against human papillomavirus (HPV) can prevent six types of cancer in women and men. Since 2006, three HPV vaccines have been licensed for use, and over one hundred countries have introduced HPV vaccines into their national immunization programs. The vaccine that is currently being used in the United States prevents infections with HPV types that are attributed to 32,100 cancers annually. Data from around the world provide compelling evidence of the substantial postlicensure population-level impact of HPV vaccination on reducing HPV infections and cervical precancers.[45]

Unfortunately, HPV vaccination coverage in the US remains suboptimal, at 70 percent in adolescent females and 66 percent in adolescent males.[46] This coverage is substantially lower than coverage for other adolescent vaccines, and it is also lower than in many other high-income countries that have achieved greater than 70 percent up-to-date HPV vaccine coverage among adolescent females. Reasons for low coverage in the US are myriad, and include such factors as lack of knowledge, low perceived risk, and vaccine hesitancy among patients, parents, and providers. Public health approaches can address knowledge and perceived risk through widespread educational campaigns and promoting focused messages delivered by trusted members of society, such as health-care providers. Addressing vaccine hesitancy is likely more challenging, as it involves shifting cultural and social norms, and here the role of health-care providers as trusted individuals who have the ability to immunize at point-of-care is likely paramount. Policy approaches may require training of health-care providers and/or requirements to document efforts to increase knowledge and vaccine confidence in medical records.

In addition to the individual-level barriers to HPV vaccine acceptance, another key factor that hinders higher coverage is widespread lack of middle school entry requirements for HPV vaccination. Since the first school vaccine requirement in the United States was instituted in the early 1800s, public health officials have used vaccine requirements to promote health by preventing numerous infectious diseases. School requirements are another key policy intervention that can provide long-term, widespread, and more equitable vaccine coverage among adolescents at the population level. Therefore, such statewide policies are an essential public health tool to increase coverage and ultimately save lives, with broad-reaching and impactful population-level effects. However, only three jurisdictions in the US currently require HPV vaccination for school entry, in stark contrast to the fifty-one jurisdictions requiring Tdap and the thirty-four that require the meningococcal vaccine.[47] In addition to direct effects, school entry requirements may also further increase coverage by changing the way providers recommend vaccines and by signaling the broad social and political support for vaccination.

Similar to other public health approaches more generally, the greatest challenge to this policy approach is resistance to requirements that are viewed as infringing on individual freedoms and parents' ability to choose for their children. A common reason cited for not being in favor of such policies is the limits they place on parental autonomy. This sentiment is particularly strong for the HPV vaccine because it prevents a sexually transmitted infection, increasing parents' reluctance to have their children be governed by state policies. There is further resistance to requiring the HPV vaccine for middle school entry because it is an infection that is not easily transmitted in school settings by casual contact. However, school entry requirements can function as a safety net by promoting greater coverage in vulnerable populations who might not otherwise have access or opportunity to be vaccinated. Such policies can also promote herd immunity: by raising population-level coverage, those who are not immunized (including those who cannot be immunized due to young age or medical contraindications) are protected by lower levels of community transmission due to the population that is vaccinated.

Despite the strong cultural value placed on individual liberties in the United States, the US has a long legislative history recognizing that the rights of parents are not without limits. For example, parents cannot withhold lifesaving treatments from their children, and parents are required to use booster and car seats for their children in automobiles. Regarding vaccination policies specifically, courts have consistently upheld the constitutionality of school entry requirements for vaccinations. Courts have declared that such policies do not violate the rights of individuals because they are a reasonable exercise of states' authority to protect the public's health and safety, as supported by the US Constitution.

Given that elected officials have a duty to protect their citizens, that school vaccination laws have proven effective at increasing coverage, and that such laws are deemed constitutional, it is somewhat perplexing that so few jurisdictions in the US currently have school entry requirements for HPV vaccination, even when key criteria have been met (e.g., strong safety record, adequate supply). Garnering public and political will to enact such legislation by raising awareness about the importance of the collective good will protect thousands of children from oncogenic HPV infections.

Vision for the Future

Public health approaches to cancer prevention and control represent the most cost-effective, long-term strategies for reducing the cancer burden and associated mortality at the population level. Unfortunately, we tend to invest in public health approaches only when there is a population health crisis, as with COVID-19. This reactive approach, along with sustained underfunding of public health, undermines cancer prevention efforts and exacerbates health inequities. Our vision for the future involves investing in public health policies and infrastructure as well as in our communities to confront the political, social, environmental, and behavioral determinants of cancer risk and mortality.

Specifically, geographic variation in implementation of effective tobacco control policies facilitates ongoing smoking, smoking-related mortality, and disparities therein. At the same time, one-third of adult smokers in the US report no desire to quit. Thus, our vision for the future involves a more strategic approach to tobacco control policy: ensuring that, nationwide, more harmful products are more expensive, harder to access, and less addictive, so as to both decrease smoking initiation and drive tobacco users who will not quit toward lower-risk products.

Regarding obesity and cancer, numerous gaps exist in our understanding of the relationship between obesity and cancer among racial/ethnic minorities, as well as among cancer survivors who are low-income, living in rural settings, and of older age. Additional research funding in these areas is needed. Future directions must also focus on how to change oncology practice to include weight management services. We envision a future where there is reimbursement for obesity prevention and treatment services in the oncology care clinic, with an accreditation created for cancer centers and hospitals that deliver optimal obesity care.

Even though many environmental exposures are outside individual control and thus difficult to avoid, as they are present in the air, drinking water, food, consumer products, building materials, and workplaces, the United States' regulatory system largely allows production and use of chemicals until they are demonstrated to cause harm, rather than requiring manufacturers to prove safety. We envision a future that includes federal and state policies around safety, as well as information, interventions, and actions which empower individuals to protect themselves against environmental carcinogens.

Addressing HPV vaccine hesitancy is likely more challenging as it involves shifting cultural and social norms and engaging with health-care providers. Policy approaches may require interventions in clinical settings, such as requirements to document efforts to increase knowledge and vaccine confidence in medical records. School entry requirements may also further increase coverage by changing the way providers recommend vaccines and by signaling the broad social and political support for vaccination. School entry requirements can also function as a safety net by promoting greater coverage in vulnerable populations who might not otherwise have access or opportunity to be vaccinated.

Lastly, and of relevance to tobacco control, obesity and cancer, environmental carcinogens, and HPV and cancer, there is a large gap between the volume of knowledge generated through research and the application of that research in community settings. It is critical that there is funding for the translation, implementation, and dissemination of research findings for use in community settings and to inform policy.

In summary, the absence of strong public health policies fosters health inequities. Overcoming the social, environmental, and behavioral determinants of cancer requires investment in our communities so that effective public health interventions can be delivered to all. Tackling these public health priorities requires a coordinated effort with immediate and bold action if we are to continue to see reductions in cancer mortality rates.

Notes

1. Office of Cancer Survivorship, "Statistics, Graphs and Definitions," Cancer.gov, cited March 2019, last modified December 9, 2020, https://cancer control.cancer.gov/ocs/statistics/statistics.html.

2. David U. Himmelstein and Steffie Woolhandler, "Public Health's Falling Share of US Health Spending," *American Journal of Public Health* 106, no. 1 (2016): 56–57, https://doi.org/10.2105/AJPH.2015.302908.

3. Rebecca Masters et al., "Return on Investment of Public Health Interventions: A Systematic Review," *Journal of Epidemiology and Community Health* 71, no. 8 (2017): 827–834, https://doi.org/10.1136/jech-2016-208141.

4. US Department of Health and Human Services, *The Health Consequences of Smoking: 50 Years of Progress. A Report of the Surgeon General* (Atlanta, GA: US Department of Health and Human Services, Centers for Disease Control and Prevention, National Center for Chronic Disease Prevention and Health Promotion, Office on Smoking and Health, 2014).

5. Centers for Disease Control and Prevention, "Cigarette Smoking Among Adults—United States, 1995," *MMWR: Morbidity and Mortality Weekly Report* 46, no. 51 (1997): 1217–1220, https://www.cdc.gov/mmwr/preview/mmwr html/00050525.htm; MeLisa R. Creamer et al., "Tobacco Product Use and Cessation Indicators Among Adults—United States," *MMWR: Morbidity and Mortality Weekly Report* 68, no. 45 (2019): 1013–1019, https://doi.org/10.15585/mmwr .mm6845a2.

6. David T. Levy et al., "Gauging the Effect of U.S. Tobacco Control Policies from 1965 Through 2014 Using SimSmoke," *American Journal of Preventive Medicine* 50, no. 4 (2016): 535–542, https://doi.org/10.1016/j.ampepre.2015.10 .001.

7. Abigail S. Friedman and R. J. Wu, "Do Local Tobacco-21 Laws Reduce Smoking Among 18 to 20 Year-Olds?," *Nicotine & Tobacco Research* 22, no. 7 (2020): 1195–1201, https://doi.org/10.1093/ntr/ntz123; Abigail S. Friedman, John Buckell, and Jody L. Sindelar, "Tobacco-21 Laws and Young Adult Smoking: Quasi-experimental Evidence," *Addiction* 114, no. 10 (2019): 1816–23, https://doi.org/10.1111/add.14653.

8. B. J. Casey, Rebecca M. Jones, and Todd A. Hare, "The Adolescent Brain," *Annals of the New York Academy of Sciences* 1124 (2008): 111–126, https://doi.org/10.1196/annals.1440.010.

9. Benjamin Lê Cook et al., "Trends in Smoking Among Adults with Mental Illness and Association between Mental Health Treatment and Smoking Cessation," *JAMA* 311, no. 2 (2014): 172–182, https://doi.org/10.1001/jama.2013.284985; Lisa Szatkowski and Ann McNeill, "Diverging Trends in Smoking Behaviors According to Mental Health Status," *Nicotine & Tobacco Research* 17, no. 3 (2015): 356–360, https://doi.org/ntr/ntu173.

10. Russell C. Callaghan et al., "Patterns of Tobacco-Related Mortality Among Individuals Diagnosed with Schizophrenia, Bipolar Disorder, or Depression," *Journal of Psychiatric Research* 48, no. 1 (2014): 102–110, https://doi.org/10.1016/j.psychires.2013.09.014.

11. Jamie Hartmann-Boyce et al., "Electronic Cigarettes for Smoking Cessation," *Cochrane Database of Systematic Reviews*, no. 10 (2020), https://doi.org/10.1002/14651858.CD010216.pub4.

12. Andrea S. Gentzke et al., "Vital Signs: Tobacco Product Use Among Middle and High School Students—United States, 2011–2018," *MMWR: Morbidity and Mortality Weekly Report* 68, no. 6 (2019): 157–164, https://doi.org/10.15585/mmwr.mm6806e1.

13. David T. Levy et al., "Examining the Relationship of Vaping to Smoking Initiation Among US Youth and Young Adults: A Reality Check," *Tobacco Control* 28, no. 6 (2019): 629–635, https://doi.org/10.1136/tobaccocontrol-2018-054446.

14. National Academies of Sciences, Engineering, and Medicine, *Public Health Consequences of E-Cigarettes* (Washington, DC: National Academies Press, 2018), https://doi.org/10.17226/24952; Committee on Toxicity of Chemicals in Food, Consumer Products and the Environment (COT), *Statement on the Potential Toxicological Risks from Electronic Nicotine (and Non-nicotine) Delivery Systems (E(N)NDS—E-Cigarettes)* (September 2020), https://cot.food.gov.uk/sites/default/files/2020-09/COT%20E%28N%29NDS%20statement%202020-04.pdf.

15. COT, *Statement on the Potential Toxicological Risks*.

16. Abigail S. Friedman, "How Does Electronic Cigarette Access Affect Adolescent Smoking?" *Journal of Health Economics* 44 (2015): 300–308, https://doi.org/10.1016/j.jhealeco.2015.10.003; Dhaval Dave, Bo Feng, and Michael F. Pesko, "The Effects of E-Cigarette Minimum Legal Sale Age Laws on Youth Substance Use," *Health Economics* 28, no. 3 (2019): 419–436, https://doi.org/10.1002/hec.3854.

17. Michael F. Pesko, Charles J. Courtemanche, and Johanna Catherine Maclean, "The Effects of Traditional Cigarette and E-Cigarette Tax Rates on Adult Tobacco Product Use," *Journal of Risk and Uncertainty* 60 (2020): 229–258, https://doi.org/10.1007/s11166-020-09330-9.

18. Hyuna Sung et al., "Global Patterns in Excess Body Weight and the Associated Cancer Burden," *CA: A Cancer Journal for Clinicians* 69, no. 2 (2019): 88–112, https://doi.org/10.3322/caac.21449.

19. Craig M. Hales et al., "Differences in Obesity Prevalence by Demographic Characteristics and Urbanization Level Among Adults," *JAMA* 319, no. 23 (2019): 241–229, https://doi.org/10.1001/jama.2018.7270.

20. Heather Greenlee et al., "Trends in Obesity Prevalence in Adults with a History of Cancer: Results from the National Health Interview Survey, 1997 to 2014," *Journal of Clinical Oncology* 34, no. 26 (2016): 3133–3140, https://doi.org /10.1200/JCO.2016.66.4391.

21. Béatrice Lauby-Secretan et al., "Body Fatness and Cancer—Viewpoint of the IARC Working Group," *New England Journal of Medicine* 375, no. 8 (2016): 794–798, https://doi.org/10.1056/NEJMsr1606602; Farhad Islami et al., "Proportion and Number of Cancer Cases and Deaths Attributable to Potentially Modifiable Risk Factors in the United States," *CA: A Cancer Journal for Clinicians* 68, no. 1 (2018): 31–54, https://doi.org/10.3322/caac.21440.

22. Neil M. Iyengar et al., "Obesity and Cancer Mechanisms: Tumor Microenvironment and Inflammation," *Journal of Clinical Oncology* 34, no. 35 (2016): 4270–4276, https://doi.org/10.1200/JCO.2016.67.4283.

23. Iyengar et al., "Obesity and Cancer Mechanisms."

24. Wendy Demark-Wahnefried et al., "Weight Management and Physical Activity Throughout the Cancer Care Continuum," *CA: A Cancer Journal for Clinicians* 68, no. 1 (2018): 64–89, https://doi.org/10.3322/caac.21441.

25. Lawrence H. Kushi et al., "American Cancer Society Guidelines on Nutrition and Physical Activity for Cancer Prevention: Reducing the Risk of Cancer with Healthy Food Choices and Physical Activity," *CA: A Cancer Journal for Clinicians* 62, no. 1 (2012): 30–67, https://doi.org/10.3322/caac.20140.

26. Greenlee et al., "Trends in Obesity Prevalence."

27. US Preventive Services Task Force, "Final Recommendation Statement: Weight Loss to Prevent Obesity-Related Morbidity and Mortality in Adults: Behavioral Interventions," September 2018, https://www.uspreventiveservices taskforce.org/Page/Document/RecommendationStatementFinal/obesity-in -adults-interventions1#citation1.

28. Kushi et al., "American Cancer Society Guidelines."

29. Jennifer A. Ligibel et al., "American Society of Clinical Oncology Position Statement on Obesity and Cancer," *Journal of Clinical Oncology* 32, no. 31 (2014): 3568–3574, https://doi.org/10.1200/JCO.2014.58.4680.

30. Alpa V. Patel et al., "American College of Sports Medicine Roundtable Report on Physical Activity, Sedentary Behavior, and Cancer Prevention and Control," *Medicine and Science in Sports and Exercise* 51, no. 11 (2019): 2391–2402, https://doi.org/10.1249/MMS.0000000000002117.

31. Commission on Cancer, *Optimal Resources for Cancer Care: 2020 Standards* (Chicago, IL: American College of Surgeons, 2019), https://www.facs.org /-/media/files/quality-programs/cancer/coc/optimal_resources_for_cancer _care_2020_standards.ashx.

32. "Oncology Care Model," CMS.gov, last modified February 18, 2021, https://innovation.cms.gov/innovation-models/oncology-care.

33. Jack Siemiatycki et al., "Listing Occupational Carcinogens," *Environmental Health Perspectives* 112, no. 115 (2004): 1447–1459, https://doi.org/10.1289 /ehp.7047.

34. Dana Loomis et al., "Identifying Occupational Carcinogens: An Update from the IARC Monographs," *Occupational & Environmental Medicine* 75, no. 8 (2018): 593–603, https://doi.org/10.1136/oemed-2017-104944.

35. R. Doll and R. Peto, "The Causes of Cancer: Quantitative Estimates of Avoidable Risks of Cancer in the United States Today," *JNCI: Journal of the National Cancer Institute* 66, no. 6 (1981): 1192–1308, https://pubmed.ncbi.nlm .nih.gov/7017215/.

36. David C. Christiani, "Combating Environmental Causes of Cancer," *New England Journal of Medicine* 364, no. 9 (2011): 791–793, https://doi.org/10 .1056/NEJMp1006634.

37. Suzanne H. Reuben, *Reducing Environmental Cancer Risk: President's Cancer Panel 2008–2009* (Washington, DC: US Department of Health and Human Services, 2010), https://deainfo.nci.nih.gov/advisory/pcp/annualreports /pcp08-09rpt/pcp_report_08-09_508.pdf.

38. Reuben, *Reducing Environmental Cancer Risk.*

39. David Kriebel et al., "Environmental and Economic Strategies for Primary Prevention of Cancer in Early Life," *Pediatrics* 138, no. S1 (2016): S56–S64, https://doi .org/10.1542/peds.2015-4268I.

40. Christopher P. Wild, Augustin Scalbert, and Zdenko Herceg, "Measuring the Exposome: A Powerful Basis for Evaluating Environmental Exposures and Cancer Risk," *Environmental and Molecular Mutagenesis* 54, no. 7 (2013): 480–499, https://doi.org/10.1002/em.21777.

41. Jeanette A. Stingone et al., "Toward Greater Implementation of the Exposome Research Paradigm within Environmental Epidemiology," *Annual Review of Public Health* 38 (2017): 315–327, https://doi.org/10.1146/annurev-publ health-082516-012750.

42. Richard Horton et al., "From Public to Planetary Health: A Manifesto," *Lancet* 383, no. 9920 (2014): 847, https://doi.org/10.1016/S0140-6736(14)60409-8.

43. Horton et al., "From Public to Planetary Health."

44. Paul D. Juarez et al., "The Public Health Exposome: A Population-Based, Exposure Science Approach to Health Disparities Research," *International Journal of Environmental Research and Public Health* 11, no. 12 (2014): 12866–12895, https://doi.org/10.3390/ijerph111212866.

45. Mélanie Drolet et al., "Population-Level Impact and Herd Effects Following the Introduction of Human Papillomavirus Vaccination Programmes: Updated Systematic Review and Meta-Analysis," *Lancet* 394, no. 10197 (2019): 497–509, https://doi.org/10.1016/S0140-6736(19)30298-3.

46. Tanja Y. Walker et al., "National, Regional, State, and Selected Local Area Vaccination Coverage Among Adolescents Aged 13-17 Years—United States, 2018," *MMWR: Morbidity and Mortality Weekly Report* 68, no. 33 (2018): 718–723, https://doi.org/10.15585/mmwr.mm6833a2.

47. "State Laws and Mandates by Vaccine," Immunization Action Coalition, last modified January 20, 2021, https://www.immunize.org/laws/.

CHAPTER 9

Lift Every Voice and Sing

Working for Equity for Children with Cancer

Nancy Goodman

When my son, Jacob, was eight years old, he was diagnosed with a rare pediatric brain cancer, medulloblastoma. My husband and I had never thought much about children having cancer. We watched with horror as Jacob was suddenly transformed from a noisy, studious, silly, absent-minded, sweet, happy, active boy to a seriously ill child. We were shocked to learn about the scarcity of new therapies to treat pediatric cancers and the many impediments that blocked pediatric cancer research and drug development. After two years of a debilitating illness and even more debilitating treatments, Jacob died. He was ten.

The morning after Jacob's death, I opened my laptop on the kitchen table and started Kids v Cancer. If the world as it was could not include Jacob, then the world had to change. I was determined to do whatever I could to alter the landscape of pediatric cancer research and drug development. Most cancer advocates have a moment like this. Advocates face their own illness or the illness and death of loved ones and emerge with a newly found passion and conviction to make a difference. Historically, advocates have leveraged this drive by launching awareness campaigns, pressing for increased federal research support, and privately fund-raising to support research. They have hosted runs and triathlons and walks, they have lit the White

---

Nancy Goodman is Founder and Executive Director, Kids v Cancer.

House pink, and they have pressed Congress to increase the federal budget for cancer research. Advocates have been the heart and soul of the cancer community's support of cancer research.

There are many advocates who still fund-raise, launch awareness campaigns, and press for increased federal funding. They play a key role. But recently, advocates have begun exploring other ways to effect change. In this chapter, I outline four categories where advocates have punched above their weight. While there are many such individuals I could name, here I focus on pediatric cancer advocates broadly viewed as leaders and game changers in each of these categories.

First, advocacy groups, such as Solving Kids' Cancer, have inverted the paradigm. Instead of raising private funds and deferring to their scientific advisory boards to issue research grants, they influence the research agenda and resource allocation of professional clinical consortiums to reflect patient preferences. Second, advocates, such as Thomas Gad, have tackled the so-called Valley of Death: the vast majority of promising academic compounds for cancer treatment that are never successfully commercialized. Gad created a biotech, Y-mAbs Therapeutics, to bring monoclonal antibody therapies for children's cancers—an area with significant unmet medical needs—to market. Third, using social media to amplify patient storytelling, small grassroots advocacy groups, such as Truth 365, have amplified the voices of children with cancer and given them an opportunity to communicate to a broader audience, including legislators. Fourth, policy advocates, including myself and Kids v Cancer, work in the legislative landscape. We have developed new rules of the road for pediatric drug development—new laws that introduce incentives for pediatric drug development and require pharmaceutical companies to test promising treatments being developed for adults in children as well.

Inverting the Funding Paradigm

Cancer advocates have traditionally focused on raising funds for cancer research and providing grants to hospitals and researchers who set their own research agendas. Now, there is an increasingly common view among cancer advocates that they can and should have a more active role in setting the research agenda so that the priorities of patients and their families are included in research projects. While researchers have often prioritized basic science, for example, these advocates place a greater emphasis on clinical studies that introduce novel therapies sooner, with lower toxicities, and which create near-term improvements in treatments.

Solving Kids' Cancer (SKC) is a small, New York City– and London-based nonprofit that raises under $1 million per year to support such patient-centered research on neuroblastoma and other deadly pediatric cancers. SKC was formed by John and Catherine London and Scott Kennedy when their respective children, Penelope London and Hazen Kennedy, died of high-risk neuroblastoma.

High-risk neuroblastoma is a hard illness of very young children. A cancer of the peripheral nervous system, it is rare and has a poor prognosis. It is the most common and deadliest solid tumor in children. After watching their children suffer, the parents of SKC focused not only on funding their own trials, but on influencing the high-risk neuroblastoma trials of the major consortia to reflect their goals as parents.

Their focus was threefold. Pediatric cancer treatments, including radiation, often leave survivors with long-term, chronic illness or disability. The standard approach to treating a newly diagnosed child is to add a new therapy to the current treatment protocol, as necessary, to see whether there is a survival benefit. The advantage of this is that children always receive at least the standard of care. However, every additional therapy brings additional toxicities and risks, including secondary cancers, cognitive impairments, infertility, abnormal growth, heart and lung compromises, and hearing loss. What could be done, SKC asked, to ensure that future developments in neuroblastoma research were less toxic rather than more?

Second, children with newly diagnosed neuroblastoma were not getting access to novel treatments. The US National Institute of Cancer funds the Children's Oncology Group (COG), one of the leading consortia of hospitals conducting clinical trials on pediatric cancers. Historically, COG tested novel cancer therapies

in children who had relapsed or were resistant to up-front therapies; newly diagnosed pediatric patients were not enrolled in clinical trials until the trials reached Phase 3—many years later. SKC
felt children with newly diagnosed neuroblastoma should also be
treated with novel cancer therapies.

Third, trials of pediatric cancer treatments were and often still
are exceedingly slow. Timing between the design of a COG trial
and the opening of that trial could be several years. Moreover,
COG trials of new pediatric treatments tend to begin from Phase
3 trials of older drugs that have already been studied in adult trials;
moreover, this was the only type of trial available to newly diagnosed pediatric cancer patients when SKC was founded. COG
only studied more promising novel therapies in Phase 1 and 2 trials in children who had relapsed. Furthermore, COG had taken
advantage of few international trials, which could have sped up
accrual, provided additional data, and avoided repeating trials
that were already occurring in other countries. SKC sought faster
translational research for the first trials of cancer drugs for children, before they had had a chance to relapse.

With these tasks in mind, SKC reached out to other pediatric
cancer organizations and together they raised $1.4 million—not
nearly enough for a full Phase 3 trial, but still enough for researchers to take notice. They wrote a call for proposals, asking researchers to propose a pilot of a trial with a novel therapy for children
with newly diagnosed high-risk neuroblastoma. They asked for a
trial with a faster design and an opportunity for lower toxicity.
They received no applications. The parent team took note. They
revised and reissued the call for proposals the following year. This
time, the language around the goals was more flexible, though they
intended to support the proposal that best embodied their goals.
A key innovation of the new call was a $35,000 stipend to fund the
development of a more detailed proposal for letters of intent that
they accepted. While this is a nominal amount in the world of biomedical research, it reflected the significant portion of a pediatric
cancer researcher's time spent applying for grants.

In 2019, the team received a trial proposal that achieved all
their goals. Dr. Yael Mossé, a leading neuroblastoma researcher,

proposed a trial that would build on two ongoing trials for children with newly diagnosed high-risk neuroblastoma run by COG and the European Society of Pediatric Oncology (SIOPE). The trial would introduce a novel low-toxicity therapy, lorlatinib, which targeted a mutation of a specific gene. The trial was designed at lightning speed. As an international trial, results would come quickly. And, as an international trial, COG would recognize ESPO's cancer data and not duplicate its work. Finally, since the assumed benefit of the trial would be significant, a randomized control study would not be part of the trial design.

The proposal was for a trial with a cost far in excess of the $1.4 million offered by SKC, but that initial $1.4 million and the attention and contributions of the advocates lead to a commitment to a trial that parents wanted: a trial of a novel therapy for newly diagnosed children with cancer, with a less toxic protocol and international collaboration to produce faster results. Parents and researchers alike are excited to have reached these clinical trial innovations and this trial opens a new model for future studies.

Bringing Pediatric Cancer Treatments to Market

Every step of cancer research and commercialization is fraught. The transition from the academic study of a novel therapy to its commercialization by a biotech company, however, remains particularly so. The facts are simple—few academic therapies are commercialized, even when there appears to be a strong scientific rationale. The transition for therapies designed for children is even more precarious.

The Valley of Death—the yawning gap between therapies developed in academia and those that make it to market—is daunting for any number of reasons. Academics often lack the financial resources to generate the kinds of clinical data companies would want before investing. Academics may not understand how to maximize intellectual property or position a therapy vis-à-vis other, competitive alternatives. Academics and industry may not even know one another and may have challenges meeting. Industry may find it difficult to identify a risk-adjusted return, even for medically exciting therapies and particularly for pediatric-related drugs, because the market is small, the manufacturing costly or difficult, and the path to commercialization might be especially long or too speculative.

Alternatives to industry financing present challenges as well. Researchers often lack the skill set and access to capital to commercialize therapies themselves. Nonprofit biotechs or venture funders who incorporate social impact as well as risk-adjusted returns into their calculations may have an interest in commercializing pediatric drugs; however, they too have challenges accessing capital and recruiting experienced executive teams.

One recent and wildly successful transfer from academia to industry occurred as a result of the experience and passion of a parent of a child with cancer: Thomas Gad, whose daughter was treated at Memorial Sloan Kettering (MSK) for high-risk neuroblastoma. The MSK immunotherapies Thomas's daughter received, 3F8 and 8H9, saved her life. However, these therapies were experimental and only available at Memorial Sloan Kettering. Thomas met his moment and brought 3F8 and 8H9 through the Valley of Death so that all US children now have potential access to these therapies.

At MSK, 3F8 and 8H9 had been in development for decades by Dr. Nai-Kong Cheung. Their trials were exciting: children with dismal prognoses—including brain metastases—were getting to remission. With such compelling results, Cheung was able to gather support from the National Institutes of Health, the FDA Orphan Drug Designation Program, Band of Parents (an advocacy and fund-raising group of parents), and MSK itself. However, Cheung was not able to raise the tens or hundreds of millions of dollars that would be needed to commercialize the therapies. Cheung had tried for years to find a suitable commercialization partner, but his efforts had not been successful.

The market to which Cheung had hoped to draw industry interest for his drugs was a particularly difficult one. The market for a high-risk neuroblastoma therapy is very small—four hundred children a year. Risk-adjusted returns on investment are not easy for a biotech to achieve, especially when biotechs could direct their efforts to therapies with larger markets. The Band of Parents, a nonprofit of parents whose children had been treated by Cheung, generated significant funding for Cheung's studies. However, it was led by a group of parents with full-time jobs in industries other than biotech. They did not have the capability or resources to bring the therapies to market themselves. Cheung's 8H9 and 3F8 were still in need of a partner to cross the Valley of Death.

Gad decided he should be that person. While he had extensive business experience, he had no start-up biotech experience. But he had his conviction. In 2014, he raised seed funding from friends and family. He brought in an experienced leadership team to build a company. In a highly unusual step, Gad approached MSK to acquire the licenses, and he launched his company, Y-mAbs Therapeutics.

Gad's story of commercialization is a happy one. Today, Y-mAbs Therapeutics is a publicly traded company with a market capitalization of $1.5 billion. It has a robust pipeline of over a dozen drugs for pediatric cancers in the works, including one FDA-approved drug, Danyelza, for neuroblastoma. And equally exciting, the success of Y-mAbs has drawn other companies into the pediatric cancer space. Against all odds, Gad fought a path out of the Valley of Death for some of the hardest therapies to commercialize: those for the small and overlooked markets of children with cancer.

Social Media and Storytelling

Advocates focusing on awareness campaigns and grassroots lobbying have undergone profound transformations as the social media age has given them platforms to communicate with each other, to tell their stories, and to market their ideas outside of their own communities.

Effective grassroots advocacy can now be driven by thinly capitalized start-up groups with a message and some smarts and style. One such group in the pediatric cancer space is Truth 365, which is headed by a pair of advocates who track the legislative process in real time at a level of detail that, until recently, even professional organizations could not. Truth 365 transmits this information to the pediatric cancer community, identifies and documents the views of children and young adults with cancer about legislation, and packages and delivers those views to members of Congress.

Dena Sherwood, a cofounder of Truth 365 and a successful entrepreneur with a booming court-reporting company, became an advocate one morning when her thirteen-month-old baby, Billy, was diagnosed with cancer. Billy's treatment was difficult, but ultimately, he became one of the children who achieve long-term remission. The experience moved Sherwood, and she founded several pediatric cancer organizations, including Truth 365.

Sherwood's cofounder, Mike Gillette, is an award-winning documentary filmmaker who can be reserved with adults, but is sly and humorous with kids. Gillette began working on a focused project with Sherwood: a documentary about pediatric cancer from the viewpoint of children and young adults with cancer. Could they, they asked, give patients a voice? Could they celebrate the patient and give children with cancer an opportunity to talk about their experiences? It was the ultimate grassroots effort to identify and present the voices of a community. The resulting video, *The Truth 365*, brought shocking and powerful images and testimonials to the screen. It won an Emmy. Riding the momentum, Sherwood and Gillette kept *The Truth 365* going by forming the eponymous nonprofit and a parent nonprofit, Arms Open Wide.

In the pediatric cancer community, patient voices are rarely heard. Truth 365 gives each child a chance to talk about what financial, physical, or mental health burdens they face from their cancer diagnosis and treatment. Much of what Gillette does, he does behind the camera. However, he also invites children and young adults to make home videos and send them to Truth 365's website, Facebook page, and Instagram and Twitter accounts. Truth 365 posts the videos on its many social media outlets and has created a large and robust following of millions. Gillette and Truth 365 have won numerous additional Emmys for subsequent videos and documentaries. Besides giving voice to those at the center of the pediatric cancer experience—children with cancer—the Truth 365 videos are a powerful conduit to draw other members of the community to the cause.

The impact of Truth 365 is not limited to videos. Every September, Gillette and Sherwood draw in more of the pediatric community through a fair, CureFest, in Washington, DC. This three-day event includes the participation of hundreds of pediatric cancer organizations and lots of performances, mostly by children and teens. CureFest is beautiful and lighthearted. It again gives children a voice, replacing the despair and lack of empowerment with passion and beauty. Many families of recently diagnosed children attend the events, collecting information, getting involved in programs, growing the pediatric cancer community, and generally feeling more empowered and hopeful.

And perhaps most important, Truth 365 consolidates the views of the pediatric cancer community and communicates those views through its videos to senators, congresspeople, and their staff. Traditionally, advocates communicated with their representatives and senators via letters, perhaps phone calls, and the occasional visit. In the era of iPhones and social media, Truth 365 gives families other ways to reach their representatives. It hosts Zoom calls with constituents. It creates tags and hashtags and media campaigns. Congressional offices track social media carefully now and these new avenues are effective in grabbing the attention of members of Congress. Through its social media platform, Truth 365 can find families by congressional district and encourage them to contact their members of Congress. Its most recent strategy includes finding children willing to serve as ambassadors of the pediatric cancer community in meetings with members of Congress in DC. This emotional link has been effective in raising the profile of pediatric cancer issues in Congress.

There is much work to be done to optimize Truth 365's social media presence and to use social media and video storytelling to keep pediatric cancer a priority in the age of COVID-19. Cancer groups have always vied against one another for congressional support and at times it may appear to be a zero-sum game. However, by framing their group not by a diagnosis but by an age category, children, and by amplifying and directing the voices of children, Truth 365's innovation in this space has been invaluable.

New Rules of the (Policy) Road

Traditionally, cancer advocates have pressed Capitol Hill for increased federal funding for cancer research. This strategy has been largely successful and, over time, federal funding for cancer research has increased, though funding for pediatric research remains a tiny slice of the overall pie. There is always more to do and there will always be a critical role for advocates to push for the inclusion of cancer research in the federal budget. However, Congress's role in promoting cancer research extends past appropriations. It includes legislation addressing FDA authority and the rights and obligations of academia and the pharmaceutical industry.

At Kids v Cancer, I have focused our efforts on regulatory reform to promote the commercialization of pediatric cancer drug development and to increase access to novel therapies for children with cancer and without effective treatments. The biopharmaceutical industry invests an estimated $100 billion annually in research and development. If just a small percentage of that were directed towards pediatric cancer, the landscape of pediatric cancer research would be transformed.

We began with Congress, writing and advocating for the Creating Hope Act pediatric priority review voucher program, a bill to incentivize companies to develop drugs for children with cancer and other life-threatening illnesses. I had never drafted a bill, and I did not have an FDA background. However, I had Jacob's classmates and his little brother, Ben, and eventually many other children touched by cancer. Together, they constituted a formidable advocacy front.

The goal of the pediatric voucher program was to address a market failure. Companies were not developing drugs expressly for seriously ill children because the markets were too small to achieve a risk-adjusted return on investment. The priority review voucher program changed that calculation. Under the Creating Hope Act, companies that develop drugs expressly for kids with cancer and other serious illnesses receive a voucher upon FDA approval. The voucher comes with rights to faster FDA review of a future drug, perhaps a blockbuster drug, thus getting that drug to market faster. And, the vouchers are fully transferable.

To get the Creating Hope Act passed, we built a campaign of children who wanted to talk to Congress about pediatric cancer. We went office to office, asking members of Congress to support the bill. And in 2012, Congress passed the Creating Hope Act pediatric priority review voucher program.

The priority review voucher program has been a stunning success. Now, many drug companies are prioritizing pediatric cancer and pediatric rare disease drug development in hopes of earning a voucher. In addition, more than $1 billion of incentives has been created—at no cost to the taxpayer. It has arguably led to the development of more than twenty new drugs for children, whereas prior decades had only seen one or two.

While the Creating Hope Act provides an incentive to develop drugs expressly for kids, it did not address the nine hundred drugs currently in the adult cancer pipeline. I wondered: could some of those drugs also have implications for pediatric patients? I started again, drafting another bill—the RACE (Research to Accelerate Cures and Equity) for Children Act—and again teamed with child advocates to lobby for it.

The goal of the RACE for Children Act was to address another market failure: the fact that companies do not test their promising adult cancer drugs on children to determine whether the drugs are effective, whether there are new toxicities, and what the appropriate dose and schedules might be. Even though the marginal cost of developing already approved drugs for children is small, the opportunity cost may be considerable, as staff dedicated to pediatric development plans are not then developing the next blockbuster drug. The RACE for Children Act responds to this market failure by requiring companies developing targeted cancer therapies for adult cancers to also undertake pediatric studies of those therapies. Specifically, RACE requires pharmaceutical companies to undertake pediatric studies of targeted oncology therapies when the targets are present in populations of children with cancers. After decades with very little new pediatric drug progress, this has led to a flood of new promising treatments for researchers and clinicians to explore. There are certainly other market failures in drug development and other diseases overlooked by the pharmaceutical industry. However, now companies are less likely to avoid development of cancer drugs for children's cancer.

Getting a bill passed through Congress is by turns exhausting, heartbreaking, and maddening (only 2% of all introduced bills are passed into law). Asking the pharmaceutical industry to accept a new requirement was a heavy political lift; that we did not accept donations from the pharmaceutical industry may have made this a bit more doable. We became the leading experts in FDA administrative law on pediatric drug development. We were supported by an editorial in *Nature* as well as other credentialized supporters. We worked for over four years on each bill before passage. We had over five hundred meetings with various congressional offices. We turned down the first two offers we received from industry and Congress. Ultimately, the RACE for Children Act was signed into law with all our provisions. Together, the Creating Hope Act pediatric voucher program and the RACE for Children Act have created a dramatic shift in how companies view pediatric cancer drug development. Companies have an incentive to develop drugs expressly for children with cancer; moreover, companies may face a requirement to develop their adult cancer drugs for children.

Where Do We Go from Here?

As I write this in 2021, we are facing a global COVID-19 pandemic with a new US president, Joe Biden. Biden is unique among US presidents insofar as he has recent personal experience with cancer and a strong track record for supporting cancer research. He has already made an historic promise to "end cancer as we know it." First Lady Dr. Jill Biden has also announced that she will make cancer research and treatment a priority of her tenure.

The advancement of cancer research requires new scientific insights and increased funding. It also requires structural change, a shift in how the parties of the cancer research landscape work together. How do we work to bring the great leaps in bench science—from the chemotherapy that was cutting-edge science at the time of the passage of the National Cancer Act in 1971 to what is cutting-edge science now: genomic research, bioinformatics, immunotherapy, and single cell studies—to patients? How can we ensure that translational research proceeds in a direction that reflects society's interests? How can we guarantee that good ideas that start in academia are taken up by biotechnology and pharmaceutical companies? These will be the questions on which advocates will continue to focus.

The role of the federal government in cancer research will be an especially critical task for advocates to consider. Since the National Cancer Act, the question of the National Cancer Institute's research and development budget allocation has become a subject of public debate. Does the funding of basic science help all cancer patients? It should. However, the trickle-down theory that basic science contributes to therapies for all cancers has not necessarily translated into new therapies for children with cancer, who have seen only four FDA therapies developed expressly for children's cancers since the National Cancer Act's passage. To address basic science's uneven impact, advocates must insist that federal funding for clinical trials be directed toward cancers that the private sector cannot and will not pursue without outside incentives or requirements, specifically rare and pediatric cancers.

Advocates may be the least credentialed members of the cancer research universe, but they are often the ones who bring new energy and new ideas to address entrenched challenges. As we hope for a new moonshot, the advocacy community will continue to innovate around the limitations of the existing ecosystem of cancer research and drug development so that one day, we achieve a better outcome for all cancer patients.

CHAPTER 10

Perspectives on Cancer Advocacy

Sherry Lansing

The world of cancer is vast and includes many kinds of stakeholders. Advocates impact every aspect of that world, from awareness and screening to research and patient care. Having become an advocate nearly four decades ago, I know what advocacy can accomplish. The results can be nothing short of revolutionary.

Advocates play vital roles that no other group can fill—including the federal government. I learned this firsthand while still an executive in the film industry. During those years, I partnered with leading figures on the cutting edge of treating cancer—from doctors and scientists to philanthropists and other advocates—as I worked to increase awareness and raise funds for research. Those experiences inspired me to embark on a new chapter in my life after I left Paramount Pictures—a journey that brought me to a watershed moment in 2008. That year, together with eight extraordinary women, I cofounded Stand Up To Cancer (SU2C). We set out to build a movement bringing together the general public, philanthropists, foundations, companies, and other organizations to support scientists in their groundbreaking research. As of December 2020, our efforts have raised over $660 million for cancer research. We have produced six historic, televised "roadblock" fund-raising events, with the most recent telecast carried on more than seventy broadcast, cable, streaming, and social platforms in the United States and Canada.

Sherry Lansing is Cofounder, Stand Up To Cancer.

The funds we raise support collaborative, scientifically rigorous, treatment-focused research and are designed to get better results, faster. Our signature "Dream Teams" encourage researchers to work together across institutions and disciplines in an unprecedented way, breaking down the silos that for decades have stymied progress. While SU2C did not invent the concept of "team science," we approached it differently, filling a key funding gap. The idea was to offer large enough grants so scientists could focus on research rather than continuous proposal-writing, while investing in innovative, "high-risk/high-reward" avenues that government and other institutional funders tend to avoid. Limiting grants to three-year terms helps concentrate the teams' efforts on getting new therapies to patients quickly so as to save lives now, prioritizing translational research in the process.

More than 1,950 scientists have collaborated through SU2C, representing 210 leading institutions in the US, Canada, and beyond. Their breakthroughs have contributed to the development of nine new cancer therapies approved by the FDA, including treatments for breast, colorectal, ovarian, pancreatic, and prostate cancers, and difficult-to-treat leukemias in children and young adults. SU2C-funded researchers have planned, launched, or completed more than 250 clinical trials that have enrolled over 19,000 patients. We have funded early work in immunotherapy and precision cancer treatment, and are supporting cutting-edge research meant to detect cancer at its earliest possible stage. We helped pioneer the emerging field of convergence—bringing together clinical researchers with engineers, mathematicians, and physicists to investigate how cancers respond to therapies. We also support efforts to accelerate clinical trials for combination therapies.

More cancer patients are experiencing better outcomes, thanks in part to efforts like ours. Researchers are closer than ever to discovering therapies that transform the most tenacious cancers, such as pancreatic and brain cancer, from deadly into chronic diseases. We have made breathtaking, life-saving progress, but there is still so much more work to do. COVID-19 has shown that, with sufficient resources, research can be even faster and nimbler. With that same urgency applied to cancer research, we can accelerate new treatments and even better outcomes. Thinking outside the box and approaching this challenge from many different perspectives is vital. To get there, we must ensure that a wide variety of voices, skills, and collaborators are at the table. We must also focus on equity in cancer care to ensure that the most cutting-edge treatments, diagnostics, and care benefit everyone.

Advocacy can change the world, and when advocates collaborate with one another—uniting researchers from different disciplines and institutions—it can save lives. This awareness has guided my work from the start.

Becoming a Cancer Advocate

I became a cancer advocate for the same reason so many do: the disease struck someone I loved. My mother was diagnosed with ovarian cancer when she was sixty-two. I was forty years old and not especially familiar with cancer at the time. I loved my mother deeply and believed that she was going to beat the disease. She did not. The helplessness of watching her suffer and the desire to honor her memory motivated me to act. When I lost my mother, I was determined to become a cancer advocate so that no one else would have to suffer as she did. Everything I do is in her honor.

That wrenching experience launched my cancer journey. I started working with various organizations, hoping to raise funds for research that would help lead to a cure, or at the very least, make cancer a manageable disease not unlike diabetes. I visited labs to better understand the research into treating this disease. I established several key partnerships that defined those early years. When I met with Dr. Armand Hammer, then head of Occidental Petroleum and a major supporter of cancer research, I volunteered to be his eyes and ears for identifying research projects worthy of funding. With limited background in science, I studied the literature carefully and frequently consulted with experts. They patiently explained their work and when something piqued my interest, I would share my findings with Dr. Renato

Dulbecco—winner of the 1975 Nobel Prize in Physiology or Medicine and Dr. Hammer's scientific adviser. Our efforts helped fund research in a substantial way, leading to meaningful breakthroughs. Through these efforts I was able to meet and develop partnerships with many scientists in cancer research, including Dr. Judy Gasson and Dr. Steven Rosenberg—pioneers in the study of granulocyte-macrophage colony-stimulating factor (GM-CSF) and immunotherapy, respectively.

Through my work in the film industry, I was able to add visibility to the disease and raise more money. Eventually, when I was running Paramount Pictures, I began holding my own fundraisers for cancer research. These experiences led me to the next—and most meaningful—chapter of my life.

The Origins of Stand Up To Cancer

I left Paramount Pictures to create my own foundation when I was sixty. I had been thinking about this move for years. As I approached my mid-fifties, I wanted a new chapter in my life dedicated to giving back. I wanted to start on this path while I was still young enough to have a third chapter in my life, but not so young that I could wait—sixty was the right age. By that point, I had been running Paramount for twelve and a half years, capping a career in the movie business that started when I was twenty-six. While I loved being in the industry, eventually the highs are not as high, the lows are not as low, and you find that you are repeating yourself. I realized that I was more interested in speaking with scientists about what they were doing than being in script meetings.

I began my new life after leaving Paramount and launching my own foundation with an initial focus on supporting education and funding cancer research. I was named a Regent of the University of California and appointed to the recently established California Stem Cell Agency. I immersed myself in learning about all these new projects I was taking on.

In 2007, I was fortunate enough to find myself among a group of women who, unbeknownst to us at the time, were all simultaneously working to bring to bear the extensive resources of the entertainment community in the fight against cancer. We all had entertainment-related careers and were all connected by this terrible disease—most of us having lost a loved one to cancer, and several facing their own cancer diagnosis. When the nine future cofounders of Stand Up To Cancer finally met, it felt like an arranged marriage. We hoped that by pooling our considerable contacts and resources and joining forces, we could make a radical, profound, and life-changing impact on how cancer is treated. These incredible women—including Katie Couric, Lisa Paulsen, Rusty Robertson, Sue Schwartz, Ellen Ziffren, and Kathleen Lobb, along with the amazing Laura Ziskin and Noreen Fraser— together formed SU2C with a clear mission: funding scientific breakthroughs that would end this horrible disease.

We officially launched SU2C with our first roadblock telecast in 2008 to raise funds to benefit cancer research. We asked the three major networks, beginning with NBC, for airtime. This was bold and unprecedented. Never before had the major networks joined for a simultaneously broadcast fundraising special of this kind. Jeff Zucker—then president of NBC and a cancer survivor himself—immediately agreed to it. ABC and CBS soon followed.

While we have experienced many successes since then, we also suffered immeasurable loss along the way. Both Noreen Fraser and Laura Ziskin passed away from cancer. Everything we do at SU2C honors their memories. Pam Williams, Laura's longtime producing partner, joined SU2C's Council of Founders and Advisors. Together, we continue to carry on Laura's vision and work seamlessly as a team to end this terrible disease.

Finding Our Point of View: Breaking Down Silos

To this group, there was no mystery to answering the "what" of SU2C: we were going to marshal the entertainment community to raise awareness and funds to beat cancer. The more complicated piece was the "why." Raising money was not enough; we needed a point of view, a clear message that explained how we were approaching this differently and what we were going to do with the funds.

We were knowledgeable about entertainment, media, fundraising, and production, but when it came to cancer research, we needed credibility. To help us chart a path forward, I drew on the advice of two very impressive women I had worked with as a cancer advocate. The first was Dr. Ellen Sigal, chairperson and founder of Friends of Cancer Research, who was my guru in this effort. We had first met while I was at Paramount, when we hosted an event involving all the studio heads and then–Vice President Al Gore to raise funds for cancer research. In 1998, I was also involved with Ellen in "The March: Coming Together to Conquer Cancer"—enlisting celebrities to lobby and help in the effort to double federal spending on cancer research. The second was Dr. Margaret Foti, the chief executive officer of the American Association for Cancer Research (AACR). Through their recommendations and guidance, we began meeting with leading researchers: Drs. Andy Conrad, John Glaspy, Patrick Soon-Shiong, Dennis Slamon, and many others. The broad problem they identified was clear: cancer was a siloed disease. If a cancer patient went to a hospital, it was common to find situations where the first floor didn't quite know what the second floor was doing—just as researchers in one hospital or cancer center were rarely collaborating with colleagues elsewhere.

There was another silo effect I became aware of during my years of advocacy. It was common to see breast, ovarian, colon, or any number of other disease-specific cancer groups lobbying for funding that targeted their diseases. Our aim was not to prioritize one cancer or one institution over another. We wanted to partner with everyone and to help them all speak with one voice.

Based on these conversations, our point of view became clear. We wanted to break down the silos that for decades had defined and impeded progress in cancer research and treatment. We knew the harmful impact of those silos from our experiences with the disease. Two of our founders—Laura and Noreen—were battling advanced breast cancer during those early years. Laura was our conscience—her daily struggles gave us a sense of urgency. Along with input from our incredible scientists, we developed a collaborative model that has since become the cornerstone of our approach to funding: uniting scientists from different centers for unique collaborative research, and enlisting support from pharmaceutical companies to help advance breakthrough research from laboratory to clinical trials.

Developing the Dream Team Model

When told that researchers from different, often competing, institutions would not work together, Laura's response was as visionary as it was emphatic: they will collaborate if we give them enough money. She was right. When we began, it was uncommon to find major collaborative grants receiving funding. Now the practice is commonplace, with the National Cancer Institute (NCI) supporting many multi-institutional collaborations. SU2C was a leader in this transformation.

Our Dream Team model quickly took shape. It entails grants large enough to incentivize teams to collaborate on major achievements. Initially, we set a goal for each Dream Team to receive a minimum of $10 million in funding, which was unprecedented at the time in cancer research. We select proposals submitted by top researchers from different institutions and disciplines who work together on promising new projects—competing against cancer rather than against one another. The researchers leading the grant must come from at least three institutions. The work must be genuinely collaborative—the scientists must share their data and meaningfully work across institutions.

We assembled a group of highly respected scientists to advise us on which proposals to fund. This committee also helps to shape each project at the start, promote collaboration within the team, help the investigators meet interim milestones, and assist in rethinking the goals as new scientific evidence comes to light. We also established Innovative Research Grants, which provide $750,000 to early-career scientists and clinicians to encourage innovative thinking. This is another of Laura's many vital contributions to our mission. By insisting early on that we support out-of-the-box ideas, Laura led the way in enabling the pathbreaking work of young researchers who were often consigned to the "garage" without adequate funding. Since launching our Innovative Research Grants, SU2C has supported forty-six researchers who might otherwise never have had the chance to pursue their ideas.

Beyond collaboration, SU2C's Dream Team model prioritizes two other core values: accountability and patient care. Our Scientific Advisory Committee carefully reviews grantees' projects at numerous points over their three-year duration. Every grant includes specific benchmarks to ensure that patients see results as soon as possible. Projects are flexible to allow teams to adapt to evolving science on the cutting edge of discovery. If deadlines slip for a good reason, funding continues. If underlying problems become apparent, resources are redirected. The success of this model hinges on our extraordinary Scientific Advisory Committee (SAC), which augments its deep knowledge of science with great wisdom to inform its decisions. Organizing the SAC was one of our first major accomplishments, and in many ways the one that has made all of the others possible.

Patient care, our third core research value, is a common feature of nearly all our major grants. In essence, it is a requirement that the projects we fund have the potential to quickly move from "bench to bedside"—to translate from laboratory to clinic, where it can benefit actual patients. It is the reason our major grants typically have a three-year time horizon: it conveys the "need for speed" and forces the teams to work expeditiously. If a worthy project requires more time, the team can usually find funding from other sources, based on the progress it has already made—from funders who earlier might have found the concept too risky or insufficiently proven to merit investment. In that sense, SU2C "de-risks" innovative research by enabling three years of solid progress on an idea before a more risk-averse funder steps in.

Building a Scientific Advisory Committee

Attracting the most talented researchers and innovative proposals requires both credibility and knowledge. For that, Sigal and Foti pointed us to one remarkable individual: Dr. Phillip A. Sharp, a Nobel laureate and scientist of the highest integrity, utterly incorruptible—a true genius. With Sharp on board, Sigal and Foti assured us, the world's best advisory committee would soon follow.

Our chance to make our case directly came at a meeting of the AACR, where all nine SU2C cofounders were in attendance to hear Laura speak movingly about her experience battling breast cancer—unforgettably describing herself as an "impatient patient." Sharp was also in attendance. After Laura was done speaking, we approached him with our proposal. As anyone who has ever had nine women descend on them knows, you cannot avoid saying yes. A few days later Sharp agreed to join us, and as soon as he did, I knew we were home free. True to Sigal and Foti's prediction, Sharp assembled a SAC of the highest integrity. Our scientific work has been impeccable because of Sharp and the committee he assembled.

America's Greatest Pastime Meets America's Worst Disease

As we were developing our Dream Team model and gathering our SAC, we also focused on raising as much money as possible to fund the science itself. Celebrity-packed telethons can raise significant funds, but we knew it would never be enough. We wanted to create a movement with broad appeal that would extend well beyond fans of Hollywood. The question became: whom should we go to? While cancer is America's disease, baseball is America's pastime—so we decided to start there.

We first approached Jerry Reinsdorf, owner of the Chicago White Sox. He pointed us to Bud Selig, then the ninth commissioner of baseball—the chief executive officer of Major League Baseball (MLB). At 2 P.M. on a weekend afternoon, I got a call from cofounder Rusty Robertson. The commissioner was in Los Angeles for a dinner and could meet with us for fifteen minutes, starting at 5:45 P.M. that very day. It was a Sunday afternoon and I had a lovely dinner planned with friends in from Chicago and now faced only a few hours' notice to meet the commissioner. There was no choice—I knew we had to go.

Our team settled into a hotel meeting room in Century City and prepared to make our case to Bud Selig. The commissioner walked in accompanied by his extraordinary wife, Sue Lappin, and sat at the head of the table. Each of us knew what we had to say. Laura talked about her ongoing battle with cancer—how we must find a cure and how she did not have time to wait. Lisa and Ellen talked about the upcoming fund-raising telecast, what we aimed to do, and how supporting this effort would benefit Major League Baseball. My job was easy: all I had to say to the commissioner was, "Therefore, we would like MLB to give us ten million dollars." Up until that moment, I had never asked for more than $10,000 for a charity. I was extremely nervous, so I drew on my best acting skills. Cool and calm, with all the casual assurance of someone asking for a cup of tea, I said it, and all eyes turned to Bud. He put his hands under his chin and began, "Well, ordinarily . . ." It was clear he was about to say no. But then Sue gave him a gentle elbow nudge and said, *Come on, Buddy, what are you waiting for?* He adored his wife, and he could sense how moved she was by our story. So, as much out of respect for his wife as for our proposal, he burst into laughter and said, "I'm in."

Everyone started to cry except for me. After the Seligs left the room, I turned to our group. "Don't you ever cry again," I said to them. "*Never* cry. If you cry, it shows we didn't think we were going to get what we asked for, and we will absolutely get it." Selig's support was transformational—it gave us credibility. Without Major League Baseball, Stand Up To Cancer would not exist. The next time we walked into a room looking to fund-raise, we could say that MLB had already contributed $10 million. Now we were ready for our first show.

The First Fund-Raiser

Having secured our first major funder, we focused on final preparations for the roadblock fund-raiser. SU2C had been formally launched on May 28, 2008. To introduce the initiative to the public, the three network evening news anchors—Katie Couric, Charles Gibson, and Brian Williams—appeared as a group for the first time ever on ABC's *Good Morning America*, CBS's *This Morning*, and NBC's *Today* show to announce the September 5 telecast. The big day finally arrived, and the hour-long show took place across the ABC, CBS, and NBC television networks as planned. We thought this would be a one-off event, but it was so successful—raising over $125 million—that we decided to host one every other year. Our most recent telecast was carried on more than seventy broadcast, cable, streaming, and social platforms. We did not set out thinking we would raise hundreds of millions through these events. Our efforts evolved over time, starting with one show and expanding from there. What was always present—what makes SU2C unique—is passion. All of us have been impacted by cancer. If I go into a room like Laura used to do and say, "Raise your hand if you've been touched by cancer," every hand will go up. We were passionate. We were women who did not understand the word *no*.

Thirteen Years of SU2C

SU2C grew quickly after our initial successes. We have now hosted roadblock telecasts in 2010, 2012, 2014, 2016, and 2018. To date, more than eight hundred celebrities supporting SU2C's efforts have participated in these telecasts and in additional awareness efforts. With the help of people across the US and Canada as well as corporate, philanthropic, and organizational donors, we have raised over $660 million as of this writing to support SU2C's portfolio of innovative cancer research. Over that time, our funded research has contributed to the development of nine new cancer therapies approved by the FDA, including treatments for breast, colorectal, ovarian, pancreatic, and prostate cancers, and difficult-to-treat leukemias in children and young adults—actively extending the lives of many cancer patients. Our efforts continue to thrive under the extraordinary leadership of our CEO, Dr. Sung Poblete, who joined us ten years ago. Under Sung's stewardship, SU2C has continued to fund innovative science and develop cutting-edge approaches to research. Sung's many initiatives include SU2C Convergence, which brings together the medical, physical, and computer sciences to explore how cancers respond to therapies; SU2C Catalyst, which is dedicated to rapidly accelerating clinical trials of combination therapies; and "cancer interception," which aims to find and treat a cancer at the earliest possible point, perhaps even before a cancer cell has fully formed. Sung also spearheaded the launch of one of our new core initiatives to address the underlying health inequities in cancer research.

Health Equity and the Path Forward

As we look to the future of SU2C, we are committed to increasing health equity. Today, certain groups are underserved by the health-care community, not receiving the same amount or quality of care as others do. Nor have researchers been as inclusive as they should be when developing and testing treatments. In January 2020, we announced the SU2C Health Equity Initiative aimed at reducing racial and ethnic inequities in cancer research as well as improving outcomes for members of underserved populations. This initiative aims to increase minority representation in cancer clinical trials by requiring that future research grant proposals address recruitment and retention of patients from various ethnic groups to bolster diverse patient representation in cancer clinical trials. We have already committed over $15 million to Health Equity grants, which will fund research on cancers affecting underrepresented populations. Funded proposals may address cancers that have a higher prevalence in a specific racial or ethnic population or those that are more deadly among specific minority populations, or may address the need for more effective treatments for specific cancers for patients of diverse backgrounds.

Our continuing efforts will play out against the backdrop of a new administration. President Biden has made it clear that finding a cure for cancer is a top priority. If he sets the agenda by prioritizing several key principles, we can make real progress. Funding for research could be expanded in a way that only the federal government can do. For all our successes, neither we nor any other non-governmental group can match the federal purse. New funding policies could encourage breaking down the various silos that define and, in many cases, limit cancer research and care. Our model offers a path forward. By strongly encouraging multi-institutional collaboration so as to receive grants, for example, the federal government could help accelerate a trend we have encouraged over the past thirteen years. Tackling health inequities should animate the federal response to cancer. Until care is more equitably available and research meets the needs of every group, our work will remain unfinished. A sharper focus on translational research should likewise be encouraged, following our mantra: "Don't just get science—get science to the patient faster." This imperative guides our approach to funding grants. We favor research that is likely to benefit patients sooner rather than later. The Biden administration should also work to expand education about prevention and early detection. Lastly, outreach to such organizations as SU2C that fund cancer research—to create a coalition stretching from the White House across the country—could help coordinate our various efforts in an unprecedented way, potentially transforming the way cancer is treated in America for the next fifty years and beyond.

There will be a time when cancer is no longer a killer. That time is not far off. New treatments will emerge, and collaboration will be vital for their discovery. I have decades of experience as a cancer advocate and have seen firsthand both the costs of this disease as well as the promise of efforts to treat it. I believe that in my lifetime, we will transform cancer from a deadly disease into a manageable condition through the work of patients, advocates, and the extraordinary scientists and clinicians leading the way.

PART THREE

SCIENCE AND TREATMENT TRANSFORMED

CHAPTER 11

The Frontier of Cancer Care

Aphrothiti J. Hanrahan, Gurshan S. Gill, and David B. Solit

Cancer is a genetic disease resulting from mutations in genes that regulate cell differentiation, growth, survival, and/or immune evasion. For decades, cytotoxic chemotherapies were the mainstay of systemic cancer treatment (Table 11.1). These drugs kill cancer cells, and some normal cells, by damaging DNA or by interfering with the machinery of DNA replication or cell division. Despite their often severe toxicities, which include hair loss, nausea, nerve damage, and an increased risk for serious infection, combinations of cytotoxic chemotherapy drugs can cure some blood cancers and metastatic germ cell tumors and reduce the likelihood of disease recurrence when used as an adjuvant to curative intent surgery or radiation therapy. However, for most metastatic cancer patients, cytotoxic chemotherapy is minimally effective and at best palliative.

The past two decades have witnessed a paradigm shift in cancer drug development. Cancer treatments are now rationally designed to disrupt the molecular alterations and dysregulated pathways

Aphrothiti J. Hanrahan is Assistant Lab Member, Memorial Sloan Kettering Cancer Center.

Gurshan S. Gill is Research Assistant, David Solit Lab.

David B. Solit is Geoffrey Beene Chair in Cancer Research; Director, Marie-Josée and Henry R. Kravis Center for Molecular Oncology at Memorial Sloan Kettering Cancer Center.

TABLE 11.1 Pillars of Systemic Cancer Therapy

Cytotoxic Chemotherapy	• Drugs that damage, interfere with, or bind to and disrupt DNA • Antimetabolites • Microtubule inhibitors
Targeted Inhibitors	• Kinase inhibitors (RTK, non-RTK, mutant- or isoform-specific) • Lineage-specific dependencies (AR, ER, B-cell machinery) • Nonkinase, small molecule oncogene inhibitors (RAS G12C, BCL-2) • PROTACs • Synthetic lethal combos (BRCA1/2+PARP) • Proteosome inhibitors
Immunotherapy	• Passive immune therapy (monoclonal antibodies: naked, antibody-drug conjugates, bispecific, BiTE) • Active immune therapy (personalized cancer vaccines, costimulatory immune agonists) • Immune checkpoint inhibitors (anti-CTLA-4, PD-1, PD-L1, LAG3, TIM3, TIGIT) • Inhibitors of immunosuppressive factors in the tumor microenvironment • Innate immune modulators (STING agonists) • Oncolytic viruses
Cellular Therapy	• Tumor-Infiltrating Lymphocyte Therapy (TIL) • T cell Receptor Therapy (TCR) • Chimeric Antigen Receptor T cell Therapy (CAR T)

Abbr: RTK-receptor tyrosine kinase; AR-androgen receptor; ER-estrogen receptor; PROTAC-proteolysis targeting chimera; BiTE-bispecific T cell engager; STING-stimulator of interferon genes.

Note: Some drugs could fit into more than one class (e.g., anti-HER2 monoclonal antibody trastuzumab or VEGF/angiogenesis inhibitors could be considered both targeted therapy and immunotherapy).

responsible for cancer development and/or immune evasion. As many "targeted" and immune-based therapies are most effective in molecularly defined subsets of patients, therapy selection is increasingly guided by real-time testing for the genetic mutations or other molecular changes responsible for cancer development in individual patients. This approach, referred to as precision oncology, relies on technological innovations in DNA sequencing that have enabled the rapid analysis of hundreds of cancer-associated genes at low cost.

In this chapter, we highlight recent innovations in systemic cancer therapy that have resulted in improved clinical outcomes, including increased survival rates. While many newer targeted and immune-based cancer therapies are significantly more effective than the cytotoxic chemotherapies they have replaced, intrinsic and acquired drug resistance are major barriers to disease cure. We therefore predict that future improvements in cancer care will require both the identification of new drug targets as well as laboratory and clinical research designed to elucidate the molecular mechanisms mediating drug resistance. These bench-to-bedside translational research studies will be critical to achieving the promise of precision oncology, as they will form the basis for combinatorial approaches designed to prevent or delay the emergence of drug resistance. Given the heterogeneity of human cancers, progress will also require innovative clinical trial designs and regulatory flexibility to facilitate the testing of more personalized targeted, immune-based, and cellular therapies in the molecularly defined subsets of cancer patients most likely to benefit.

Kinase Inhibitors and Other Molecularly Targeted Therapies

Kinases are enzymes that transmit signals from the cell surface or within cells that influence the rate of cell division or determine whether cancer cells survive, invade surrounding normal tissues, or spread to distant organs (metastasize). Cancer cells are frequently dependent on hyperactivated kinases or other mutated proteins for growth or survival, a phenomenon known as oncogene addiction.

Historically, it took decades to translate novel biologic insights from the laboratory into new cancer drugs, but this process is now rapidly accelerating. As an example, in 1960, an abnormally small chromosome (known as the Philadelphia chromosome) was first observed in the cancer cells, but not the normal blood cells, of patients with chronic myelogenous leukemia. Subsequent research revealed that this abnormal chromosome resulted from a type of mutation known as a translocation, an exchange of DNA segments between two regions of the human genome. In chronic myelogenous leukemia, the cancer cells are "addicted" to the fusion protein, called BCR-ABL1, which is encoded by parts of the BCR and ABL1 genes, which are normally located on different chromosomes. This insight into the molecular cause of chronic myelogenous leukemia prompted the development of drugs that selectively inhibit ABL1 kinase (e.g., imatinib), the enzymatic portion of the fusion protein. This first-in-class molecularly targeted therapy has since supplanted older cytotoxic chemotherapies, transforming a previously life-threatening disease into an often manageable chronic condition with an overall survival rate approaching that of age-matched control patients.[1]

While the success of imatinib in patients with chronic myelogenous leukemia led to the hope that most cancer patients would soon be treated with therapies designed to selectively inhibit the mutations responsible for inducing their cancer, two decades later, only a minority of cancer patients (<30%) benefit from targeted therapies. To hasten the identification and development of additional targeted therapies, comprehensive molecular profiling studies were initiated to catalog the full spectrum of genomic alterations in both common and rare cancers. Lung cancer has been one of the most impacted cancer types with drugs that selectively inhibit several mutated genes, namely EGFR, ALK, ROS1, RET, MET, BRAF, KRAS, and NRTK1-3, now approved by the US Food and Drug Administration (FDA) for the treatment of patients with tumors harboring activating mutations in these oncogenes. However, some patients, including those with mutations in targetable cancer genes, never experience tumor shrinkage following treatment with kinase inhibitors (primary resistance), whereas others develop resistance to therapy after an initial response (acquired resistance). Furthermore, many cancer patients have tumors caused by mutations in genes that have proven to be "undruggable" to date. With the goal of increasing the fraction of patients who benefit from precision oncology, the following novel approaches are being pursued (Table 11.1).

Kinase Inhibitors with Greater Selectivity

Kinase inhibitors are generally viewed as having fewer side effects than cytotoxic chemotherapies because they are designed to inhibit mutated proteins present in cancer, but not normal, cells. However, most targeted therapies have adverse effects resulting from "off-target" toxicities (inhibition of proteins other than the desired target) or "on-target, off-tumor" effects (inhibition of the intended drug target in normal cells). One way to limit off-target toxicity is through the development of more selective kinase inhibitors. For example, early attempts to develop PI3 kinase inhibitors targeting the commonly mutated kinase, PI3 kinase-alpha, were limited by severe toxicities resulting in part from concurrent inhibition of all four structurally related PI3 kinase family members (PI3K-alpha, -beta, -delta, -gamma). Thus, alpelisib was designed to have greater selectivity for the PI3K-alpha isoform versus the other PI3 kinase family members and has greater efficacy and reduced toxicity as compared to older, less selective PI3 kinase inhibitors. In 2019, alpelisib was FDA-approved for the treatment of breast cancers that harbor mutations in the PIK3CA gene (which encodes PI3K-alpha).[2]

Greater selectivity can also be achieved by designing drugs that are more potent inhibitors of a mutated kinase versus its normal, nonmutant version. For instance, the BRAF inhibitor vemurafenib only inhibits BRAF activation in cancer cells that express a specific mutated version of the BRAF protein.[3] In the past, many pharmaceutical companies were leery of pursuing mutant-selective drugs over concern that the potential market size would be too small to justify the costs of drug development and clinical testing. However, the ubiquity with which patients are now molecularly profiled, advances in structure-based drug design, the development of novel clinical trial designs, and the willingness of regulators to consider tumor-agnostic drug approvals have made the economics of developing mutant-selective drugs more favorable.

Cancer researchers are also trying to reduce on-target, off-tumor side effects through targeted delivery of kinase inhibitors or other drugs to tumor cells only, thus avoiding damage to normal cells. One method involves coating or wrapping a cancer drug in tiny particles (e.g., nanocapsules) that shield the drug from degradation while more specifically directing it to the cancer cells. Drugs can also be injected directly into some tumors, or they can "piggyback" on antibodies or peptides that bind to proteins over-expressed on cancer cells (e.g., antibody-drug conjugates, as will be discussed).

Kinase Inhibitors That Retain Potency in the Setting of Acquired Resistance Mutations

The paradigm of cataloging the most common mechanisms of drug resistance as a guide to the development of second- and third-generation kinase inhibitors or combinations of kinase inhibitors that overcome or delay the emergence of drug-resistant tumor cells, is now firmly established. Osimertinib, a third-generation EGFR inhibitor, was developed to treat EGFR-mutant lung cancers that had acquired a resistance mutation in EGFR that reduces the binding of older EGFR inhibitors, such as erlotinib, to the EGFR protein.[4]

Drug treatment may also force cancer cells to undergo other types of adaptations to survive. Targeting these changes, or "acquired vulnerabilities," to induce the death of resistant cells is termed "collateral sensitivity." As an example, BRAF-mutant melanoma cells resistant to BRAF inhibitors were found to have increased reactive oxygen species, natural molecules highly damaging to DNA and RNA. To exploit this observation, drugs are being designed that further induce reactive oxygen species to lethal levels, selectively killing BRAF inhibitor resistant cells.[5]

Combinations of Targeted Inhibitors

Combining cytotoxic chemotherapies with different mechanisms of action and non-overlapping toxicities was critical to the development of curative regimens for childhood leukemias and germ cell tumors. The hope is that the development of more selective kinase and other targeted inhibitors together with the increasing adoption of tumor genomic profiling will facilitate the development of personalized, combination strategies that engender complete responses or even disease cures. Critical to the testing of drug combinations will be large cooperative studies, such as the National Cancer Institute's ComboMATCH trial, that seek to overcome many of the logistical challenges of testing drug combinations (e.g., the need to coadminister drugs developed by competing pharmaceutical companies).

Identification of Lineage-Specific Targets
An alternative to targeting mutationally activated signaling pathways is the inhibition of signaling pathways critical for the normal development or maintenance of the cell type from which the tumor cells arose, a concept referred to as lineage addiction. An underappreciated example of lineage addiction is the dependence of prostate and breast cancer cells on androgen and estrogen receptor signaling, respectively. Tamoxifen, which blocks the binding of estrogen to its receptor, has been used for decades to treat estrogen receptor-expressing breast cancers. More recent examples include idelalisib, a selective PI3 kinase delta inhibitor, and ibrutinib, an inhibitor of Bruton's tyrosine kinase (BTK). Many B cell cancers are addicted to these kinases, which are mediators of normal B cell maturation and proliferation.[6]

Drugging the "Undruggable"
Novel approaches are being pursued to target cancer-causing oncogenes and tumor suppressor genes that have proven to be "undruggable" to date. Several innovative drugs in late-stage clinical testing take advantage of a specific mutation (G12C) in the difficult-to-target KRAS gene, which is mutated in approximately 15 percent of all human cancers. These novel drugs, including the recently FDA-approved drug sotorasib, lock the mutated RAS protein in its "off" position by binding to the resultant cysteine (C) commonly introduced by DNA mutation.[7] Another

novel class of experimental drugs called PROTACs (proteolysis targeting chimera) are engineered to bind a mutated protein of interest and link it to the cell's internal enzymes responsible for destroying unwanted proteins (e.g., the ubiquitin-proteasome system).[8]

Researchers are also seeking to indirectly exploit the presence of an undruggable mutation through a process called synthetic lethality, which refers to cell death resulting from inactivation of two or more genes, where inactivation of only one of the genes does not compromise cell viability. Notably tumors with mutations in the DNA repair pathway genes BRCA1 and BRCA2 are frequently sensitive to olaparib, an inhibitor of the DNA damage repair protein PARP.[9] Because BRCA1 and BRCA2 are only fully inactivated in the tumor cells, drug inhibition of a second DNA repair pathway (PARP) creates a double hit to DNA repair that only occurs in the tumor cells. This leads to a buildup of irreparable DNA damage resulting in cancer cell–specific death.

The Need for Better Diagnostic Tests as a Guide to Precision Oncology
The success of precision oncology rests on the development of diagnostic tests that allow clinicians to identify those patients most likely to benefit from a particular therapy.[10] Cancers, even those arising in the same organ, can result from a diversity of genetic alterations that are impossible to distinguish by morphologic examination under a light microscope. Thus, diagnostic assays that can quickly identify mutations in actionable cancer genes, such as BRAF mutations in melanoma, are needed to guide treatment selection. Over the past decade, diagnostic tests that can detect a single genetic mutation have been replaced by tests that can screen for mutations in hundreds of cancer-associated genes or even the whole genome. It is hoped that future advances in tumor molecular profiling will give rise to diagnostic tests that incorporate measurements of gene expression, protein activation, and immune cell activation that will allow greater personalization of cancer care. Newer diagnostic tests may also be able to detect precancerous cells before they transform into invasive cancers (i.e., cancer inter-

ception), allowing for curative treatment before the development of lethal metastatic progression.

Novel Clinical Trial Designs to Test Treatments for Rare Mutations
Given the low prevalence of some targetable mutations or mutation combinations, novel clinical trial designs are needed to efficiently test new targeted drugs or drug combinations in the small subset of cancer patients most likely to benefit. Traditionally, late-stage clinical trials restricted eligibility to only a single cancer subtype (e.g., lung or breast cancer). Eligibility for basket studies, on the other hand, is based on the presence of a specific targetable mutation in the patient's tumor or normal cells (e.g., BRAF or HER2 mutation) irrespective of cancer subtype. Basket studies of BRAF, HER2, and NTRK inhibitors have established that both mutation type and cancer subtype can influence drug response. For example, response rates to the BRAF inhibitor vemurafenib differ widely as a function of cancer type, ranging from >80 percent in BRAF-mutant histiocytosis to 50 to 60 percent in BRAF-mutant melanoma and less than 5 percent in BRAF-mutant colorectal cancer. In contrast, larotrectinib, a selective inhibitor of the three related NTRK genes, was shown to be effective in patients with NTRK fusion tumors, irrespective of cancer type, and was granted the first tumor-agnostic approval by the FDA.[11]

The Cancer Immunotherapy Revolution

Attempts to harness the immune system for therapeutic benefit date to the late nineteenth century when treatments with heat-killed bacteria (called Coley's toxin) and later with live-attenuated bacteria (bacillus Calmette-Guerin [BCG]) were shown to have antitumor effects. A century of scientific advances has clarified the critical role played by the immune system in cancer suppression. In response to bacteria, viruses, or other entities deemed "foreign," the body initiates an "innate" immune response, which involves the rapid mobilization of immune cells to prevent the foreign entity from damaging normal cells or spreading within the body. This is followed by a slower "adaptive" immune response, which results in the expansion of specific white blood cells called T cells and B cells, which can recognize and attack specific foreign invaders.

In the 1950s, Nobel laureate F. Macfarlane Burnet and noted immunologist Lewis Thomas reasoned that the immune system is able to identify cancerous cells as foreign based on differences in cell surface protein fragments called antigens, and eliminate them before lethal tumors become apparent. The critical role played by immune surveillance in suppressing cancer development is highlighted by the cancer predisposition of patients with immune deficiencies, such as acquired immunodeficiency syndrome (AIDS). Laboratory and clinical research studies have established that a dynamic interaction exists between cancer cells and the immune system, known as immunoediting, which drives the selection for tumor cells that have acquired the ability to evade natural immune defenses.[12] Modulating immune function to block this "tumor escape" is a cornerstone of modern cancer immunotherapy (Table 11.1).

Antibodies as Cancer Drugs

Acquired immunity gives rise to antibodies, which are Y-shaped proteins that bind to distinct antigens on the surface of a foreign entity and serve to flag the foreign invader for destruction by the immune system. A critical step in the use of antibodies as therapeutics was the development of laboratory methods to produce, at scale, antibodies capable of binding with high affinity to a single antigen, called monoclonal antibodies. In 1997, rituximab became the first monoclonal antibody to be FDA-approved as an anticancer drug. Rituximab binds to the CD20 protein present on the surface of B cell lymphomas, triggering the body's immune system to kill CD20-expressing cancer cells. Antibodies can also disrupt the activation of kinases or other cell surface proteins. For example, trastuzumab binds to the cell surface protein HER2 and kills cancer cells by both inhibiting HER2-mediated survival signaling as well as by enhancing immune-mediated cell death.

While most monoclonal antibodies have modest activity when used alone, their antitumor effects can be significantly enhanced when they are coadministered with chemotherapy. Another strategy to increase the antitumor effects of antibodies is the chemical linkage of a toxin to a therapeutic antibody (antibody-drug conjugates [ADCs]), which enables the selective delivery of a lethal payload to the cancer cells. As a further enhancement, antibodies have been engineered to cotarget two antigens (bispecific antibodies), which can boost efficacy by simultaneously inhibiting two pathways critical for tumor growth and survival. Amivantamab, an EGFR/MET bispecific antibody, was recently FDA-approved to treat lung cancer patients whose tumors express EGFR mutations resistant to older EGFR inhibitors, and is being further tested in lung cancers with EGFR inhibitor resistance caused by MET tyrosine kinase pathway activation.[13] A related strategy called bispecific T cell engager (BiTE) cotargets a protein expressed on tumor cells and a second expressed on immune cells, which facilitates the physical interaction of cytotoxic T cells with tumor cells. Some researchers believe that BiTEs will prove to be a cost-efficient alternative to cellular therapies (discussion follows).

Immune Checkpoint Inhibitors:
Anti-CTLA-4 and Anti-PD1/PD-L1 Therapy

To say that immune checkpoint inhibitors have revolutionized cancer treatment over the past decade is not an overstatement. In the context of cancer, T cells use surface proteins, called T cell receptors (TCRs), to recognize and bind protein fragments, called tumor antigens, expressed on the surface of cancer cells. However, T cells will only kill a target cell if antigen engagement is accompanied by a co-stimulatory signal. T cells also express inhibitory proteins, or "checkpoint proteins," such as CTLA-4 and PD-1, which function to limit immune cell activation and thereby minimize nonselective attack of nearby normal tissues.

Tumor cells can hijack CTLA-4 and PD-1 inhibitory signaling to trigger T cell exhaustion or death, so as to avoid immune surveillance. Pioneering work by James Allison and colleagues revealed that inhibiting these immune checkpoint proteins can "release the brakes" on the immune system, resulting in immune-mediated killing of cancer cells.[14] The anti-CTLA-4 antibody ipilimumab was first shown to prolong the survival of patients with metastatic melanoma, leading to its FDA approval in 2011.[15] Several years later, anti–PD-1 antibodies were demonstrated to have antitumor activity, but with a toxicity profile more favorable than that of anti–CTLA-4 antibodies. Antibodies that bind to PD-1 (nivolumab, pembrolizumab, and cemiplimab) or its ligand PD-L1 (atezolizumab, avelumab, and durvalumab) are now FDA-approved for a variety of cancer types.[16] Despite sometimes severe immune-mediated side effects, immune checkpoint inhibitors targeting CTLA-4, PD-1, and PD-L1 can cure a subset of patients with metastatic melanoma, renal cancer, and lung cancer, which were historically among the cancer subtypes most refractory to cytotoxic chemotherapies.

As with other therapies, the response of cancer patients to immune checkpoint inhibitors is highly variable. Three classes of immunotherapy resistance have been identified: (1) primary resistance, defined as a lack of a host immune response; (2) adaptive resistance, defined as an ineffectual host immune response due to rapid evasion of the immune response by the tumor; and (3) acquired resistance/secondary escape, defined as an initial effective immune response followed by cancer progression. Novel immunotherapy combinations seek to overcome immune checkpoint inhibitor resistance by targeting the cancer cell and host adaptations that allow tumor cells to evade immune surveillance at different points within the "cancer-immunity cycle."[17]

Enhancing Immune Checkpoint Inhibitor Response
Tumors that have a scarcity of T cells within the tumor microenvironment are called cold tumors, noninflamed tumors, or immune deserts, and often exhibit primary resistance to immunotherapy. These cold tumors foster invisibility because they lack potent tumor antigens, have suppressed antigen expression, or because they actively produce factors that block antigen presentation. Concurrent or sequential administration of cytotoxic chemotherapies,

radiation therapy, or targeted therapies is being studied for their ability to turn cold tumors "hot" through the release of tumor antigens or pro-inflammatory molecules following induction of cancer cell death. Another approach to enhance immune checkpoint blockade is the use of engineered oncolytic virotherapies that selectively infect and kill tumor cells, thereby enhancing antigen release and presentation. Lastly, it is hoped that advances in tumor genomics and RNA vaccine technology will allow for a priming of the immune system via administration of personalized cancer vaccines directed toward neoepitopes—mutant antigens expressed exclusively on the patient's tumor but not on normal cells.[18]

Colorectal, ovarian, and pancreatic cancers are often referred to as immune-excluded or immune-privileged tumors, as T cells are trapped just outside the tumor. This phenomenon is believed to be mediated, at least in part, by the tumor stroma, a specialized matrix of secreted proteins and supportive cells derived from normal tissue, which surround and permeate the tumor and evolve to promote tumor growth, altered metabolism, invasion, metastasis, and immune suppression. For example, fibroblasts (cells that make up normal connective tissue) in the stroma can differentiate into cancer-associated fibroblasts (CAFs) that express an enzyme called indole 2,3-dioxygenase (IDO), which breaks down an amino acid essential for T cell viability. Strategies are being developed to block immunosuppressive factors enriched in the tumor microenvironment, such as IDO, with the goal of enhancing immune checkpoint inhibitor response.

Inflamed, or "hot," tumors are those with activated T cells and pro-immune factors robustly infiltrating the tumor. While this phenotype is predictive of immune checkpoint inhibitor response, many patients with inflamed tumors still fail to respond, or eventually relapse following treatment with immune checkpoint inhibitors. To address this unmet clinical need, the combination of anti–CTLA-4 and anti–PD-1 antibodies was tested, resulting in a modest improvement in survival versus single-agent therapy in melanoma, albeit with greater toxicity.[19] Alternative approaches to enhancing immune checkpoint inhibitor response include modulation of gut bacteria, a healthy diversity of which is predictive of immunotherapy response, and concurrent inhibition of additional immune checkpoints, including LAG3, TIM3, and TIGIT.[20] Another strategy entails the coinhibition of oncogenes that promote not only tumor growth and survival but also immune evasion.[21] When mutated, RAS or BRAF can impair antigen presentation, and alterations in the PTEN or CTNNB1 genes can impair T cell infiltration into tumors. Certain cancer mutations also cause increased PD-L1 expression on the cancer cell surface, which can then bind PD-1 on T cells and turn them off. Studies combining targeted inhibitors and checkpoint inhibitors are thus under way and represent a convergence of two pillars of cancer treatment.

Additional approaches to enhancing immune checkpoint inhibitor response include boosting T cell stimulation and trafficking to the tumor. Tumors actively release immunosuppressive factors that reduce costimulatory signals, resulting in only partial T cell activation, induction of an anergic state (alive, but functionally unresponsive), or T cell death. Drugs designed to mimic and enhance costimulatory signals, such as agonists (activators) for the costimulatory receptors ICOS and 4-1BB, are being tested both as single agents and in combination with anti–PD-1/PD-L1 antibodies. Further, the journey of an activated T cell from a lymph node into the blood circulation and then through the blood vessel wall at the site of a tumor is a choreographed sequence controlled by proteins that stimulate cell movement and adhesion. To avoid being identified by T cells, tumors can release proteins (e.g., VEGF and ANG2) that make it harder for T cells to exit the bloodstream. These factors also promote the formation of new blood vessels, which can increase intratumoral oxygen and nutrient sources and provide new avenues for tumors to escape and invade tissues. Antibodies and kinase inhibitors that target VEGF, its receptor VEGFR, and ANG2 are being tested in combination with anti–PD-1 therapy, with recent success in kidney cancer.

Harnessing the Innate Immune Response
Immune mediator proteins, such as the Toll-like receptors and stimulator of interferon genes (STING), can sense foreign or mu-

tant DNA or RNA particles released from tumors or infectious pathogens, and trigger an innate immune response to contain the foreign entity. To leverage this innate immune response, synthetic DNA analogs that mimic the types of aberrant DNA or RNA released from tumors are being developed to bind to and agonize Toll-like receptors and STING.

Cellular Immunotherapy: Adoptive Cell Transfer

Adoptive cell transfer is an umbrella term for cell-based immunotherapies that utilize a patient's own T cells for therapeutic use (Table 11.1). All three approaches developed to date extract T cells from the patient, and then grow, expand, activate, and/or genetically modify the T cells in a laboratory, followed by reinfusion. Current cellular therapies differ in the degree to which the patient's T cells are genetically altered. TIL therapy expands tumor-infiltrating lymphocytes (TILs) extracted from a tumor biopsy or resection, without any engineered changes. TIL therapy has been shown to induce durable complete responses in melanoma and cervical squamous cell carcinoma patients, among other tumor types. A major limitation to the broader adoption of TIL therapy is the difficulty of extracting adequate tumor-infiltrating T cells for expansion in the laboratory. As an alternative, T cell receptor (TCR) therapy involves isolation of T cells from the patient's blood, followed by introduction of a T cell receptor into the patient's T cells that recognizes an antigen expressed by the patient's tumor. As an example, TCR therapy targeting Wilms' tumor antigen 1, a protein often expressed by acute myeloid leukemias, has shown promise.[22]

Chimeric antigen receptor (CAR) T cells, which are T cells derived from a patient's blood and then engineered to express a synthetic receptor, is the cell-based immunotherapy that has had the greatest impact to date. CARs designed to target the CD19 antigen (Kymriah, Yescarta, Tecartus, and Breyanzi) or the B cell maturation antigen (BCMA, Abecma) are now FDA-approved.[23] Induction of cell death can be so rapid following CAR T cell infusion that it can result in a severe, but usually treatable, excessive immune reaction referred to as cytokine storm. CD19-directed CAR T cell therapy can also significantly increase the risk of infection due to the clearance and long-term suppression of normal CD19-expressing B cells. It has also proven challenging to develop cellular therapies for solid cancers. The major difficulty lies in identifying tumor antigens expressed by common solid tumors that are also not expressed by critical normal tissues. Thus, the following strategies are being pursued to enhance the safety and efficacy of cellular therapies.

Innovations in Cell Therapy

Similar to kinase inhibitors, CAR T cells can have on-target, off tumor toxicities, as exemplified by the death of a colon cancer patient who received a HER2-directed CAR T cell therapy that resulted in lethal damage to HER2-expressing normal lung tissue.[24] Therefore, several CAR modifications are being tested that seek to limit toxicity.[25] First, CARs have been designed to allow clinicians to rapidly induce CAR self-destruction via administration of a second drug (e.g., SMASH or suicide CARs). Gene editing technologies are also being used to delete cytokine genes in T cells or to engineer the release of anti-inflammatory proteins to prevent cytokine storm. Another strategy to reduce on-target, off tumor toxicities is to design CARs that require the binding of two tumor antigens to initiate T cell activation (e.g., split or SynNotch CARs) or CARs that disengage if an antigen on a normal cell is bound (iCAR). Alternatively, researchers are trying to couple CAR activation with microenvironmental conditions more frequently observed in tumors, such as hypoxia (lack of oxygen).

Leveraging their ability to selectively home to antigen-expressing tumor cells, "armored CARs" are designed to carry cargo, such as bispecific antibodies, immune checkpoint inhibitors, or pro-immune factors that are released at the tumor site and aid in immune activation and tumor attack. "SUPRA CARs" can be reprogrammed during the treatment course to address tumor adaptations that cause acquired drug resistance.[26] Finally, there would be significant logistical and cost benefits to the development of universal or "off-the-shelf" cell therapies in which T cells could be collected from donors (akin to donating blood) and engineered to bypass immune rejection, as it would be a "non-self" therapy.[27] Scientists are also looking to engineer other types of immune cells to express CARs. Advantages of using alternate cell types, such as natural killer (NK) cells, which are the cytotoxic cells of the innate immune response, include easier sourcing (e.g., umbilical cord blood) and decreased toxicity profiles (due to shorter half-life and less cytokine release).

Future Directions

In the closing remarks of his 1957 publication on the biology of cancer, F. Macfarlane Burnet, a Nobel laureate for his theories on acquired immune tolerance, wrote, "There is little optimism about cancer . . . A final solution will probably never be possible."[28] Although we continue to struggle to fully decipher the biologic complexity and heterogeneity of human cancer, we are confident that ongoing laboratory and translational research will identify new drug targets and therapeutic approaches that will increase the likelihood of cancer cure with less acute and long-term toxicity.

Critical to recent progress has been the recognition that cancer is not a single entity; rather, a collection of diseases characterized by dysregulated growth, cell survival, and immune evasion. As such, we cannot reasonably expect a single solution or "magic bullet" to be effective in all cancer patients. As cancers, even those arising in the same organ, are both genetically and biologically heterogeneous, it is not surprising that progress toward cure has been uneven. In the past several decades, targeted and immune-based therapies have dramatically improved cure rates and/or survival in some cancers, such as chronic myelogenous leukemia and melanoma, whereas progress has been minimal for others, such as pancreatic cancer.

We predict that future improvements in cancer care will result from greater personalization of treatment. Progress will require the identification of new therapeutic vulnerabilities and the development of more selective and less toxic targeted, immune, and cellular therapies. This would allow for concurrent or sequential administration of combinations of therapies with different mechanisms of action and nonoverlapping toxicities, a strategy key to the development of curative cytotoxic combinations for leukemias and germ cell tumors. Recent advances in RNA vaccine technology and genetic sequencing methods may also allow for the development of precision immunotherapies, such as personalized cancer vaccines and cellular therapies that target mutated antigens expressed exclusively on an individual patient's cancer cells.

As more personalized therapies will, by definition, be effective in only small subsets of cancer patients or even in a single individual, it will not be feasible to evaluate such treatments using traditional randomized clinical trial designs. Therefore, regulatory flexibility will be needed to fully realize the potential of precision oncology. Finally, given the need for combinatorial approaches, collaboration between academia and multiple pharmaceutical companies will be necessary, as will pricing structures that reduce the financial toxicity that currently restricts access to expensive cancer therapies. In sum, continued progress in the war on cancer will require both scientific discovery as well as regulatory and structural changes to our health-care system to facilitate the rapid testing of innovative ideas and access for all patients to the most promising diagnostic technologies and local and systemic treatments.

Notes

1. A. Hochhaus et al., "Long-Term Outcomes of Imatinib Treatment for Chronic Myeloid Leukemia," *New England Journal of Medicine* 376, no. 10 (2017): 917–927.

2. F. André et al., "Alpelisib for PIK3CA-Mutated, Hormone Receptor-Positive Advanced Breast Cancer," *New England Journal of Medicine* 380, no. 20 (2019): 1929–1940.

3. P. Lito, N. Rosen, and D. B. Solit, "Tumor Adaptation and Resistance to RAF Inhibitors," *Nature Medicine* 19, no. 11 (2013): 1401–1409.

4. S. S. Ramalingam et al., "Overall Survival with Osimertinib in Untreated, EGFR-Mutated Advanced NSCLC," *New England Journal of Medicine* 382, no. 1 (2020): 41–50.

5. L. Wang et al., "An Acquired Vulnerability of Drug-Resistant Melanoma with Therapeutic Potential," *Cell* 173, no. 6 (2018): 1413–1425 e14.

6. A. K. Gopal et al., "PI3Kdelta Inhibition by Idelalisib in Patients with Relapsed Indolent Lymphoma," *New England Journal of Medicine* 370, no. 11 (2014): 1008–1018.

7. D. S. Hong et al., "KRAS G12C Inhibition with Sotorasib in Advanced Solid Tumors," *New England Journal of Medicine* 383, no. 13 (2020): 1207–1217.

8. G. M. Burslem and C. M. Crews, "Proteolysis-Targeting Chimeras as Therapeutics and Tools for Biological Discovery," *Cell* 181, no. 1 (2020): 102–114.

9. M. Robson et al., "Olaparib for Metastatic Breast Cancer in Patients with a Germline BRCA Mutation," *New England Journal of Medicine* 377, no. 6 (2017): 523–533.

10. D. Chakravarty and D. B. Solit, "Clinical Cancer Genomic Profiling," *Nature Reviews Genetics* 22, no. 8 (August 2021); 483–501. doi: 10.1038/s41576-021-00338-8. Epub 2021 Mar 24.PMID: 33762738.

11. A. Drilon, et al., "Efficacy of Larotrectinib in TRK Fusion-Positive Cancers in Adults and Children," *New England Journal of Medicine* 378, no. 8 (2018): 731–739.

12. J. S. O'Donnell, M. W. L. Teng, and M. J. Smyth, "Cancer Immunoediting and Resistance to T Cell–Based Immunotherapy," *Nature Reviews Clinical Oncology* 16, no. 3 (2019): 151–167.

13. J. Yun et al., "Antitumor Activity of Amivantamab (JNJ-61186372), an EGFR-MET Bispecific Antibody, in Diverse Models of *EGFR* Exon 20 Insertion-Driven NSCLC," *Cancer Discovery* 10, no. 8 (2020): 1194–1209.

14. D. R. Leach, M .F. Krummel, and J. P. Allison, "Enhancement of Antitumor Immunity by CTLA-4 Blockade," *Science* 271, no. 5256 (1996): 1734–1736; A. Ribas and J. D. Wolchok, "Cancer Immunotherapy Using Checkpoint Blockade," *Science* 359, no. 6382 (2018): 1350–1355.

15. F. S. Hodi et al., "Improved Survival with Ipilimumab in Patients with Metastatic Melanoma," *New England Journal of Medicine* 363, no. 8 (2010): 711–723.

16. J. D. Wolchok et al., "Nivolumab Plus ipilimumab in Advanced Melanoma," *New England Journal of Medicine* 369, no. 2 (2013): 122–33.

17. D. S. Chen and I. Mellman, "Oncology Meets Immunology: The Cancer-Immunity Cycle," *Immunity* 39, no. 1 (2013): 1–10.

18. P. A. Ott et al., "An Immunogenic Personal Neoantigen Vaccine for Patients with Melanoma," *Nature* 547, no. 7662 (2017): 217–221.

19. J. Larkin et al., "Five-Year Survival with Combined Nivolumab and Ipilimumab in Advanced Melanoma," *New England Journal of Medicine* 381, no. 16 (2019): 1535–1546.

20. R. E. O'Neill and X. Cao, "Co-stimulatory and Co-inhibitory Pathways in Cancer Immunotherapy," *Advanced Cancer Research* 143, no. (2019): 145–194.

21. P. Sharma et al., "Primary, Adaptive, and Acquired Resistance to Cancer Immunotherapy," *Cell* 168, no. 4 (2017): 707–723.

22. A. G. Chapuis et al., "T Cell Receptor Gene Therapy Targeting WT1 Prevents Acute Myeloid Leukemia Relapse Post-transplant," *Nature Medicine* 25, no. 7 (2019): 1064–1072.

23. N. C. Munshi et al., "Idecabtagene Vicleucel in Relapsed and Refractory Multiple Myeloma," *New England Journal of Medicine* 384, no. 8 (2021): 705–716.

24. R. A. Morgan et al., "Case Report of a Serious Adverse Event Following the Administration of T Cells Transduced with a Chimeric Antigen Receptor Recognizing ERBB2," *Molecular Therapy* 18, no. 4 (2010): 843–851.

25. S. Rafiq, C. S. Hackett and R. J. Brentjens, "Engineering Strategies to Overcome the Current Roadblocks in CAR T cell Therapy," *Nature Reviews Clinical Oncology* 17, no. 3 (2020): 147–167.

26. J. H. Cho, J. J. Collins, and W. W. Wong, "Universal Chimeric Antigen Receptors for Multiplexed and Logical Control of T Cell Responses," *Cell* 173, no. 6 (2018): 1426–1438 e11.

27. S. Depil et al., "'Off-the-Shelf' Allogeneic CAR T Cells: Development and Challenges," *Nature Reviews Drug Discovery* 19, no. 3 (2020): 185–199.

28. M. Burnet, "Cancer: A Biological Approach, III. Viruses Associated with Neoplastic Conditions, IV. Practical Applications," *British Medical Journal* 1, no. 5023 (1957): 841–847.

CHAPTER 12

Oncologist Perspectives on the Evolution of Clinical Care Since the National Cancer Act of 1971

Neal J. Meropol and Eric P. Winer

Since the passage of the National Cancer Act of 1971, the practice of oncology has undergone a revolutionary transformation. As we look back over our careers as medical oncologists, we have observed a multitude of changes. Many were incremental, but taken as a whole, there has been a fundamental shift in our approach to the patient with cancer. These collective advances have altered what it means for patients to have a cancer diagnosis, including expectations regarding possible outcomes, the application of science and technology to clinical practice, and how and where care is delivered.

We began our careers in the late 1980s as two oncologists working at major academic hospitals, one of us at Duke and the other at the University of Pennsylvania. At that time, no matter what hospital you went to for treatment, a cancer diagnosis was still commonly viewed as a death sentence. We can recall some patients

---

Neal J. Meropol is Vice President, Head of Medical and Scientific Affairs, Flatiron Health.

Eric P. Winer is Chief Clinical Strategy Officer, Chief of the Division of Women's Cancers, and Director of the Breast Oncology Program in the Susan F. Smith Center for Women's Cancers at Dana-Farber Cancer Institute.

insisting on secrecy, which led to isolation. Cancer was more likely to be diagnosed at a late stage, and highly effective treatments were restricted to a few types of cancer. Disfiguring surgery was often the only hope for a curative approach; in other cases, only highly toxic drugs or radiation could prove lifesaving. The tools available to oncologists were limited, crude, and mostly focused on short-term palliation of symptoms or modest extension of survival.

Fast-forward to 2021, and approximately seventeen million cancer survivors in the US testify to advances in screening, early detection, and treatment.[1] Multimodality treatment, including combinations of surgery, radiation, and systemic approaches, is now common. Scientific and technologic advances have led to the development of highly targeted therapies, so-called precision oncology, with greater effectiveness and fewer side effects. Immunotherapy and cellular therapies, only experimental or wholly theoretical early in our careers, are now standard practice. Most cancer care today is delivered in the outpatient setting by teams of clinicians and support personnel. A cancer diagnosis, while still traumatic and dreaded, is no longer commonly expected to be a terminal event by patients and their loved ones. Cancer is now often curable, and when it is not, treatment may result in long-term survival with remarkably good quality of life.

In the next fifty years, we expect science and technology to continue driving reductions in cancer mortality through improvements in prevention, early detection, treatment, and surveillance—each enhanced by greater personalization. Approaches to behavior and biology will be refined, reducing the incidence of cancer and improving survival. Future diagnostics and therapeutics will be less invasive and toxic. Our growing understanding of the social determinants of health will hopefully address existing disparities in care and outcomes. The practice of oncology will evolve as team-based care expands. The development of new evidence will be enhanced by information technologies, as will its accessibility at the point of care.

Future advances will build on the transformative changes of the past thirty years, including our revolutionized understanding of the genetic basis for cancer risk. Genetic risk assessments have expanded the meaning of a cancer diagnosis for patients. Certain types of cancer have long been recognized as possibly "running in families." The precise definition of that risk and the ability to identify its genetic underpinnings with simple blood tests has only become available in recent decades. Cancer patients now routinely receive genetic testing based on personal or family history or young age of diagnosis, among other factors. Common cancers, such as breast and colorectal, may be associated with hereditary conditions, and genetic testing is now available for risk stratification. Identifying an altered gene that predisposes a patient or their family member to certain cancers may now impact cancer follow-up, surveillance, screening, prevention strategies, prophylactic surgical decisions, reproductive decision-making, and, at times, identify unique cancer therapeutic options. This information may also impact insurability and have significant psychosocial effects on individuals and families, including anxiety and guilt.

Recent decades have seen the emergence of so-called targeted therapies. These are more directed to cancer tissues, often less toxic, and frequently administered over an extended time. Certain cancers have been converted into chronic conditions as a result, creating a large survivorship population. Cancer survivors may have medical and psychological sequelae (aftereffects) related to the long-term effects of treatment, including risk for other cancers, cardiac or other organ damage, psychosocial challenges, sexual health problems, and employment or insurance dilemmas. Cancer survivors also serve as prominent advocates for advances in cancer research.

In this context of dramatic changes in our field, there has been one constant: the privilege of the doctor-patient relationship. As oncologists, we are entrusted with helping our patients navigate a threat to their mortality in a setting filled with ever-increasing complexity and uncertainty. As our profession looks ahead, we can and must adapt to the breakneck speed of scientific advancements, dramatic shifts in social norms around doctor-patient relationships and patient advocacy, and a health-care ecosystem that threatens to bankrupt our patients while overloading physicians with administrative, rather than medical, work.

The Doctor-Patient Relationship

A cancer diagnosis raises existential questions. The importance of the doctor-patient relationship and the effective communication between oncologists and their patients in oncology is magnified as patients ask themselves and their physicians "Am I going to die?" "What are the possible outcomes of treatment, both good and bad?" and "Will I suffer?" They are often making treatment decisions for themselves, their families, and their caregivers in a context characterized by a high level of uncertainty. In this setting, the relationship between an oncologist and their patient can be both intense and rewarding.

In the past decades, social and ethical norms around treatment have shifted firmly to what is known as shared decision-making. Within the medical model, there is a spectrum of patient engagement that ranges from pure paternalism ("Doctor, just tell me what to do") to independent patient decision-making ("Give me the facts and I'll decide"). In the center of this continuum is the concept of shared decision-making, where the physician conveys medical information, the patient expresses their values and goals, and together they arrive at a preference-sensitive treatment decision.[2] Over the past half century, the benefits of shared decision-making have been increasingly recognized. This is especially true where treatment may not be curative, multiple options exist, quality of life may be impacted, and the probability of various outcomes (e.g., cure, length of survival, side effects) is uncertain. Given the multiple outcomes of relevance to both quality and length of life in oncology, patient preferences take on added importance. Different patients may have varied goals, leading to different treatment decisions. For example, some patients may prioritize surgery avoidance, staying close to home for treatment, or out-of-pocket expense minimization, whereas others may prioritize the possibility of a cure, however unlikely, at all costs. Some patients may value maintaining quality of life and freedom from discomfort, or perhaps the ability to attend an important event, such as a family wedding. In our own work, we have found that the vast majority of cancer patients prefer a shared decision-making model.

Shared decision-making requires a set of communication tools that were historically not taught in medical school when we were students. The elicitation of patient values and goals takes patience and skills that may not be intuitive for medical students. This is especially challenging given our societal norms where the "war" or "battle" metaphor may make it difficult for patients to feel comfortable expressing their personal preferences, especially when family members are encouraging a "never give up at any cost" mentality. Likewise, medical information is often technical, requiring extensive experience to explain to patients and their families in lay terms. Statistical or probabilistic information can be especially challenging. As an example, in our own research we found that the statement "This new treatment controls cancer in 40 percent of cases like yours" was not understood by 28 percent of cancer patients.[3] Further, even patients likely to be cured may overestimate their risk of recurrence and death, which may adversely affect decision-making and psychological health.[4] Conversely, studies have documented that patients approaching the end of their life may vastly overestimate their prognosis.[5]

Research over the past several decades has also highlighted that attention to end-of-life care in oncology is an important measure of high-quality care, as aggressive intervention in terminal phases of disease has been demonstrated to result in impaired quality of life and dehumanizing and painful intensive care unit (ICU) utilization without reversal of the underlying medical condition or prolongation of survival. These data have led to expert guideline recommendations that promote early "goals of care" discussions, including ascertainment of preferences regarding aggressive life-extending but uncomfortable interventions (e.g., mechanical ventilation or ICU admission) for which the potential for recovery is low.[6] For example, patients who have had goals of care discussions with their physicians receive less aggressive medical care at the end of life and earlier hospice referrals, which are both associated with better quality of life near death.[7] These conversations are now routine during the care of oncology patients. In fact, between 2003 and 2012, the proportion of cancer patients enrolling in hospice programs before death increased from 54.6 to 63.4 percent.[8] A strong doctor-patient relationship facilitates these difficult conversations consistent with patient-centered care. Yet, current trends in care have made maintaining a quality doctor-patient relationship challenging.

While the influence of technology, such as electronic health records (EHRs), has streamlined certain aspects of care and improved access to (and legibility of!) clinical documentation, an increase in documentation requirements for administrative and reimbursement purposes has in some cases interfered with the direct interactions between patients and their oncologists. For example, clinical documentation required for billing purposes, but not essential for provider communication or care coordination, is commonly cited as interfering with face-to-face time between a patient and the oncologist. The rapid adoption of EHRs may be viewed as a legislative accomplishment, with both the Health Information Technology for Economic and Clinical Health Act of 2009 and the 21st Century Cures Act of 2016 (Cures Act) incentivizing the use of EHR technology. In addition to improving communication between care team members and also between the care team(s) and patients, EHRs are now recognized as a rich source of real-world data that can be used to derive new evidence about the impact of cancer treatments. In fact, the Cures Act required the US Food and Drug Administration (FDA) to address the potential use of real-world evidence in regulatory decision-making.

Finally, the accelerating cost of oncology care, related to new innovations, has burdened patients and added a new complexity to the doctor-patient relationship. Out-of-pocket costs now require patients to integrate considerations of "financial toxicity" into their treatment decisions. Even cancer patients with "good" health insurance report making trade-offs between medical care and other expenditures, and many report borrowing money and using savings to pay for cancer care. Bankruptcies among cancer patients are higher than among patients with other chronic conditions.[9] Furthermore, an evolving payment landscape is altering how practices provide care, with increased patient volumes and team-based approaches to care delivery. Recognition of these emerging influences is essential as we seek to optimize the patient experience and the quality of their care.

The Impact of Science and Technology on the Practice of Oncology

Since the war on cancer began fifty years ago, scientists have made huge strides in our knowledge of cancer biology. The Human Genome Project, which was completed in 2003, led the way to a full-scale interrogation of the genetic drivers of cancer and potential targets for new treatments.[10] This research demonstrated the remarkable genomic heterogeneity of individual cancers (e.g., all colorectal cancers are not alike) and across different malignancies. It also resulted in the realization that certain malignancies shared a number of basic genetic changes. In laboratory systems, we have an understanding of the molecular changes that lead to the development of cancer, its growth, and its ability to metastasize. We have also learned much about host factors that can fuel or inhibit cancer growth.

These advances informed new therapies targeting specific molecular drivers of cancer growth. Whereas in 1990 we treated most patients with a certain "type" of cancer simply based on the organ of origin, we now treat patients with lung, colon, breast, and many other types of cancer based upon the specific genomic changes in their tumors. In essence, what we used to think of as "lung cancer" is now more than ten different diseases, each with a different recommended treatment approach.

The revolution in cancer immunology and immunotherapy in the past decade has leveraged an individual's innate immune system to control and even eradicate cancer. Immunotherapy and other highly targeted approaches are contributing to a meaningful decrease in cancer death rates in the US.[11] In certain circumstances, these treatment advances have resulted in cures for previously fatal cancers, such as advanced melanoma. Even when a cure is not possible, many common cancers such as colon, lung, and breast cancer are now manageable even in advanced stages—this has furthered the view of "cancer as a chronic disease." While advances are not evenly distributed across cancer types, the pace of discovery, especially in the past two decades, has increased in what often seems to be an exponential fashion, leading all of us to anticipate where we will be in another decade.

Today's treatment landscape would not be possible without novel technologies that have given rise to new diagnostics, drugs, and cellular therapies with specific cancer targeting. Genomic sequencing, once restricted to the research setting, is now a routine component of cancer care. Sequencing genes in tumors to identify targetable alterations initially took days. Now, it can be completed in hours. Not surprisingly, associated costs have also plummeted. Expert clinical guidelines now recommend genomic testing—the sequencing of hundreds of relevant cancer genes—in most patients with advanced cancers, identifying targetable mutations for which effective therapies exist. Within the past five years, the FDA rendered its first "tumor agnostic" drug approvals for treatments based upon genomic changes, rather than the organ of origin. Whereas genomic testing was initially restricted to tumor-based testing, the recent ability to identify minute fragments of tumor DNA in blood has opened the door to noninvasive serial blood monitoring for cancer patients, as well as future potential for cancer screening.

Monoclonal antibody therapies have also revolutionized care. Antibodies were long recognized by researchers for their target specificity in the innate response to infectious diseases. A natural question arose as to whether this specificity could be leveraged against cancers. Nearly fifty years ago, the ability to produce high quantities of a uniform population of antibodies (so-called monoclonal antibodies) in the laboratory was described. It was not until 1997 that the first monoclonal antibody treatment for cancer, rituximab, was FDA-approved for patients with non-Hodgkin's lymphomas that had the relevant target on their surface. Since that time, more than thirty-five monoclonal antibodies for cancer treatment have entered routine clinical practice.[12]

Whereas monoclonal antibodies are proteins that mimic an immune response, more recently cellular therapies have been introduced that employ a patient's own T cells (a type of white blood cell) to target cancers. This technologic feat requires removal of a patient's T cells with a filtration process called pheresis, growing and processing these T cells in the laboratory to engineer them to recognize the target cancer, and then reinfusing them back into the patient. This chimeric antigen receptor T cell (CAR-T) therapy is now available in specialized centers for the treatment of certain leukemias and lymphomas. This remarkable advance represents the first cell-based therapy (rather than drugs to kill cancer cells) to prove curative and garner FDA approval. It is a treatment approach that can result in serious toxicities, however, and efforts in the coming years will focus on both expanding the use of CAR-T therapy and making it safer.

When we were oncology trainees, patients who were cured of Hodgkin's disease with radiation had a 1 percent chance per year of developing a second malignancy, a very high rate over the course of one's lifetime. In addition, chest radiation increased the risk of cardiac disease. Fast-forward to 2020, and radiation oncologists have the ability to treat cancers with high doses of precisely targeted radiation based on three-dimensional imaging and computer-modulated delivery that minimizes effects on normal tissues. Radiation therapy may now be delivered as photons or protons, each with characteristics that can guide appropriate selection. During our careers, we have also witnessed an evolution in surgical techniques, with the introduction of less-invasive procedures with lower morbidity. Robotic approaches that permit augmented dexterity and laparoscopic surgeries that do not require large excisions have both been shown to maintain tumor control with faster patient recovery from abdominal surgery.

The field of cancer diagnostic imaging is another area replete with examples of technologic progress since the 1980s. Computed tomography (CT) scanning was already well established early in our careers. This represented an incremental extension of X-ray radiology that provided cross-sectional anatomic information. Now, the selection of an imaging modality is more complex, with the availability of magnetic resonance imaging (MRI) that utilizes magnets and radio waves to generate images, and positron emission tomography (PET) that measures tumor metabolism. Additional diagnostic modalities, often with an enhanced ability to track changes in the cancer over time, are in development. These assorted methods are complementary and their selection is based on the specific clinical context.

This cascade of life-extending developments, however, has dramatically increased the complexity of cancer care, its cost, and the decision-making processes for oncologists and patients. To partially address this issue, professional organizations and commercial entities have begun to develop clinical practice guidelines for oncology, including automated applications within physician workflow.[13] Moreover, these advances have been accompanied by escalating drug, diagnostic, and other medical costs. New genetic discoveries may affect patient insurability—or even the insurability of their families—in future medico-legal environments. In addition, the costs associated with conducting clinical trials has skyrocketed. While the financial challenges, both societal and personal, are beyond the scope of this chapter, it is critical to underscore that the high price of cancer treatment represents a major challenge and compounds existing health-care disparities.[14]

Autonomy, Burnout, and Professionalism

The oncologist of the twenty-first century is facing an emerging threat to our profession: physician burnout. Burnout is a constellation of symptoms that include "emotional exhaustion, depersonalization, and reduced sense of personal accomplishment."[15] The National Cancer Policy Forum of the National Academies of Sciences, Engineering, and Medicine convened a workshop in 2019 to consider careforce resilience.[16] As summarized by Samuel Takvorian and colleagues, a variety of factors that bear on today's practice of oncology create a setting conducive to burnout.[17] The aging US population is resulting in growth in cancer diagnoses that outstrips careforce growth, challenging practices to provide high-quality care to more patients. As noted earlier, the complexity of care has increased, and this requires new approaches to care coordination and navigation, as well as decision support. In addition, the administrative burden for oncologists has increased dramatically over the past several decades. A substantial portion of the oncologist's time is devoted to documentation that will support billing requirements and payment preauthorization. Cost and administrative burdens have led many oncologists to sacrifice their practice autonomy; the proportion of physicians in an employment model setting rather than independent practice has increased dramatically since the 1980s, and continues to increase.[18] Each of these influences represents a threat to our profession in terms of both the personalized care we deliver to our patients and maintenance of an adequate workforce.

Addressing the threat of burnout in an evolving cancer care landscape requires rethinking the ways in which we provide care to patients and to ourselves. Meeting the needs of increased patient volume and complex care is now more commonly accomplished with integrated teams involving oncologists, advanced practice clinicians (e.g., nurse practitioners, physician assistants), social and mental health services, palliative care experts, and so on. Oncologists now require new leadership skills to ensure the commitment to high-quality patient care and research. There is a need to work closely with varied stakeholders including hospital or practice administrators, purchasing groups, EHR vendors, payers, and representatives of pharmaceutical companies. Protecting our profession also mandates an appreciation of policies and regulations that impact our practice and patients, and active involvement in advocacy beyond our local environment. Working through our professional organizations is an essential and powerful tool to ensure that the current challenges are opportunities to influence our future state.

The Impact of Patient Advocacy on Research and Patient Care

For much of the twentieth century, a diagnosis of breast cancer was hidden in the closet. Few women revealed their struggles with breast cancer publicly, as this disease was associated with fear and shame. Surgery, such as the radical mastectomy, was disfiguring. Systemic therapy was barely in its infancy. Most women suffered in silence and often lost their lives to the disease. Pioneers, such as Rose Kushner, spoke out in the mid-1970s about mutilating surgical procedures and the need for research.

A group of like-minded individuals gathered around her, and the modern breast cancer advocacy movement was born. In the early 1980s, others in the vanguard, such as Nancy Brinker, spoke about the pain that breast cancer inflicted on her sister. She went on to establish the Susan G. Komen Foundation, with a focus on awareness, early detection, advocacy, support for women living with breast cancer, and research.[19] Fran Visco founded the National Breast Cancer Coalition in 1991 with an eye toward scientific investigation, policy, and the role of advocates as equal partners in the research enterprise.[20] Since 1995, the coalition has been training research advocates in its highly respected program, Project LEAD (Leadership, Education, and Advocacy Development). Finally, in the mid-1990s, Evelyn Lauder, a staunch supporter of breast cancer research, founded the Breast Cancer Research Foundation with the goal of raising funds solely for breast cancer research.[21]

Breast cancer advocacy, as well as highly visible AIDS advocacy organizations, led to the development of similar groups that have focused on virtually all types of cancer. Cancer advocates are key members of the National Cancer Institute–sponsored cancer clinical research cooperative groups, government grant review panels, and research programs around the country. They attend scientific meetings, serve on program planning committees, and participate in scientific programs. Many granting agencies require the inclusion of advocates on the research team. As team members, advocates provide the patient voice in research deliberations and also serve as the "honest broker." Over the past two decades, cancer researchers have come to appreciate the value that cancer advocates bring to the table and welcome them enthusiastically. It is widely accepted that advocates improve the overall quality of research.

Advocates have also played a role in the clinical setting, accelerating the development of patient-centered care. In the clinical arena, advocates have also promoted access to clinical trials and changes in trial eligibility to make them more available to the majority of patients who are recently diagnosed or living with cancer. Finally, cancer patient advocates are an important voice in national policy discussions regarding all cancer-relevant deliberations, providing a key perspective in decisions regarding new drug approvals, regulations, payment, access, and research funding.

The Future of Oncology Practice

The National Cancer Act and associated marketing of the "War on Cancer" have transformed the meaning of a cancer diagnosis and the care of cancer patients. We now understand that cancer is not a single disease, but rather hundreds of different conditions driven by specific molecular alterations in normal genes. Cancer is often curable, and when not, it may sometimes be rendered a chronic condition. The era of precision oncology has arrived. As of 2017, the death rate from cancer had decreased by 31 percent since 1991,[22] but we still have a long way to go. Advances in science and technology have driven an explosion in new evidence to support regulatory approval of 238 new drug treatments for patients with cancer over the past quarter century.[23] Today's oncologist faces an onslaught of clinical and molecular information related to their individual patients, as well as daily publications of new research results that must be incorporated into our decision-making and recommendations. In our view, the pace of innovation distinguishes oncology from other fields in medicine, and this rapid evolution leads to unique challenges.

When we entered the field in the 1980s, a day in the clinic focused on face-to-face interactions with patients and their families, review of diagnostic information, discussion with colleagues, and written clinical documentation. We would go to the library searching for journal articles or book chapters, and would consult with colleagues to inform our recommendations. Treatment options were often limited. It was uncommon to speak with payers and the cost of care rarely entered into consideration. It felt easy to keep up with the latest information relevant to clinical care.

In the 2000s, there is a greater sense of optimism when we meet with patients and their families. Nonetheless, there is less time for face-to-face patient interaction, as patient volumes have increased, and more time-consuming documentation is required at point of care, largely driven by payer mandates. While many aspects of care are unchanged, the complexity of treatment decision-making has increased, as the flow of new evidence has accelerated. We are able to manage this onslaught thanks to the internet and the development of clinical practice guidelines. As treatment options have expanded, our personal connections with our patients and our ability to communicate clearly are more important than ever. While these connections can be satisfying, they are threatened by administrative burdens, burnout, and the huge challenge of remaining knowledgeable about the latest advances.

With increased recognition of the link between practice variation, more costly care, and inferior clinical outcomes has come more research into measures of care quality, with practices and institutions eager to reduce variation in clinical care. Metrics about one's clinical practice abound, including clinical volume and patterns of practice. It is critical that oncologists participate in the development and selection of these metrics to ensure that they serve practice efficiency and patient care. The business of oncology now affects all oncologists, regardless of their practice setting. This constant culture of surveillance and documentation threatens clinician autonomy, increases burnout, and can only be addressed by a commitment of physician leaders to gain the requisite skills to share in business leadership.

In spite of the challenges we have described, we remain optimistic about the future. In the next fifty years, we believe that cancer will no longer be feared. The survivor population will continue to grow, and their medical and psychosocial needs will require a new skill set for primary care clinicians who may ultimately provide the bulk of their care.

In the past five years alone, dozens of new treatments for cancer have been approved by the FDA.[24] Many of these treatments not only control cancer, but prolong survival. The development of new treatments requires a robust clinical trials infrastructure and is dependent upon patients who agree to participate in research studies. Unfortunately, only a small percentage of cancer patients currently take part in clinical trials, which reflects both logistical challenges and societal attitudes. We are hopeful that these challenges may be overcome, and we can achieve a future state where clinical research opportunities are available wherever cancer care is delivered, and care and research are seamlessly integrated for the benefit of cancer patients, now and in the future.

We believe that technology will transform clinical practice. Emerging evidence will be rapidly incorporated into clinical guidelines, and computer applications will make these readily accessible at the point of care. These applications driven by artificial intelligence will also seamlessly integrate with clinical systems, pulling relevant clinical information and applying this to expert-developed algorithms. EHRs will increasingly fulfill the promise of improving efficiency as the pendulum swings toward aligning documentation requirements with high-quality care. The EHR will become more of a digital assistant, organizing information in a manner that is consistent with clinical decision-making and efficient workflow. We also anticipate that patients and health-care organizations will increasingly see the value in data-sharing to enable a learning health-care system that provides feedback and is able to continuously generate new knowledge to inform clinical care. Although cancer patient participation in research has not met the demands for the testing of all the important questions that can be answered through clinical trials, emerging solutions to enable research wherever care is provided, with technology supporting data capture and oversight, promise to close the divide between research and practice. Within ten to fifteen years, we should certainly be learning from the experience of every cancer patient.

The practice of oncology is driven by science and filled with humanity, optimism, hope, and realism. Cancer research and cancer care are team activities. Cancer researchers need to collaborate on complex scientific problems. Clinical cancer care involves diverse specialties in medicine as well as many other disciplines. By working closely together, we can accelerate progress in research for the future and deliver the very best cancer care that is available today.

While so much about the delivery of cancer care has changed during our careers, it remains a privilege and an honor to care for patients with cancer and share their journeys, while striving for improvements in cancer care.

Notes

1. *Cancer Treatment & Survivorship Facts & Figures 2019–2021* (Atlanta, GA: American Cancer Society, 2019), https://www.cancer.org/research/cancer-facts-statistics/survivor-facts-figures.html.

2. Lesley F. Degner, Jeff A. Sloan, and Peri Venkatesh, "The Control Preferences Scale," *Canadian Journal of Nursing Research* 29, no. 3 (Fall 1997): 21–43, https://pubmed.ncbi.nlm.nih.gov/9505581/.

3. Kevin P. Weinfurt et al., "Understanding of an Aggregate Probability Statement by Patients Who Are Offered Participation in Phase I Clinical Trials," *Cancer* 103, no. 1 (2005): 140–147, https://doi.org/10.1002/cncr.20730.

4. Ann Partridge et al., "Risk Perceptions and Psychosocial Outcomes of Women with Ductal Carcinoma in Situ: Longitudinal Results from a Cohort Study," *Journal of the National Cancer Institute* 100, no. 4 (2008): 243–251, htps://doi.org/10.1093/jnci/djn010.

5. J. C. Weeks et al., "Relationship Between Cancer Patients' Predictions of Prognosis and Their Treatment Preferences," *JAMA* 279, no. 21 (1998): 1709–1741, https://doi.org/10.1001/jama.279.21.1709.

6. Timothy Gilligan et al., "Patient-Clinician Communication: American Society of Clinical Oncology Consensus Guideline," *Journal of Clinical Oncology* 35, no. 31 (2017): 3618–3632, https://doi.org/10.1200/JCO.2017.75.2311.

7. Alexi A. Wright et al., "Associations Between End-of-Life Discussions, Patient Mental Health, Medical Care near Death, and Caregiver Bereavement Adjustment," *JAMA* 300, no. 14 (2008): 1665–1673, https://doi.org/10.1001/jama.30.14.1665.

8. "Care for Chronically Ill (Last 2 Years)," Dartmouth Atlas of Health Care, accessed December 14, 2020, https://atlasdata.dartmouth.edu/downloads/eol_chronic.

9. Scott Ramsey et al., "Washington State Cancer Patients Found to Be at Greater Risk for Bankruptcy Than People Without a Cancer Diagnosis," *Health Affairs* 32, no. 6 (2013): 1143–1152, https://doi.org/10.1377/hlthaff.2012.1263.

10. "The Human Genome Project," National Human Genome Research Institute, accessed December 14, 2020, https://www.genome.gov/human-genome-project.

11. Rebecca L. Siegel et al., "Cancer Statistics, 2021," *CA: A Cancer Journal for Clinicians* 71, no. 1 (2021): 7–33, https://doi.org/10.3322/caac.21654.

12. David Zahavi and Louis Weiner, "Monoclonal Antibodies in Cancer Therapy," *Antibodies (Basel)* 9, no. 3 (2020): 34, https://doi.org/10.3390/antib9030034.

13. Robin T. Zon et al., "American Society of Clinical Oncology Criteria for High-Quality Clinical Pathways in Oncology," *Journal of Oncology Practice* 13, no. 3 (2017): 207–210, https://doi.org/10.1200/JOP.2016.019836; Barbara McAneny et al., "Supporting Optimal, Value-Based, and Sustainable Cancer Care Delivery," *Journal of Clinical Pathways* 6, no. 8 (2020): 58–61, https://doi .org/10.25270/jcp.2020.10.00002.

14. Junaid Nabi and Quoc-Dien Trinh, "New Cancer Therapies Are Great— But Are They Helping Everyone?" *Health Affairs* Blog, April 12, 2019, https://doi .org/10.1377/hblog20190410.590278.

15. Christina Maslach, Susan E. Jackson, and Michael P. Leiter, *Maslach Burnout Inventory*, 3rd ed. (Palo Alto, CA: Consulting Psychologists Press, 1996).

16. National Academies of Sciences, Engineering, and Medicine, *Developing and Sustaining an Effective and Resilient Oncology Careforce: Proceedings of a Workshop* (Washington, DC: The National Academies Press, 2019).

17. Samuel U. Takvorian et al., "Developing and Sustaining an Effective and Resilient Oncology Careforce: Opportunities for Action," *Journal of the National Cancer Institute* 112, no. 7 (2020): 663–670, https://doi.org/10.1093/jnci /djz239.

18. Tanya Albert Henry, "Employed Physicians Now Exceed Those Who Own Their Practices," American Medical Association, May 10, 2019, https:// www.ama-assn.org/about/research/employed-physicians-now-exceed-those -who-own-their-practices.

19. Susan G. Komen Foundation, accessed April 14, 2021, https://www .komen.org/.

20. National Breast Cancer Coalition, accessed April 14, 2021, https://www .stopbreastcancer.org/.

21. Breast Cancer Research Foundation, accessed April 14, 2021, https://www .bcrf.org/.

22. Siegel et al., "Cancer Statistics, 2021."

23. Julia A. Beaver et al., "A 25-Year Experience of US Food and Drug Administration Accelerated Approval of Malignant Hematology and Oncology Drugs and Biologics: A Review," *JAMA Oncology* 4, no. 6 (2018): 849–856, https://doi.org/10.1001/jamaoncol.2017.5618.

24. "Hematology/Oncology (Cancer) Approvals & Safety Notifications," FDA.gov, accessed January 21, 2021, https://www.fda.gov/drugs/resources -information-approved-drugs/hematologyoncology-cancer-approvals-safety -notifications.

CHAPTER 13

Responsible Open-Source Data Sharing for Precision Oncology

Cynthia Jung, Kenna Shaw, Arjun Mody,
Barrett J. Rollins, and Charles L. Sawyers

As a disease of the genome, cancer is particularly well suited to genome-tailored treatment. Affordable and ready access to genomic sequencing has made it relatively easy to test for genomic alterations in cancer patients and is now routine clinical practice for many common tumor types. While researchers have championed genetic sequencing to advance science and inform cancer treatment, genomic data alone offer limited clinical value. Pairing genomics with clinical outcome data is essential to advancing precision oncology and to treating more forms of cancer.

Sequenced genomes from >100,000 cancer patients are currently available publicly, yet only a fraction of these are linked to

Cynthia Jung is Scientific Research Manager, Human Oncology and Pathogenesis Program, Memorial Sloan Kettering Cancer Center.

Kenna Shaw is Executive Director of the Cancer Genomics Laboratory, MD Anderson Cancer Center.

Arjun Mody received his JD from Yale Law School in 2020.

Barrett J. Rollins is Linde Family Professor of Medicine, Harvard Medical School.

Charles L. Sawyers is an Investigator of the Howard Hughes Medical Institute and Chair of the Human Oncology and Pathogenesis Program at Memorial Sloan Kettering Cancer Center.

longitudinal clinical outcomes records despite the clear scientific and medical value of correlating these data. Widespread adoption of tumor sequencing into current clinical oncology practice has provided the opportunity to create such linked registries, but this has not happened at the scale and pace needed to power precision medicine. In conversations with physicians, scientists, and legal experts working in the cancer field, we notice two primary barriers at play: perceived privacy risks, and concerns about feasibility and real-world applicability. Health-care institutions are often reluctant to join such registries because of concerns about potential patient reidentification from genomic data, perceived institutional legal risk, and the impact on their subsequent ability to monetize their data. Even where this barrier is overcome, there is skepticism about the feasibility of maintaining multi-institutional registries of this size and scope and whether the data will be relevant to real-world community oncology patients.

A third barrier is the fact that the largest repositories of genomic data from cancer patients now reside within molecular diagnostic companies that provide tumor genome sequencing services as a diagnostic test. Although there is one precedent in which some of this commercially collected data has been contributed to a public repository,[1] these data cannot be accessed by the research community. In fact, there are huge incentives to keep the data siloed because of the significant revenue that can be generated by providing biopharma companies access to these data to guide their internal decisions regarding drug targets, biomarker development, and the prevalence of new subgroups of patients defined by genomic testing. An example of the value of these data: Roche spent over $5 billion to acquire Foundation Medicine (which provides genomic sequencing tests) and Flatiron (which collects longitudinal clinical data). The inability to access these rapidly growing private data repositories for research purposes is a lost opportunity to accelerate progress in precision medicine, but it is difficult to envision a scenario in which these companies, which invest substantially in their generation, could risk their revenue potential by contributing the data to public repositories.

In this chapter, we address the first two concerns by providing examples of how genomic and clinical outcome data from tens of thousands of cancer patients are currently shared in an open-source manner, with tangible outcomes relevant to broad populations of patients. We hope these examples can help overcome these privacy- and application-based misperceptions and pave the way to even larger-scale clinical genomic data registries that will serve public health. We acknowledge, however, that current data privacy protections are imperfect, and so review practices that can further secure confidence in the privacy of protected health information (PHI), including revised data management protocols. These privacy protections, while clearly important, add additional layers of complexity and expense to the process of clinical genomic data collection that can only be addressed at larger medical centers with the resources to implement such procedures. Consequently, the diversity of individuals represented in these registries is limited to those seen at larger tertiary care institutions. We need additional solutions to democratize clinical genomic data sharing more broadly and suggest potential routes though policy making (e.g., liberalize sharing of data for research purposes under the Health Insurance Portability and Accountability Act [HIPAA]) and changes to the legal system (establish laws that prohibit reidentification of patients from clinical genomic registries).

Sharing Oncology Data: Precedent for Large-Scale Sharing of Genomic and Clinical Data

In 2005, several years after the completion of the human genome sequence, the National Cancer Institute (NCI) partnered with the National Human Genome Research Institute (NHGRI) to launch the Cancer Genome Atlas Project (TCGA)—a large-scale project to map the genome of various cancer types. At program completion twelve years later, TCGA generated comprehensive genomic maps of the key genomic changes in thirty-three types of cancer in addition to releasing data pertaining to almost eleven thousand patients. The TCGA program drew upon a global network of 161 tissue source sites to enroll and collect consent from the patients who provided samples and, in some cases, clinical data. Twenty collaborating institutions across North America coordinated TCGA genomic data analyses, providing the curated datasets that remain publicly available for research use through the National Institutes of Health (NIH) Genomic Data Commons (GDC). The TCGA initiative supported several important conceptual advances, including the classification of tumors based on genomic subtype, and the idea that tumors found at different organ sites can share similar molecular features and may therefore be sensitive to common therapeutic approaches. With the success of TCGA, investment in personalized oncology has continued to grow. In 2015, President Obama announced the Precision Medicine Initiative (PMI), which dedicated almost one-third of its $215 million budget to the NCI as part of its near-term goal to support precision oncology.[2] In 2016, also as part of the PMI, the NIH announced its All of Us Research Program, a long-range plan which seeks to "extend precision medicine to all diseases by building a national research cohort of one million or more US participants."[3]

The TCGA datasets have revealed enormous and necessary insight into the common and distinct genetic features of many cancers. However, TCGA was not designed to collect patient clinical outcomes (e.g., treatment history, treatment response/resistance, predictors of response/resistance to therapy, clinical trials enrollment) associated with genomic features. Understanding the associations between genomic sequence and clinical outcomes is essential for adopting precision medicine into clinical practice. To overcome this limitation, in 2015, the American Association for Cancer Research (AACR) launched Project Genomics Evidence Neoplasia Information Exchange (GENIE). GENIE is a public, regulatory-grade registry of genomic data associated with clinical outcomes. The GENIE consortium comprises eighteen independently operating institutions, including many of the world's leading academic centers in cancer genomics, molecular pathology, clinical trials leadership, and informatics.[4] In the GENIE model, participating institutions have agreed to provide clinical-grade (i.e., CLIA-/ISO-certified) tumor sequencing data and the longitudinal treatment

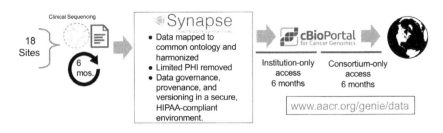

The AACR Project GENIE Consortium, *Cancer Discovery*, 2017

FIGURE 13.1 How the Registry Operates:
Baseline Date (The AACR Project GENIE Consortium)

and outcomes data associated with these tumors, primarily obtained during routine clinical practice from patients with metastatic cancer. The data are held in electronic health records (EHRs) at the host institutions and made available for analysis ("abstracted" in a de-identified form) after institutional review board (IRB) approval. As of January 2021, the GENIE registry contained over 100,000 de-identified sequencing records representing one hundred major cancer types, including data from greater than 14,000 patients with lung cancer, nearly 12,000 patients with breast cancer, and nearly 9,500 patients with colorectal cancer. The ability to amass a dataset this large becomes extremely valuable and powerful when studying rare cancers, since several institutions can pool scant data to analyze rare cancers at statistical power.

Approaches to Address Privacy Concerns

How was this level of clinical genomic data sharing accomplished without violating privacy regulations? Federal laws governing human subjects research and the privacy of individual health information, the Common Rule and HIPAA Privacy Rule, respectively, established frameworks for the secondary use and sharing of health information with third parties. Under the Common Rule (now the Final Rule), research using individually identifiable data or biospecimens is subject to IRB oversight, and requires either the informed consent of the subject or a determination by the IRB that consent may be waived. Similarly, under HIPAA, use and disclosure of individually identifiable health information (also known as PHI) for research purposes is permitted with the individual's written HIPAA authorization, or pursuant to a waiver of authorization approved by a duly constituted IRB or privacy board. Under this framework, investigators have long been able to conduct research on clinical test samples, and to collect and analyze relevant information from the subject's medical records. Strict patient-record de-identification protocols further enable sharing with other researchers—including sharing through the establishment of databases—while safeguarding individual subjects' privacy.

Under Section 164.514(a) of the HIPAA Privacy Rule, "health information is not individually identifiable if it does not identify an individual and if the covered entity has no reasonable basis to believe it can be used to identify an individual."[5] To satisfy the Privacy Rule, HIPAA outlines two acceptable methods of data de-identification: (1) Expert Determination, and (2) Safe Harbor (which names eighteen types of identifiers that must be removed, often referred to collectively as PHI). Use of either method would demonstrate that a covered entity has met the Privacy Rule standard for de-identification.

Working within these frameworks, TCGA and Project GENIE have both laid robust groundwork for effective and safe patient data sharing. As described in 2014, TCGA set out three guiding policies governing its practices for Human Subjects Protection and Data Access Policies: (1) patient informed consent and IRB approval, (2) the types of data collected and their transfer, and (3) ensuring HIPAA compliance. Following similar principles, Project GENIE has successfully relied on participating centers to share data in a manner consistent with each center's specific patient consent and IRB policies. The exact approach varies by institution, but generally falls into one of three categories: (1) IRB-approved patient consent to sharing of de-identified data captured at the time of molecular testing, (2) IRB waivers, and (3) IRB approvals of GENIE-specific research proposals. Additionally, all data in GENIE are de-identified via the HIPAA Safe Harbor Method.

One often cited barrier to cross-institutional data sharing is the need for uniform, standardized consent forms approved by a central IRB. Although this could eventually be a preferred solution, our experience demonstrates that existing frameworks are sufficient to achieve the desired goals. Project GENIE and TCGA each serve as scalable models. Both rely on well-established IRB infrastructures at individual institutions, rather than a single or central IRB. The local IRB of each participating institution provides ethical oversight to determine whether such research studies would proceed. Memorial Sloan Kettering Cancer Center (MSK) and Dana-Farber Cancer Institute (DFCI), two GENIE-founding institutions, use institution-wide consent protocols for all patients who undergo their in-house clinical sequencing assays (MSK-IMPACT and Profile, respectively). Centralized operational and regulatory teams at these institutions develop and update (electronic) consent forms and training modules, facilitate interdepartmental database use, and support the IRB process, helping MSK and DFCI manage vast collections of information.

Diversity and Access: Novel Insights Emerge from Ethnically Diverse Datasets

Despite the number of participants recruited to existing registries, precision oncology databases are far from complete, particularly with regard to ethnic diversity and data from rare tumors. Current germline and cancer genomic databases contain an overly high proportion (~80%) of individuals of European descent.[6] One reason for this overrepresentation is the fact that academic research institutions have been the primary contributors of data to such registries as TCGA and GENIE. These tertiary care centers offer novel or investigative treatments and technology and therefore attract patients with the educational and financial resources needed to access such care. This is an important distinction because non-White patients are underrepresented in the patient pools of most academic cancer centers (AMCs). Furthermore, AMCs treat a larger fraction of patients with more advanced cancers, often with investigative therapies, who are not necessarily representative of the ~80 percent of patients who receive treatment in a community oncology setting not affiliated with a hospital, academic, or medical teaching institution. Finally, less than 5 percent of adult cancer patients are treated as part of a clinical trial,[7] further underscoring the importance of establishing broadly representative clinical genomic data registries.

This call for greater diversity in cancer genomic registries is not just a matter of equity. Novel medical insights can emerge, as illustrated by three recent examples, with important treatment implications. First, analysis of 2,393 prostate cancer genomic profiles in the GENIE registry revealed that Black men have a higher frequency of mutations in genes that would influence treatment selection (DNA repair genes, BRAF) compared to White or Asian men.[8] Conversely, mutations in the TMPRSS2 and ERG genes, widely regarded as the most common genomic alteration in prostate cancer,[9] are nearly twice as frequent in White patients compared to Black patients. A second example, also through analysis of the GENIE database, underscores the importance of both race and sex in the prevalence of the newly actionable $KRAS^{G12C}$ mutation. The frequency of this mutation, which predicts for sensitivity to a novel precision medicine therapy called sotorasib,[10] is five to ten times higher in White and Black women with non-small-cell lung cancer compared to Asian women.[11] Finally, a third example, based on genomic analysis of a Latin American lung cancer cohort, documents a strong association of Native American ancestry with the frequency of mutations in KRAS and in the clinically actionable EGFR gene.[12] Each of these examples reinforces the importance of incorporating tumor sequencing into clinical practice across ethnicities to ensure access to effective therapies that might otherwise not be considered. There are additional implications for more efficient conduct of precision medicine trials, focusing enrollment on ethnicities with high prevalence of the relevant mutation. Finally, it is worth noting that the first two examples emerged from a database overrepresented with individuals of European descent, but with results made possible only due to a large sample size. Imagine the power of future datasets enriched for diversity: improved cancer diagnosis, treatment, and clinical trial design, and access to therapeutic trials of *all* cancers for all patients.

Strategies to Capture Greater Diversity in Cancer Registries

Recent societal events have resulted in a long overdue focus on diversity and inclusion, and this has extended into the cancer genomics arena. One example is the Polyethnic 1000 project coordinated by the New York Genome Center, which has the goal of sequencing the tumors of one thousand African American, Latinx, and Asian cancer patients from the ethnically diverse New York metropolitan area at the whole genome level.[13] This and similar efforts should be applauded as a means of helping to rectify current deficiencies, but we should also consider another approach: expanding data collection into the community setting, where increasing numbers of patients already undergo genomic sequencing, but the data are never captured. Moving into the community practice setting addresses two key problems linked with the current AMC model: underrepresentation of non-European patients, and data collection limited to the 20 percent of cancer patients referred to AMCs versus the 80 percent seen in the community. The challenge is that community practitioners lack the infrastructure needed to share these data in a safe and effective way.

To empower data sharing by practitioners in community health settings, we look to some existing models for guidance. The MSK Cancer Alliance is a clinical care network of smaller community hospitals who have partnered with MSK to enable their patients to have access to MSK-IMPACT sequencing, data resources, and clinical trials. With guidance from MSK, Alliance hospitals manage patient informed consent locally and employ dedicated clinical study coordinators to identify potential clinical trial matches while relying on MSK as the IRB of record. Significantly, patients at these smaller hospitals can access emerging standards of care and therapeutic trials for which they might otherwise be overlooked. This type of partnership also illustrates how, in this case, working with the IRB from an academic center can help community hospitals comply with regulations regarding use and disclosure of health data with outside parties for research purposes. A similar cooperative model is used by NCI's Community Cancer Centers Program, which has played a key role in accrual of patients to the

NCI-MATCH trial. Here, patients are assigned to clinical trials of targeted therapies that are based on genetic changes rather than organ type, and which are conducted at public and private institutions included in the National Clinical Trials Network. To enroll in a MATCH trial, a patient must be under the care of an oncologist at a participating MATCH site, of which there are about 1,100 in the US including Puerto Rico, and agree to have their tumor profiled by genomic sequencing at an approved laboratory. Finally, the Oncology Research Information Exchange Network (ORIEN), a partnership among academic and industry researchers from about eighteen cancer centers, uses a common consent form for tissue profiling branded as "Total Cancer Care," which is accompanied by access to the ORIEN Clinical Trials Network. However, one key difference between ORIEN and the other partnerships is that it has a for-profit component that restricts open-access data sharing. The Cancer Alliance, NCI-MATCH, and ORIEN illustrate how existing data sharing consortiums might partner with community-based oncology practices to share patient clinical-genomics data and participate in clinical trials.

Safeguards Against Reidentification

The examples of TCGA and GENIE demonstrate that genomic and clinical data from cancer patients can be shared in an open-access, scalable format and remain compliant with current health information privacy laws. This compliance includes ethical oversight of the institutions contributing the data, performed by IRBs, and strict control of access to de-identified patient data by the registries. Furthermore, the costs of creating and maintaining these registries and/or the research conducted using registry data is often funded by US federal agencies, such as the NCI, which requires explicit disclosure of plans for how genomic data will be shared. However, despite this level of oversight, the specter of potential reidentification from de-identified genomic data registries remains, as illustrated by recent examples that have attracted media attention. Fortunately, these examples have not, to our knowledge, impacted genomic data sharing in the research setting, but nonetheless deserve serious consideration. Here we frame recent issues surrounding data privacy in the genomic era[14] and suggest a path forward to maximize the societal benefits from data sharing while balancing the risk of breaching data privacy.

While data breaches reported in the popular media have been alarming, their actual impact on health data sharing appears to be low.[15] Importantly, the majority of publicized attacks have occurred with databases that did not use HIPAA or statistical disclosure limitation (SDL) de-identification methods,[16] and therefore do not provide a reliable measure of reidentification risk. In a rare instance, the Heritage Health Prize analytics competition, a concerted attempt to reidentify individuals from HIPAA-compliant de-identified data, failed: the demonstrated reidentification risk was effectively zero from 113,000 samples.[17] In a different case (not reported by the general media), onerous data wrangling and advanced computational skills were required to arrive at the alleged identity of two individuals from fifteen thousand records.[18] This reidentification exercise demonstrates how time-consuming, expensive, and difficult such an attempt would be, leading most to conclude that the current standards of PHI de-identification under the Privacy Rule are robust in the current data technology environment.

These examples are comforting, but current privacy regulations were established prior to the genomic era and still contain gaps that could leave people vulnerable to inappropriate *downstream* use of their genomic data. The HIPAA Privacy Rule was established in 1996 with the intention of protecting consumer health information privacy in the health-care market, largely governing interactions between health insurance companies and health-care providers, at a time when routine personal genomic sequencing was science fiction. When it was written and implemented, HIPAA set forth reasonable guidelines for de-identification and sharing de-identified data such that "de-identified health information created following these methods is no longer protected by the Privacy Rule because it does not fall within the definition of PHI."[19] This left "de-identified" genomic sequences, which by nature are potentially individually identifying, unprotected by HIPAA, since they were no longer defined as PHI. In 2013, Congress passed two important amendments to the HIPAA Privacy Rule: it clarified that "health information" includes genetic information and, as a means to implement the Genetic Information Nondiscrimination Act (GINA) of 2008, it prohibited the use of genetic information by health plans for underwriting purposes. For the purposes of ensuring fair access to and distribution of health insurance coverage, GINA was an important step toward protecting personal privacy and preventing discrimination by employers. However, GINA serves only as a privacy patch, since the Final Rule does not specify clear protections for individuals' genetic data outside the healthcare provider or federally funded research environment.

As database infiltration techniques become more sophisticated, it remains possible that successful, targeted reidentifications will occur, especially outside of the regulated environment. Better data privacy safeguards are needed to not only protect individuals but also protect public acceptance of precision medicine since patients could become reluctant to share their genomic data if breaches were to become more common. Recently, data scientists undertook an academic exercise to examine the likelihood of a data breach, using various forms of patient-derived genomic data reflecting gene expression (RNA-seq) and chromatin landscapes (ATAC-seq) (collectively referred to as functional genomic data) that are increasingly found in data repositories.[20] The authors conducted "linked attacks" combining private information and publicly available data records to reidentify individuals, revealing unnecessary vulnerabilities in current modes of data access. They propose data sanitation strategies that would effectively mask identifying genetic variants by partitioning variant data under controlled access while preserving access to the valuable information provided in the original records.

As we grapple with the COVID-19 pandemic, crowdsourced contact-tracing and associated genomic data might be valuable for public health studies and guiding future pandemic responses. For this public health emergency, the Department of Health and Human Services relaxed enforcement of certain HIPAA provisions for sharing PHI, demonstrating that HIPAA possesses the authority and flexibility to regulate medical information sharing if there is a critical public health need. Current HIPAA regulations provide sufficient oversight to protect the sharing of heath information as long as the records remain with HIPAA covered entities, their named business associates, and public health authorities, but once the records leave that regulated environment, the protections cease. The COVID-19 pandemic poses real-time concerns about patient reidentification that parallel those in precision medicine.

Toward Newer Models of Genomic and Clinical Data Sharing

The collective experience of genomic and clinical data sharing through such academic consortia as GENIE and TCGA clearly documents the enormous public good that comes from these efforts. These examples also show that the concerns many have raised about patient privacy when sharing such data openly can be overcome through use of informed consent, data-use agreements, and existing de-identification methods. However, many questions in precision medicine remain to be solved and will require much larger repositories than currently exist in the academic community. The academic consortia model has the potential to scale but will still be encumbered by the costs associated with building robust infrastructure for informed consent and by the skewed diversity of patients with the resources to travel to AMCs for their care.

In addition to the academic model, we suggest a complementary scenario whereby the rapidly growing private data repositories within companies, such as Foundation Medicine, Tempus, Guardant, and others, could be leveraged for public good, but this will require significant efforts by policy makers and by Congress. For example, it should be possible to liberalize current HIPAA restrictions that place limits on the use of clinical data for research purposes (similar to changes enacted early in the COVID-19 pandemic, as mentioned earlier). Such a policy change would reduce the personnel and infrastructure cost needed to include such patients in public genomic data repositories because a separate informed consent process would no longer be required. In addition, the diversity of patients in these cancer registries would expand substantially, because all patients receiving cancer sequencing tests, regardless of where they receive their care, could be included. Of course, safeguarding patient privacy must remain of paramount importance, requiring further protections to ensure that data is only accessed by responsible individuals, as well as legal solutions to deter misuse of data, as summarized in the recommendations that follow.

Coupled with a change in HIPAA policy that expands the use of clinical data for research, we encourage the development of new intellectual property policies that could incentivize data sharing by clinical sequencing companies. The patent system rewards investments in innovation by granting a period of exclusivity for marketing a product, but the scientific knowledge that led to the innovation is made public at the time the patent is filed and/or issued. A similar paradigm might be used to protect investments made in the generation of private cancer databases while simultaneously mandating their public release, through mandatory licensing fees if the data is used for commercial purposes, coupled with severe legal penalties for failure to comply. This is an admittedly aspirational and ambitious vision, but it has enormous potential to enhance the public good.

Recommendations

To our knowledge, there have been no data privacy breaches using precision oncology registries. The likelihood of data theft remains theoretical and even if successful, efforts to reidentify such records would be inefficient and therefore impractical using current technologies. Yet we know that perfect, lasting data anonymity is an illusion, especially as health informatics systems evolve rapidly. Meanwhile, we must ensure that the current momentum behind precision oncology continues to grow. Patient consent remains integral to genomic data sharing and we should do everything possible to protect patient trust.

Data registries and consortiums should regularly reevaluate data sanitation approaches and choose the data restriction level most suitable for their intended research audience. Another way to approach data protection is through data federation, a familiar practice in consumer banking and credit card data transactions. In a precision oncology context, data would appear as a single (virtual) database to researchers, but the original data records and their storage would be fragmented into multiple separate databases, making it difficult for anyone outside that particular data query to understand. Typically, data travels in packets through encrypted channels and would be stored across separate collections so that data points would be meaningless at face value. Project GENIE has adopted a form of data federation as a practical solution to harmonize the disparate data elements and database formats submitted by multiple participating institutions, as well as to standardize clinical abstraction of patient records. The data federation approach could also incorporate data masking and controlled access levels to minimize data linkage attacks.

Finally, support for legal protection of genomic data is growing. Executive orders from the White House to prevent genetic discrimination among health insurers and employers resulted in GINA. In 2015, the NIH PMI Working Group recommended that Congress pass several protections to regulate the privacy, misuse, and security of patient health data, including penalties for those who reidentify or inappropriately use someone's genetic data.[21] Making it illegal to reidentify patients whose data resides in de-identified registries would immediately enhance patient confidence to participate in such projects. It could also lower the barriers that currently limit contributions of patient data from community practices, which lack the resources needed to obtain informed consent and remain compliant with the HIPAA Privacy Rule.

A View Toward the Next Fifty Years

There is immense excitement and patient support for cancer genomics sequencing. Large cancer centers possess everyday institutional strategies for collaborative research and can pay it forward to broaden participation by community practitioners. Including more patients in open-access, clinical genomic databases across these different practice settings creates a virtuous cycle benefiting the greater good: a wider patient population provides representative data, allows for statistically powered studies of rare cancers and extends improved standards of care to more patients. Advances in natural language processing technology and machine learning are likely to greatly simplify and accelerate the collection of longitudinal clinical data from EHRs. Parallel advances in data encryption should facilitate widespread sharing of primary genomic data with minimal risk of reidentification, as is currently the case in the banking and credit card industries. Policymakers should consider modifying current HIPAA restrictions on use of clinical data for research purposes, as such changes could substantially increase the size and utility of existing cancer registries and broaden the diversity of patients included. As technologies will surely evolve and public sources of personal data proliferate, concerns about the ability to reidentify patients from genetic sequencing data must be continuously assessed and addressed—but this should not obstruct the vital insights achievable through these collaborations. We believe additional legal safeguards that penalize efforts to misuse these data and/or reidentify patients are a necessary next step.

Acknowledgments

The authors wish to thank Kristin Kim, Chief Regulatory Counsel, MSK, for her invitation to C.L.S. to speak at the American Health Care Lawyers Educational Program for Academic Medical Centers in January 2020 and the helpful discussions that followed, as well as Jessica Roberts, University of Houston Law Center, and Nicholson Price, University of Michigan Law School, for discussions at the "Policy, Politics and Law of Cancer" conference held at Yale Law School, February 2018. We also thank Joanna Halpern and Jorge Lopez, Office of General Counsel, MSK, and Eugene Rusyn and Abbe Gluck, Solomon Center for Health Law and Policy, Yale Law School, for critical input and feedback.

Notes

1. Ryan J. Hartmaier et al., "High-Throughput Genomic Profiling of Adult Solid Tumors Reveals Novel Insights into Cancer Pathogenesis," *Cancer Research* 77, no. 9 (2017): 2464–2475, https://doi.org/10.1158/0008-5472.CAN-16 -2479.

2. Francis S. Collins and Harold Varmus, "A New Initiative on Precision Medicine," *New England Journal of Medicine* 372 (2015): 793–795, https://doi.org /10.1056/NEJMp1500523.

3. "All of Us Research Program," accessed April 9, 2021, allofus.nih.gov.

4. AACR Project GENIE Consortium, "AACR Project GENIE: Powering Precision Medicine Through an International Consortium," *Cancer Discovery* 7, no. 8 (2017): 818–831, https://doi.org/10.1158/2159-8290.CD-17-0151.

5. https://www.hhs.gov/hipaa/for-professionals/privacy/special-topics/de -identification/index.html#standard.

6. Alice B. Popejoy and Stephanie M. Fullerton, "Genomics Is Failing on Diversity," *Nature* 538, no. 7624 (2016): 161–164, https://doi.org/10.1038/538161a; Giorgio Sirugo, Scott M. Williams, and Sarah A. Tishkoff, "The Missing Diversity in Human Genetic Studies," *Cell* 177, no. 1 (2019): 26–31, https://doi.org /10.1016/j.cell.2019.02.048.

7. Vineeta Agarwala et al., "Real-World Evidence in Support of Precision Medicine: Clinico-Genomic Cancer Data as a Case Study," *Health Affairs* 37, no. 5 (2018): 765–772, https://doi.org/10.1377/hlthaff.2017.1579.

8. Brandon A. Mahal et al., "Racial Differences in Genomic Profiling of Prostate Cancer," *New England Journal of Medicine* 383 (2020): 1083–1085, https://doi.org/10.1056/NEJMc2000069.

9. Cancer Genome Atlas Research Network, "The Molecular Taxonomy of Primary Prostate Cancer," *Cell* 163, no. 4 (2015): 1011–1025, https://doi.org/10 .1016/j.cell.2015.10.025.

10. David S. Hong et al., "KRASG12C Inhibition with Sotorasib in Advanced Solid Tumors," *New England Journal of Medicine* 383 (2020): 1207–1217, https://doi.org/10.1056/NEJMoa1917239.

11. Amin H. Nassar, Elio Adib, and David J. Kwiatkowski, "Distribution of KRASG12C Somatic Mutations across Race, Sex, and Cancer Type," *New England Journal of Medicine* 384 (2021): 185–187, https://doi.org/10.1056/NEJM c2030638.

12. Jian Carrot-Zhang et al., "Genetic Ancestry Contributes to Somatic Mutations in Lung Cancers from Admixed Latin American Populations," *Cancer Discovery* 11, no. 3 (2021): 591–598, https://doi.org/10.1158/2159-8290.CD-20-1165.

13. Emma Goldberg, "Cancer Projects to Diversify Genetic Research Receive New Grants," *New York Times*, September 11, 2020, https://www.nytimes .com/2020/09/11/science/genetic-cancer-research-race.html.

14. W. Nicholson Price Jr. and I. Glenn Cohen, "Privacy in the Age of Medical Big Data," *Nature Medicine* 25 (2019): 37–43, https://doi.org/10.1038/s41591 -018-0272-7.

15. National Committee on Vital and Health Statistics, "Agenda of the May 24–25, 2016, NCVHS Subcommittee on Privacy, Confidentiality & Security Hearing," accessed April 9, 2021, https://ncvhs.hhs.gov/meetings/agenda-of -the-may-24-25-2016-ncvhs-subcommittee-on-privacy-confidentiality-security -hearing/; Daniel C. Barth-Jones, "Improving HIPAA De-identification Public Policy," presented at the NCVHS Hearing: De-identification and HIPAA, May 24, 2016, https://ncvhs.hhs.gov/wp-content/uploads/2016/04/BARTH -JONES.pdf.

16. John Czajka et al., *Minimizing Disclosure Risk in HHS Open Data Initiatives* (Washington, DC: Mathematica Policy Research, 2014), https://aspe.hhs gov/report/minimizing-disclosure-risk-hhs-open-data-initiatives.

17. Khaled El Emam et al., "De-identification Methods for Open Health Data: The Case of the Heritage Health Prize Claims Dataset," *Journal of Medical Internet Research* 14, no. 1 (2012): e33, https://doi.org/10.2196/jmir.200.

18. Peter K. Kwok et al., "Harder Than You Think: A Case Study of Re-identification Risk of HIPAA-Compliant Records," presented August 2, 2011, at Joint Statistical Meetings, Miami Beach, Florida.

19. "Guidance Regarding Methods for De-identification of Protected Health Information in Accordance with the Health Insurance Portability and Accountability Act (HIPAA) Privacy Rule," HHS.GOV, last modified November 6, 2015, https://www.hhs.gov/hipaa/for-professionals/privacy/special-topics /de-identification/index.html#:~:text=De%2Didentified%20health%20informa tion%20created,health%20information%20in%20certain%20circumstances.

20. Gamze Gursoy et al., "Data Sanitization to Reduce Private Information Leakage from Functional Genomics," *Cell* 183, no. 4 (2020): 905-17.e16, https:// doi.org/10.1016/j.cell.2020.09.036.

21. Precision Medicine Initiative Working Group, *The Precision Medicine Initiative Cohort Program—Building a Research Foundation for 21st Century Medicine* (2015), https://acd.od.nih.gov/documents/reports/DRAFT-PMI-WG-Report -9-11-2015-508.pdf.

CHAPTER 14

(Over-)Paying for Cancer Care

Cary Gross, Stacie B. Dusetzina,
and Ezekiel J. Emanuel

The High Cost of Cancer Care

The cost of cancer care in the United States is staggering. Overall national costs related to cancer care in 2015 were $183 billion, and are projected to increase to $246 billion by 2030.[1] The rise in cancer costs can be attributed to a "cancer cost trifecta": more cancers diagnosed, high utilization of cancer-related care, and more expensive testing and treatment options.

The aging of the population is a major driver of trends in cancer diagnosed in the United States each year. The size of the sixty-five years of age and older population is expected to double, from approximately thirty-five million to over seventy million between

---

Cary Gross is Professor of Medicine (General Medicine) and Epidemiology (Chronic Diseases) as well as Director of the Cancer Outcomes Public Policy and Effectiveness Research (COPPER) Center at Yale School of Medicine and Yale Cancer Center.

Stacie B. Dusetzina is Associate Professor of Health Policy and Ingram Associate Professor of Cancer Research, Vanderbilt University Medical Center.

Ezekiel J. Emanuel is the Vice Provost for Global Initiatives, the Diane v.S. Levy and Robert M. Levy University Professor, and Chair of the Department of Medical Ethics and Health Policy at the University of Pennsylvania.

2010 and 2030. Because cancer is largely an aging-related disease, this demographic shift has a profound impact on the number of people diagnosed with cancer—and the associated costs of care.

Modern treatment plans include numerous advanced technologies—new screening tests, genetic profiles, supportive measures, radiation and surgical modalities, and, most important, drugs and biologics. There has been a meteoric rise in the cost of cancer drugs—both in the launch price of novel drugs and increases in the price of existing drugs over time. Every new cancer drug approved in 2017 had a launch price higher than $100,000 per year, with some exceeding $450,000.[2] Even with these high initial prices, the US routinely sees price increases well above inflation, with price increases unrelated to either changes in market size for the drug (e.g., new US Food and Drug Administration [FDA] approvals) or the entry of competitors into the market.[3]

Complex technologies, such as chimeric antigen receptor T cell (CAR-T) therapy, proton beam radiation therapy, and surgical robots, are also contributing to the cost burden. In some cases, these therapies provide important advances over the standard of care. In others, however, there are no additional benefits relative to the added cost. For example, the cost of the newer proton beam therapy (over $115,000) is substantially higher than the current standard radiation therapy treatment ($59,000)[4] for men with prostate cancer, but there is no proven additional benefit of using proton beam therapy. Similarly, surgical robots have become commonplace for prostate tumor removal, despite the lack of evidence supporting improved outcomes.[5] And in some cases, such as cervical cancer, robotic surgery is proven to lead to worse outcomes—more recurrences and deaths—and yet continues to be paid for and used.

The status quo prompts several fundamental questions: What are the medical, psychological, financial, and other impacts of higher cancer care costs on patients? Does the US achieve better cancer care outcomes for the higher costs? Why are US costs for cancer care so high? How can these spiraling financial costs of cancer care be controlled without sacrificing high-quality cancer care?

Impact on Patients

In 2018, patients with cancer in the US paid $5.6 billion in out-of-pocket costs for their cancer drug or biologic treatments.[6] The detrimental effects of these high out-of-pocket costs are known as financial toxicity, a nod toward its likeness to physical toxicity in its adverse impact on mental and emotional health, and quality of life. Third-party payers are shifting more of the expenses on to individuals through higher premiums, deductibles, co-payments, and coinsurance. Although commercial health plans have out-of-pocket limits, these limits are high: $8,550 for individuals or $17,100 for families in 2021. Currently, there is no out-of-pocket limit for Medicare Part D, and beneficiaries have to pay a percentage of the drug's price with every prescription filled. This can mean that patients pay over $10,000 out-of-pocket per year for a single drug.

Financial toxicity has a powerful and sometimes unrecognized impact on patients. The direct financial impact can be devastating. In one study, a quarter of colon cancer patients were in debt due to treatment-related expenses, with debts averaging to $26,860.[7] Not only are patients with cancer more likely to require bankruptcy protection, but those who do declare bankruptcy have a higher risk of death.[8] Higher out-of-pocket costs are associated with lower adherence to cancer treatments, and forgoing physician visits.[9] Ultimately, financial toxicity not only increases stress while decreasing access to cancer treatment; it can also divert resources from fundamental living expenses, such as housing, utilities, and food.[10]

Are We Getting Our Money's Worth?

In an ideal world, as exists in many wealthy countries outside the United States, there would be a substantive relation between the cost of a new treatment and the clinical benefit it provides to patients. A first step in assessing this "value" relationship is determining the amount of clinical benefit associated with a new drug relative to a standard of care. Because many new drugs are initially approved through the FDA's Accelerated Approval program, evidence regarding risks and benefits are limited at the time of approval. Even when there is enough evidence to allow for an assessment of clinical benefits compared with other treatments, the results have been unimpressive. Using objective, explicit frameworks that were promulgated by professional oncology societies for evaluating clinical benefit, a recent analysis found that only about one-third of thirty-seven new cancer drugs evaluated actually conferred a clinically meaningful benefit such as increase in overall survival or improved quality of life.[11] The researchers also found no meaningful relationship between clinical benefit and drug price, a finding corroborated by other studies.[12]

International Comparisons

Compared to other countries, the US has substantially higher health-care spending, without achieving commensurate health outcomes. Cancer is no exception. Americans pay up to twice as much for the same cancer treatments.[13] At the aggregate level, in 2020 the direct medical spending on cancer care in the US exceeded $600 per capita, compared to a median of $300 per capita across other wealthy countries. And while the population-level cancer mortality rate in the US is lower than most of these countries (see Figure 14.1), there is little correlation between cancer-related spending and survival.

In terms of survival across specific cancer types, five-year survival after a diagnosis in the United states is not consistently better, despite higher costs. For cervical cancer, US survival rates are 62.6 percent, which lags behind the 66 percent average survival in Organisation for Economic Co-operation and Development (OECD) countries. Survival after a diagnosis of colorectal cancer or childhood leukemia is similar in the US and OECD countries. For breast cancer, the US is the best in the world, with five-year survival of 90.2 percent, compared with 87.7 percent in OECD countries. However, rather than a marker for superior treatments, this may be related to the fact that American women tend to be diagnosed at an earlier stage.

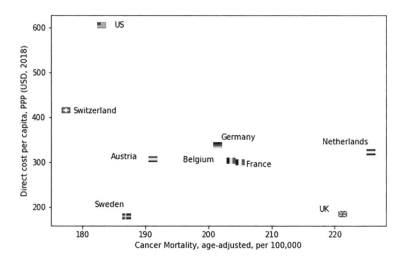

FIGURE 14.1 Cancer Mortality vs Direct Cost of Cancer for Countries
in the Global North

Why Are Cancer Costs High?

Misguided Prevention Efforts

Missed Opportunities for Prevention

While the United States has made impressive strides in terms of cancer prevention, there are still many preventable cancers, and cancer deaths, each year. Tobacco continues to be a major contributor; as described in Chapter 17, tobacco control efforts vary substantially across states, resulting in needless excess cancer burden. In addition, the tax on tobacco products—a proven effective prevention measure—has not increased in over a decade. Similarly, screening is markedly underused among eligible patients, according to widely accepted guidelines. Black and Latinx patients undergo cancer screening at even lower rates, as do patients who have fewer economic resources or lack insurance.[14] The chronic underscreening plaguing already marginalized communities results in preventable late-stage cancers and substantive disparities in cancer mortality.

Overscreening

Cancer screening efforts also play an important role in the increasing number of patients diagnosed with cancer. Overscreening occurs when screening tests are used in patient populations in whom the test is highly unlikely to provide a net benefit. For example, an elderly patient with a life expectancy of five years is unlikely to reap benefits from screening and detection of an early-stage cancer that might otherwise have gone undetected before the patient died from their other health problems. Because of concerns about overscreening, many professional guidelines recommend against routine cancer screening above specific age cutoffs, given the notable risk of harm. Despite this, many older persons continue to undergo cancer screening.

Even in young and otherwise healthy persons, not all detected cancers would necessarily have led to health problems. Finding a cancer in this setting is known as overdiagnosis.[15] Population-level data underscore the strong association between screening and overdiagnosis. In the absence of overdiagnosis, the rollout of a cancer screening program would lead to an increase in the number of cancers diagnosed at an early stage, with a subsequent decrease in the incidence of late-stage cancers. Yet increased breast cancer screening did not have this effect. As mammography use increased in the 1990s, there was a dramatic increase in detection of early-stage breast cancers—with only a minimal drop in detection of metastatic cancers. This discrepancy between the rise in early-stage cancers—and the lack of a drop in late stage—can be attributed to overdiagnosis (see Figure 14.2). This pattern has been noted in other cancer types as well. Hence, while widespread screening is helpful in some instances, it also results in a substantial increase in the number of cancers, increased costs, and questionable health benefits. Overdiagnosis of breast cancer alone could cost as much as $4 billion per year.[16]

Treatment Costs

Although spending on cancer treatment has grown across nearly all treatment modalities over time, prescription drug spending is a

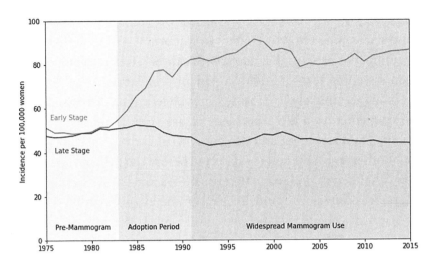

FIGURE 14.2 Breast Cancer Incidence per 100,000 (age-adjusted)

substantial and growing component of cancer treatment. For example, the average price for orally administered cancer treatments offered under Medicare Part D increased from approximately $7,500 per fill in 2010 to nearly $14,000 per fill in 2019. Several factors contribute to high spending on prescription drugs and biologics in the United States, including a lack of negotiating power due to policies that require coverage for virtually all cancer treatments, regardless of their clinical benefit, and payment systems that reward physicians for prescribing more expensive over less expensive drugs, even when products are equally effective.

A major contributor to the United States' overpayments for cancer treatments is related to the mandatory coverage policies for anticancer treatments, regardless of value. For example, anticancer drugs are part of the "protected classes" on Medicare and Medicaid and virtually all of these treatments must be available to individuals insured by these programs. This leaves very little opportunity for prescription drug plans to negotiate for lower prices. Because they are unable to exclude drugs for which prices are too high, the plans cannot negotiate for discounts or other price reductions.

Cancer drugs are somewhat unique in the US, given their broad and immediate coverage by payers for FDA approved indications. In many other high-income nations, regulatory approval for marketing (similar to that granted by the FDA) does not necessarily ensure that payers will cover the new cancer drug. In these countries, a critical next step after marketing approval is a health technology assessment (HTA). The HTA employs comparative and cost-effectiveness methods to help inform decisions about whether the new agent should be covered—allowing payers to decide how best to allocate limited health-care resources. In the US, insurance regulations and market fragmentation limit the viability of HTA to inform drug decision-making. Furthermore, laws in many states mandate private health insurance companies cover any FDA-approved cancer therapy, and large federal payers (e.g., Medicare and Medicaid) have similar mandatory coverage provisions for drugs listed in published guidelines, known as "Compendia." However, listing in a Compendia is not based upon rigorous proof of clinical benefit. Indeed, there are valid concerns about the Compendia's lack of transparency, financial conflicts of interest, and lack of systematic methods to review or update evidence.

Another reason for high cancer drug and biologic costs is the fact that many cancer drugs and biologics are approved through regulatory pathways, particularly the FDA's Accelerated Approval (AA) program, that allow for approval without proof of actual medical benefit. The AA was created in 1992 to address concerns that rigorous regulatory requirements that new treatments must have demonstrated clinical benefit—such as proof of prolonged survival or improved quality of life—were delaying the public's access to potentially lifesaving treatments for serious conditions, such as cancer. The AA pathways were intended to strike a balance between the need for clear evidence of clinical benefit and the need for quicker public access. Yet the actual implementation of these pathways falls far short of the desired balance. Through the AA pathways, industry sponsors obtain approval based on studies showing improvement in surrogate outcome measures—such as shrinking tumor size or lower biomarker levels—but are required to conduct postmarketing studies that assess more clinically meaningful endpoints, such as survival or quality of life.

Unfortunately, subsequent trials are not always conducted so oncologists lack evidence of cancer drug efficacy. For example, one analysis found that only nineteen of the ninety-three indications had clear evidence that they extended patient lives, and one-third of postmarketing confirmatory trials used the same surrogate outcome measures used in the preapproval trials. Notably, even when cancer drugs that have been approved through the Accelerated Approval regulatory pathway fail to measure up in subsequent studies (i.e., the follow-up studies show no survival benefit or improvement in quality of life), their approved indication is not withdrawn by the FDA.

It Is the Price, Stupid
In the United States, there is no current mechanism to manage prices of drugs when they are first approved or to limit price increases for most payers. This allows companies to set prices as high as they believe the market will bear, and they have taken advantage of this market failure. Although companies are likely to consider competitors in these decisions, the lack of demonstrably effective treatment options available for many cancer types or subtypes, combined with mandatory coverage policies, typically allow companies to command very high prices even if clinical benefits are minimal. A recent study that assessed cancer drug prices and value in the US and several other countries found that there was no difference in the price the US paid for drugs that were deemed high value and those deemed low value.

Many patients with cancer receive physician-administered infused or injected chemotherapies. Three peculiarities of the US market also incentivize using higher-cost infused or injected chemotherapies. First, under traditional fee-for-service Medicare, physicians have historically received an "average sales price plus 6 percent" markup for infused drugs. This reimbursement practice incentivizes physicians to prescribe more expensive drugs over less expensive drugs when there is a relevant choice to make. While commercial payers can require use of less expensive options (e.g., biosimilars over brands), the fee-for-service Medicare program does not limit prescribing of these products, and instead "rewards" physicians who choose the more expensive option.

Second, until the passage of the Affordable Care Act (ACA) in 2010, the FDA approval pathway for generic biosimilar agents was not developed. There are now biosimilar versions of several key anticancer therapies. However, uptake of these biosimilars has been somewhat slower than expected. Finally, spending has also increased for physician-administered cancer treatments as the site of care has shifted over time from the office setting to the more expensive hospital outpatient departments. For commercially insured patients, spending on the same drug in an outpatient hospital-affiliated practice is approximately twice that of spending in physician office settings—a finding not seen in the Medicare program, where drug payment is standardized across settings.

Aggressive Care

Aggressive care is a hallmark of the US health-care system in general, and is emblematic of cancer care in particular. For example, several professional organizations recommend that men with low-risk prostate cancer can be appropriately treated with active surveillance because the benefits of treating with surgery and radiation (known as cancer-directed therapy) do not outweigh the complication risks. While the rate of prostatectomies and radiation therapy has been declining in recent years, the majority of men with low-risk prostate cancer still receive cancer-directed therapy. The excess expenditures associated just with treating Medicare beneficiaries with low-risk prostate cancer has been estimated to exceed $300 million annually.[17]

The overuse of cancer-directed therapy also plagues cancer patients nearing the end of life, with many receiving chemotherapy or undergoing hospital care in settings where there is little clinical benefit. The use of futile and toxic therapies at the end of life increases costs and frequently reduces quality of life. For instance, in the last six months of life, over 40 percent of US patients are admitted to the ICU, while in other countries it is under 20 percent. Similarly, nearly 44 percent of US patients with lung cancer receive one or more chemotherapy treatments in the last six months of life compared to 30 percent in Norway and less than 20 percent in Canada.[18] Aggressive treatment plans are costing patients and the nation's health-care system significantly with average costs for the end-of-life phase of care exceeding $100,000 per decedent. Hospice and palliative care are important interventions that align care with patients' wishes, improve comfort and patient satisfaction, and decrease costs. Several studies have demonstrated that hospice use has been increasing over time, but frequently patients are referred to hospice very late in their disease course—even a few days prior to death—limiting the impact of hospice referral on end-of-life care.

Conflicts of Interest in Clinical Care

Two areas have raised substantive concerns over financial conflicts in cancer care: the fee-for-service health-care system, and payments from large pharmaceutical and medical device companies directly to providers. The fee-for-service health-care system plays a major role in perpetuating high utilization and costs. Multiple studies have found that physician self-referral, as well as profitability of specific anticancer therapies, are associated with oncologists' treatment selection. One study reported a 20 percent relative reduction in use of chemotherapy at the end of life after reductions in Medicare reimbursement for chemotherapy were implemented in 2006.[19]

Physicians' financial relationships with pharmaceutical companies have been shown to impact their practice and prescribing behaviors. Drugs and devices are marketed to physicians through various practices, including drug samples, sponsored meals, and education subsidies. From 2014 to 2019, medical oncologists received more than half a billion dollars in payments across 2.2 million instances. Studies have also found substantial payments from industry for members of professional guideline committees, leaders of academic institutions, patient advocacy organizations, journal editors—nearly every imaginable stakeholder group. Studies throughout medicine, and in oncology in particular, have shown that these monetary physician-industry relationships shift the prescribing patterns of the physician to one that will benefit the prescriber, or the industry partner, rather than one that necessarily provides maximum benefit to the patient.[20]

The Cancer Clinical Research Ecosystem

The cancer research ecosystem neither prioritizes nor facilitates research that addresses clinically relevant questions efficiently. As discussed earlier, pivotal trials used for FDA approval frequently do not assess clinical benefit using meaningful outcomes. But even when they do, it is unclear whether these findings are generalizable to the broader population. Patients in real-world practice tend to be substantially older, and with a greater burden of chronic conditions (in addition to their cancer) than patients in the pivotal clinical trials leading to FDA approvals. Although individuals aged sixty-five or older account for about two-thirds of new cancer diagnoses, they constitute less than one-third of oncology clinical trial participants. These differences have profound clinical implications, as Medicare beneficiaries receiving FDA-approved cancer drugs tend to survive for a substantially shorter period, and have a higher risk of complications, than participants in the clinical trials used to approve the drugs.[21]

Pharmaceutical companies are incentivized to focus on cancer care research due to the lower threshold of evidence required for approval of cancer drugs through the accelerated approval program, combined with high prices for cancer drugs and biologics. Thus, there are over six hundred cancer chemotherapies in human trials. Many new cancer treatments will make it to market without proof that they improve longevity or quality of life. Moreover, given that reimbursement is essentially mandated—even for therapies of marginal benefit—there is little incentive to develop therapies with substantive benefits.

Another important pitfall of the current research ecosystem is the increasing reliance on industry funding. In the 1970s and 1980s, trials were predominantly government-funded (60%), whereas in more recent years, almost 90 percent were industry-funded.[22] To be sure, industry funding is critical for innovation. Yet industry funding can introduce bias in study design such as selecting sub-optimal control groups, as well as in the conduct, analysis, and dissemination of results. Industry tends to focus on studies that evaluate—and hopefully, from the shareholder's perspective, demonstrate—that their new agent is superior to a comparison treatment. There are opportunities to elevate the quality of industry-sponsored studies in terms of selection of control groups, including representative samples (at least in postmarketing studies).

Our Recommendations

Reinvigorate Research & Practice of Cancer Prevention

A first step in decreasing the cost of cancer care is to increase investments in areas where there is strong evidence of benefit: increasing tobacco taxes, funding tobacco cessation programs, and evidence-based prevention strategies, such as cervical cancer vaccination and colorectal cancer screening. States, payers, health systems, and providers should be incentivized to reduce the incidence of preventable advanced or metastatic disease by being held accountable to the populations they serve. And, as a commitment to equity, they should be required to improve their screening and other prevention measures for all populations, with a particular focus on minoritized, rural and low income communities. They should be measured not just on overall screening and prevention, but on achieving goals for these relatively underserved subpopulations.

Second, more rigorous research is urgently needed to identify strategies to increase rates of evidence-based screening, and to distinguish which screening tests are truly helpful in which clinical settings, and which tests are simply contributing to overdiagnosis. Mass screening is an expensive endeavor, considering not only the cost of the tests themselves and the downstream evaluation of positive tests, but also the evaluation of treatment of overdiagnosed cancers. Continuing screening efforts in the absence of clear evidence is risky and wasteful. A substantive, national effort to bolster evidence around cancer screening is critical.

Finally, screening practices that are not helpful should not be reimbursed. For instance, Medicare, Medicaid, and private insurance companies should not pay physicians or facilities for prostate, colorectal, or breast cancer screening in men and women over the age of seventy-five.

High-Yield, Pragmatic Research on Cancer Treatments

The current clinical cancer research enterprise is uncoordinated, industry dominated, and not focused on identifying and addressing clinically relevant questions in a timely manner. A new approach to clinical research is needed: a substantial investment in platform trials. Platform trials, which have been employed to a limited extent in oncology, enroll patients with a specific cancer type, and randomize them to several different treatments. The platform trial should become the norm, using standardized endpoints that are meaningful to patients, building on a sound infrastructure with longitudinal funding. As new treatments come to market, platform trials could evolve, incorporating the new treatment and comparing it to other existing options. Large national platforms could be created for each cancer type, creating a never-ending effort to continually evaluate different alternatives, often within biomarker-defined subgroups, adapting its treatment allocation design as new information becomes available. The substantial investment required to support national platform trials across multiple cancer types could be borne by multiple stakeholders including the federal government as well as private insurance payers, who have a strong interest in bolstering the objective evidence-base. An independent body could coordinate this national effort.

Second, clinical research must become more efficient. Greater transparency around the cost of trials would not only inform efforts to understand how industry sets prices, but also provide valuable data to help identify strategies that can make research more efficient. Enrollment is a large expense that could be reduced with different incentives for academic institutions and practicing oncologists to enroll in larger trials. Large platform studies, for example, could provide substantive efficiencies in trial costs rather than re-creating infrastructure for single studies across multiple sites. Incorporating prospective clinical trials with robust electronic medical record and genomic data, with patient consent, could also greatly reduce trial costs. A unified "national cancer care databank" that potentially could be linked to clinical trial data, decreasing the cost of outcome ascertainment and facilitating observational research. As fewer than 5 percent of adult patients with cancer are enrolled in research studies, there is a sense of urgency—a tremendous amount of knowledge regarding treatment effects—from the other 95 percent—is being lost.

Addressing Drug Prices

There are four key strategies to reduce spending on prescription drugs in the long run. First, expedite generic and biosimilar entry and encourage adoption of these lower-cost products over their brand-name counterpart. Second, patients should be held harmless based on the price of the therapies they received since they are chosen by physicians. Thus, for cancer patients, deductibles and co-pays should be decoupled from the cost of their cancer care. Third, prices for new and existing therapies should be based on their clinical benefits ("value-based pricing"). Finally, payer reimbursement should be decoupled from the FDA approval process.

For cancer care, there are some concerns that generic entry may be less promising as a solution to spending, given rapid advances and changes in practice that favor newer over older drugs. Physicians should not be incentivized to prescribe higher-cost or brand-name drugs when equally effective, less costly options are available. The current ASP+ reimbursement, in particular, provides a financial disincentive for physicians to choose less costly drugs. This system should be corrected. Oncologists should be paid for caring for the patient and their payment should not be connected to the cost of the prescription drug dispensed. Patient out-of-pocket costs should also be lower when higher-value options are selected.

Patients do not choose the chemotherapies they receive to treat their cancers. Oncologists do. Thus, the major rationale for deductibles and co-pays does not apply to cancer chemotherapy.

Deductibles and co-pays are meant to decrease patients' excessive use of treatments and choosing expensive, discretionary treatments. But as relates to cancer, patients do not choose between different regimens. Yet these deductibles and co-pays lead to financial toxicity. The best way to eliminate this toxicity is to eliminate deductibles and co-pays when patients have a diagnosis of cancer and instead provide incentives to physicians to order the most cost-effective proven chemotherapy for the patient's type of cancer.

Value-based pricing requires consideration of the evidence base available at the time that a drug is approved and how this evidence could be used to decide a "fair" price. Unfortunately, evidence of treatment benefit relative to a standard of care is unavailable for many drugs at the time that they are available on the US market. Although the FDA's Accelerated Approval program has allowed for early access to prescription drugs with promising—yet uncertain—early results while longer-term outcome data are collected, the clinical benefits of these drugs often remain unclear for years—if they are ever determined. To improve the evidence base for assessing treatment value, drug manufacturers should be required to measure outcomes that matter to patients. This includes overall survival and patient-reported outcomes (e.g., quality-of-life measures), and these studies should compare the new treatment relative to the current standard of care. For studies that are approved through an AA pathway based on surrogate endpoints, these manufacturers should be required to pay rebates to public payers that reflect the uncertainty related to the product's overall benefits for patients. This discounted price could then be adjusted to reflect the product's value once longer-term studies are complete. Demonstration projects to assess the impact of this approach on cost, access, and outcomes could be managed by the Center for Medicare and Medicaid Innovation (CMMI). Finally, in instances where postmarketing studies do not clearly demonstrate clinical benefit—as defined in advance of beginning the study—the FDA's response should be robust and clear: the indication should be removed.

Finally, payers should not be required to provide coverage for all new therapies that are approved for an indefinite period of time.

Ultimately, prices should be set to reflect the value that the product provides to patients. Drugs for which the prices greatly exceed the benefit to patients should not be subject to mandatory formulary coverage. For instance, Medicare could provide coverage for therapies approved through the AA pathways through a modified "Coverage with Evidence in Development" process that will allow beneficiaries to receive the new and unproven therapies in the context of clinical trials to assess their risks and benefits in the Medicare population.

Health System—Align Incentives to Improve Quality/Equity and Decrease Waste

Alternative payment models are critical to accelerate the shift from a fee-for-service to a value-based reimbursement approach. For example, the Oncology Care Model (OCM) is a multipayer alternative payment model that was implemented in 2016 with a goal of transforming oncology care for patients undergoing systemic cancer therapy. Established by the CMMI, this five-year voluntary model aimed to improve quality and lower expenditures, primarily through reductions in acute care utilization. Participating practices received their traditional Medicare fee-for-service payments as well as a supplemental $160 monthly care coordination payment. However, a recent evaluation found that the OCM had no significant impact on hospitalizations, emergency department use, hospice utilization, or patient satisfaction.[23] Moving ahead, alternative payment models will certainly have a place in efforts to improve the value of cancer care—but to be successful, they must address drug costs directly and unambiguously, and incorporate more novel approaches to care redesign. One example would be adopting a Hospital at Home (HaH) model that provides inpatient-level services in patients' homes, substituting for inpatient admissions or facilitating early discharge for stable, hospitalized patients who still require some degree of hospital-level care, but can safely be monitored at home.

The outcome of another proposed payment innovation underscores one of the major challenges to addressing the cost of cancer care. The Obama administration attempted to limit drug costs and curtail physician financial interests in 2016. They proposed a Medicare Part B Drug Payment Model experiment that would lower physician drug reimbursements from "average sales price + six percent" to "average sales price +2.5 percent + a flat $16.80 administration fee." Despite the potential cost-savings for Medicare, over three hundred groups representing physicians, drugmakers, and patient advocacy groups effectively killed the proposal. This demonstrates a key challenge for addressing costs in a multibillion-dollar industry: vested interests will aggressively—and in many cases effectively—defend their interests. Future work should identify strategies to align goals when possible, and to act definitively, yet transparently and fairly, even when all interests cannot be aligned. Efforts must be put into place to hold oncologists, and provider networks, accountable for the cost of care they provide, using mandatory payment or delivery reform that is implemented in a manner such that rigorous assessment of outcomes can be tracked.

Stop Aggressive Treatment

Overly aggressive cancer treatment, particularly at the end of life, results from a combination of the misaligned incentives of the American health-care system and the cultural reluctance to discuss and address dying. The policy aspect is easier to address, by increasing reimbursement—and availability—of palliative and hospice care. The Medicare Care Choices Model (MCCM) is also instructive. The MCCM addresses the short-sighted decision that Medicare will not reimburse for hospice care when patients are also undergoing active cancer treatment. Initial analyses found that the MCCM led to an increase in hospice use, as well as a 25 percent decrease in total Medicare expenditures, mostly driven by a reduction in inpatient care. Further expansion of similar models will likely lead to even greater savings, and more patient-centered care. The cultural aspect of end-of-life care is admittedly more difficult to change. Further education of the lay public, medical professionals, and rigorous incentives to discuss care goals are warranted.

Centering Equity in Cancer Cost Reforms

The high cost of cancer care itself exacerbates entrenched racial disparities that adversely impact people of color by adding additional barriers to accessing preventive services and treatment. The exorbitant costs of cancer care stems from, and exacerbate, systemic racism that has permeated the US health-care system. Black patients as well as other minoritized groups face delayed diagnosis, disproportionately higher cancer burden, and higher mortality rates, which further increase the economic burden of cancer care at the individual and population level. An equity lens should be applied to all efforts to control cancer costs, focusing on the distribution of health, access, burdens, and costs across the health system.

Notes

1. Angela B. Mariotto et al., "Medical Care Costs Associated with Cancer Survivorship in the United States," *Cancer Epidemiology, Biomarkers & Prevention* 29, no. 7 (2020): 1304–1312, https://doi.org/10.1158/1055-9965.EPI-19-1534.

2. IQVIA, *Global Oncology Trends 2018* (2018), https://www.iqvia.com/insights/the-iqvia-institute/reports/global-oncology-trends-2018.

3. Noa Gordon et al., "Trajectories of Injectable Cancer Drug Costs After Launch in the United States," *Journal of Clinical Oncology* 36, no. 4 (2018): 319–325, https://doi.org/10.1200/JCO.2016.72.2124.

4. Hubert Y. Pan et al., "Comparative Toxicities and Cost of Intensity-Modulated Radiotherapy, Proton Radiation, and Stereotactic Body Radiotherapy Among Younger Men with Prostate Cancer," *Journal of Clinical Oncology* 36, no. 18 (2018): 1823–1830, https://doi.org/10.1200/JCO.2017.75.5371.

5. Bec Crew, "Worth the Cost? A Closer Look at the da Vinci Robot's Impact on Prostate Cancer Surgery," *Nature Index*, April 23, 2020, https://www.natureindex.com/news-blog/a-closer-look-at-the-davinci-robots-impact-on-prostate-cancer-surgery.

6. Rebecca L Siegel, Kimberly D. Miller, and Ahmedin Jemal, "Cancer Statistics, 2020," *CA: A Cancer Journal for Clinicians* 70, no. 1 (2020): 7–30, https://doi.org/10.3322/caac.21590.

7. Veena Shankaran et al., "Risk Factors for Financial Hardship in Patients Receiving Adjuvant Chemotherapy for Colon Cancer: A Population-Based Exploratory Analysis," *Journal of Clinical Oncology* 30, no. 14 (2012): 1608–1614, https://doi.org/10.1200/JCO.2011.37.9511.

8. Scott D. Ramsey et al., "Financial Insolvency as a Risk Factor for Early

Mortality Among Patients with Cancer," *Journal of Clinical Oncology* 34, no. 9 (2016): 980–986, https: doi.org/10.1200/JCO.2015.64.6620.

9. Stephanie B. Wheeler et al., "Cancer-Related Financial Burden Among Patients with Metastatic Breast Cancer," *Journal of Clinical Oncology* 36, no. 30S (2018): 32–32, https://doi.org/10.1200/JCO.2018.36.30_suppl.32.

10. Alex Berenson, "A Cancer Drug's Big Price Rise Is Cause for Concern," *New York Times*, March 12, 2006, https://www.nytimes.com/2006/03/12/business/a-cancer-drugs-big-price-rise-is-cause-for-concern.html.

11. A. Vivot et al., "Clinical Benefit, Price and Approval Characteristics of FDA-Approved New Drugs for Treating Advanced Solid Cancer, 2000–2015," *Annals of Oncology* 28, no. 5 (2017): 1111–1116, https://doi.org/10.1093/annonc/mdx053.

12. Sham Mailankody and Vinay Prasad, "Five Years of Cancer Drug Approvals: Innovation, Efficacy, and Costs," *Journal of the American Medical Association Oncology* 1, no. 4 (2015): 539–540, https://doi.org/10.1001/jamaoncol.2015.0373.

13. Daniel A. Goldstein et al., "A Global Comparison of the Cost of Patented Cancer Drugs in Relation to Global Differences in Wealth," *Oncotarget* 8, no. 42 (2017): 71548–71555, https://doi.org/10.18632/oncotarget.17742.

14. Ahmed T. Ahmed et al., "Racial Disparities in Screening Mammography in the United States: A Systematic Review and Meta-analysis," *Journal of the American College of Radiology* 14, no. 2 (2017): 157–165.

15. H. Gilbert Welch, Barnett S. Kramer, and William C. Black, "Epidemiologic Signatures in Cancer," *New England Journal of Medicine* 381, no. 14 (2019): 1378–1386.

16. Mei-Song Ong and Kenneth D. Mandl, "National Expenditure for False-Positive Mammograms and Breast Cancer Overdiagnoses Estimated at $4 Billion a Year," *Health Affairs* 34, no. 4 (2015): 576–583, https://doi.org/10.1377/hlthaff.2014.1087.

17. Justin G. Trogdon et al., "Total Medicare Costs Associated with Diagnosis and Treatment of Prostate Cancer in Elderly Men," *Journal of the American Medical Association Oncology* 5, no. 1 (2019): 60–66, https://doi.org/10.1001/jamaoncol.2018.3701.

18. Justin E. Bekelman et al., "Comparison of Site of Death, Health Care Utilization, and Hospital Expenditures for Patients Dying with Cancer in 7 Developed Countries," *Journal of the American Medical Association* 315, no. 3 (2016): 272–283, https://doi.org/10.1001/jama.2015.18603.

19. Carrie H. Colla et al., "Impact of Payment Reform on Chemotherapy at the End of Life," *Journal of Oncology Practice* 8, no. 3S (2012): e6s–e13s, https://ascopubs.org/doi/full/10.1200/JOP.2012.000539.

20. Stanford C. Taylor et al., "Physician-Industry Interactions and Anti-Vascular Endothelial Growth Factor Use Among US Ophthalmologists," *Journal of the American Medical Association Ophthalmology* 134, no. 8 (2016): 897–903, https://doi.org/10.1001/jamaophthalmol.2016.1678.

21. Angela K. Green et al., "Assessment of Outcomes Associated with the Use of Newly Approved Oncology Drugs in Medicare Beneficiaries," *Journal of*

the American Medical Association Network Open 4, no. 2 (2021): e210030, https://doi.org/10.1001/jamanetworkopen.2021.0030.

22. Joseph C. Del Paggio et al., "Evolution of the Randomized Clinical Trial in the Era of Precision Oncology," *Journal of the American Medical Association Oncology* (2021), https://doi.org/10.1001/jamaoncol.2021.0379.

23. Jackson T. Bowers et al., "The CMS Oncology Care Model Is Falling Short of Its Promise. Could Oncology Hospital at Home Be the Remedy?," *Health Affairs* Blog (2020), https://www.healthaffairs.org/do/10.1377/hblog2020 1221.830917/full/.

PART FOUR

GOVERNING
CANCER

CHAPTER 15

FDA and Cancer R&D

The Engine for Future Cures

Gideon Blumenthal

The Landscape of Cancer R&D

Creating new cancer drugs is a long, expensive, and risky endeavor. Each step of the process is highly intricate and capital-intensive. First, scientists must discover which new chemicals or biologics may kill cancer cells—either through screening multiple chemicals and seeing how well they kill cancer cells on a dish, or through designing drugs based on our knowledge of a specific protein or pathway that is activated in cancer. But once a candidate emerges from this process, years of preclinical testing remain. The drug's toxicity in other species such as rats, monkeys, and dogs must be tested. Scientists must also understand how the new drug might be metabolized in the body and develop a stable formulation that can be reliably manufactured. No patient has even an experimental chance to be treated by the drug until Phase 1 clinical trials.

In these initial trials, cancer patients that have failed all non-experimental treatment options take small doses of the drug. The dose is slowly increased until the clinical staff titrate a dose that may appear to be active, yet not excessively toxic. If a drug passes its Phase 1 trials, it moves on to Phase 2 testing. Here, roughly

---

Gideon Blumenthal is Vice President of Global Regulatory Affairs for Oncology at Merck.

fifty patients with a given tumor type are treated with the dosage determined in the Phase 1 trial, so as to ascertain the antitumor activity of the drug. Next, a Phase 3 study (typically four hundred to one thousand patients) begins. Such a trial usually consists of a randomized trial of the new drug against the standard of care, concluding this premarketing stage of successive human trials.

On average, it takes $1 billion and a decade to take a drug from initial human studies to FDA approval. At every stage of the process, promising drugs drop out of the pipeline. For example, a drug entering a Phase 1 trial has less than a 10 percent chance of gaining US Food and Drug Administration (FDA) approval. Drugs that reach Phase 3 testing, however, have been more likely to gain approval in recent years, with success rates upward of 50 percent. Despite the time, expense, and risk involved, the number of cancer drugs in the FDA approval pipeline in 2020 increased to 17,737. That increase represents a 9.6 percent growth rate over the previous year. The sheer number of potential new cancer drugs represents both an increased scientific understanding of cancer and a more predictable and engaged regulatory environment.

As the number of drugs in development has increased, the primary drivers of research and development (R&D) have changed. Currently, the private sector, made up of large multinational pharmaceutical companies as well as well-funded venture-backed biotechnology companies, funds the lion's share of cancer R&D. In the 1970s and 1980s, however, roughly 60 percent of pharmaceutical development was funded and conducted by the US government. Today, almost 90 percent of the clinical development of cancer drugs is conducted and funded by the private sector. That private sector, too, looks vastly different than its 1980s predecessor.[1] Smaller biotech companies have emerged in the past decade, leading to a slow decline in the share of the total number of drugs in the pipeline for the top twenty-five pharmaceutical companies. Meanwhile, the share of drugs in the pipeline for companies with only one or two drugs in development has slowly increased over the last five years.

In earlier eras, diabetes, cardiovascular disease, and asthma were the major therapeutic areas in drug development (with blockbuster small molecule drugs, such as Lipitor, Januvia, and Advair, dominating). Yet, cancer is now the main therapeutic area driving R&D budgets, with more research dollars and drug approvals than any other therapeutic area, as well as heavy investment in biologic therapies, such as monoclonal antibodies, antibody drug conjugates, and cell and gene therapies. Yet paradoxically, cancer drugs are the most expensive to develop: the average R&D expenditure for cancer drugs was $4.46 billion between 2009 and 2018, as compared to $1.43 billion for gastrointestinal and metabolic drugs and $1.15 billion for cardiovascular drugs.[2]

Cancer is considered a relatively de-risked therapeutic area, as the science of cancer is relatively well understood, patients and doctors are willing to take more risks in terms of toxicity to derive a therapeutic benefit, and regulators tend to embrace innovation. For this reason, the focus on cancer drugs in the R&D pipeline is intense: across the top ten pharmaceutical companies, between 15 and 55 percent of drugs in development have an anticancer focus. With over nine thousand active trials, oncology has almost four times as many trials currently under way as any other therapeutic area, or a stunning 46 percent of all trials.[3] Overall, 37 percent of the entire pharmaceutical industry's pipeline consists of cancer candidates. Cancer's share of the pipeline grew a whopping 14 percent from 2019 to 2020.

How did this tectonic shift in the entire field American pharmaceutical R&D come to be? This chapter surveys the history of cancer R&D from the first days of the War on Cancer to the present, then moves to sketch a vision of the future. In the end, streamlining regulation and encouraging the development of novel technologies provides the best pathway to improve outcomes for cancer patients.

A Brief History of Cancer R&D: From the 1970s to the Modern Era of Precision Medicine and Immuno-Oncology

Government-Funded Cancer R&D

In 1971, when President Richard Nixon signed the National Cancer Act and the US government officially declared war on cancer,

cancer R&D was largely driven by the federal government. Much of the early research in cancer, beginning with Sidney Farber's work on folic acid antagonists to combat childhood leukemia, was empiric, as the underlying molecular pathogenesis of cancer was poorly understood. Many early clinical trials used combinations of cytotoxic chemotherapy, testing drugs with discreet mechanisms of action in a multitude of different tumor types to look for early signs of clinical activity.

In the 1960s, the development of combinatorial regimens, such as MOPP (mechlorethamine, vincristine, procarbazine, and prednisone), was a major breakthrough for the treatment of Hodgkin's lymphoma, demonstrating that systemic therapy could meaningfully cure cancer. This was followed by another cytotoxic chemotherapy drug, cisplatin, approved by the FDA in 1978 based on overall response rate (ORR) data in a single-arm Phase 2 trial in combination with vinblastine and bleomycin in disseminated testicular cancer.[4] This approval was consistent with the FDA's approach to single arm trials at the time.

Following the successes with cisplatin and such combinations as MOPP, in the late 1970s, the National Cancer Institute (NCI), with an influx of funding from the National Cancer Act, poured money into its drug discovery program. The program began screening hundreds of thousands of chemicals to discover new cancer drugs. The strategy was empirical—finding compounds that killed cancer cells in vitro—as the biology of cancer was not well understood. Paclitaxel, adriamycin, etoposide, and bleomycin[5]—all important chemotherapy drugs for combination regimens—were discovered at this time. The funding from the National Cancer Act also stimulated the organization of large multi-institutional clinical trials, the organization of the Coalition of Cancer Cooperative Groups (CCCG), and the creation of NCI Comprehensive Cancer Centers.

Beginning in the 1980s, the Oncologic Drug Advisory Committee (ODAC) recommended that criteria for patient benefit be changed from simply shrinking tumors to more substantial and clinically meaningful measures of treatment efficacy. ODAC is an external committee comprising academic experts, a patient representative, and an industry representative. Together, they provide advice to the FDA Oncology Office that reviews new therapeutics. ODAC recommended that the FDA require that a drug show improvement in overall survival or improvements in patient symptoms or function prior to granting marketing authorization. As chemotherapy reached the limits of its effectiveness, its benefit in more common cancers became more incremental and the benefit-risk could often only be reliably ascertained in very large, "all comer" randomized controlled trials. As a consequence, the pace of FDA approvals in the 1980s and 1990s for cancer drugs remained relatively slow.

Growing Private Sector Investment and Innovation

In the 1990s, private and public investment in novel biotechnology innovations began to bear fruit. Genentech, a small biotechnology company in San Francisco, invested heavily in developing proteins using recombinant DNA technology (joining together DNA molecules from different species to produce new proteins) to create a new platform of biologic therapies. Researchers began to test whether monoclonal antibodies could be used to target cancer cells. One putative target, HER2/neu, was found to be an oncogene that was amplified or overexpressed in a subset of patients with breast cancer.

Although the company initially resisted development of a drug for only a subset of cancer patients, academic researchers at UCLA persisted. Ultimately, a humanized monoclonal antibody targeting the protein HER2/neu, which became trastuzumab (Herceptin), gained FDA approval. Herceptin was FDA approved in 1998, based on the improvement in survival rates when given in combination with cytotoxic chemotherapy. This approval signaled the birth of targeted therapy and precision oncology.

Imatinib (Gleevec) also heralded the arrival of precision oncology. Imatinib is a small molecule tyrosine kinase inhibitor targeting BCR-ABL, the oncogene that is turned on to drive chronic myeloid leukemia (CML) carcinogenesis. Like trastuzumab, imatinib was championed by an academic researcher, Brian Druker of Oregon University. Dr. Druker convinced Novartis researchers to develop the drug after it demonstrated remarkable efficacy in nonclinical experiments of CML in vitro and in mice. In 2001, imatinib became the first tyrosine kinase inhibitor approved by the FDA for the treatment of patients with CML in blast crisis, accelerated phase or in chronic phase after failure of interferon-alpha therapy.

From a regulatory standpoint, the approval was notable for several reasons: this was one of the first Accelerated Approvals, an early approval based on a surrogate (in this case molecular response rate and complete hematologic response) that was reviewed by the agency in a two-and-a-half-month priority review. Accelerated Approval and priority review are expedited tools that the FDA Oncology Office, run by Richard Pazdur, would use frequently for transformative therapies in the coming decades. This approval, along with trastuzumab, began the era of precision oncology and targeted therapies.

Precision Oncology

Precision oncology, broadly defined as finding the right drug for the right patient at the right time, has advanced significantly since the approvals of trastuzumab and imatinib. Arguably, the greatest driver of this shift toward precision oncology was the revolution in high-throughput DNA sequencing. As the cost and speed of performing DNA sequencing improved exponentially through technological advancements, our understanding of the underlying molecular and genetic drivers of cancers also dramatically improved.

The precision oncology revolution presented challenges for the FDA—could the paradigm be shifted to move from enrolling patients in "all-comer" clinical trials, to selecting patients based on whether their cancer shows biomarkers making them more likely to respond to treatment? Given the renewed importance of new biomarkers, both to help stratify patients within a given tumor type and across tumor types, the agency was compelled to rethink clinical trial designs and proposed several adaptations—including master protocols, "basket trials" studying a biomarker across a number of different tumor types, and "umbrella trials" studying a number of drugs in a given tumor type.

In addition, given the rarity of some of these genomic-defined subsets, could these drugs be tested in smaller trials using earlier endpoints other than overall survival? The FDA responded to these challenges by accepting earlier endpoints when targeted drugs had dramatic effects in early clinical development. There is currently an ever-growing list of FDA-approved companion diagnostics to help oncologists decide which drug to give to patients. For example, in advanced non-small-cell lung cancer, it is standard practice at diagnosis to molecularly profile the cancer for mutations in EGFR, BRAF, and cMET as well as rearrangements in ALK, ROS1, NTRK, and RET; and to check for PD-L1 overexpression.

For many of these targets, there are now multiple therapies approved, with some given sequentially to target resistance mutations that develop over time. The precision oncology approach is also being deployed for colorectal cancer, prostate and ovarian cancer, and biliary and bladder cancer, among many others. In addition, the first "tumor agnostic" approvals occurred in 2017 and 2018. Under these approvals, adults and children could be treated for any cancer, irrespective of which body part it arose from, if it had the correct biomarker: pembrolizumab was approved for microsatellite high solid tumors and larotrectinib or entrectinib for NTRK fusion positive refractory solid tumors.

Immuno-oncology

In parallel to precision oncology, in the past decade there has been a revolution in the field of immuno-oncology—using the patient's own immune system to recognize and attack the cancer. In the 1990s, researchers discovered that immune checkpoints, such as CTLA-4 and PD-1, were expressed by the tumor to signal the immune system not to attack the cancer. Monoclonal antibodies that block CTLA-4 and PD-1 and PD-L1 were developed to inhibit these checkpoints and thus harness the immune system to reject cancer cells. The FDA approved the anti-CTLA4 monoclonal antibody ipilimumab in 2011 for the treatment of advanced refractory melanoma patients, based on improvements in overall survival.

In 2014, the FDA approved the anti-PD1 monoclonal antibodies nivolumab and pembrolizumab for the treatment of advanced melanoma, initially based on durable responses and then by demonstration of improvements in overall survival. The following year, pembrolizumab and nivolumab were approved in a tumor type that was previously not thought to be responsive to immune cell manipulation, non-small-cell lung cancer. The anti-PD1/PD-L1 success triggered an unprecedented era of drug development, with seventy-six total indications across all seven currently approved anti-PD-1/PD-L1 agents, including thirty-five accelerated approvals. Immuno-oncology was here to stay.

However, some aspects of immuno-oncology development have been challenging from a regulatory perspective, such as finding predictive biomarkers to identify which patients will respond to which agents and developing endpoints to fully capture their benefit. The FDA has worked with sponsors to help identify predictive biomarkers for immunotherapy response (such as PD-L1 expression on the tumor, microsatellite instability, and high tumor mutational burden) and to look at endpoints, such as durable response rate, that better capture the benefit of immuno-oncology agents.

Another landmark in immuno-oncology has been the advent of cell- and gene-based therapies. In 2017, the FDA approved the first chimeric antigen receptor T cell (CAR-T) therapy tisagenlecluecel, a CD19-directed genetically modified autologous T cell immunotherapy for the treatment of children and young adults with relapsed or refractory B cell acute lymphoblastic leukemia (ALL). This was followed by the approval of several more CAR-T therapies also targeting CD19 for the treatment of acute lymphocytic leukemia (also known as ALL), diffuse large B cell lymphoma, mantle cell lymphoma, and recently a BCMA targeting CAR to treat multiple myeloma.

Regulatory Innovations

The FDA Oncology Office has adapted nimbly to the changing landscape in cancer drug development. The office has grown, with approximately one hundred medical oncologists working in the office, with broad expertise across tumor types.

One of the key tools that the FDA Oncology Office has used in expediting development is the Accelerated Approval pathway. This approval pathway was initially implemented in the early 1990s to address the HIV/AIDS crisis, after patient advocates demanded that the agency bring promising drugs to market with more urgency. Since the 1990s, however, the oncology office has been the primary end user of the Accelerated Approval pathway.

Since 1992, the FDA Oncology Office has approved cancer drugs using the Accelerated Approval pathway 151 times.[6] The basis of the approval was surrogate endpoints "reasonably likely to predict clinical benefit," such as overall response rate. As a condition of approval, postmarketing studies are conducted to verify clinical benefit using longer-term outcomes, such as progression-free survival and overall survival. These early approvals stimulated biopharmaceutical investment into cancer R&D, as there was a path for an early approval while the large confirmatory clinical trials were enrolling patients and the definitive readout would occur. However, this pathway is only applicable in cases where drugs cause definitive durable responses in cancers with high unmet need.

In the majority of Accelerated Approval cases, clinical benefit goes on to be verified and the drug receives traditional or full approval. There have been a handful of cases where the postmarketing trials failed to confirm benefit and the indication was withdrawn. For example, the gefitinib second-line indication in non–small-cell lung cancer was initially withdrawn after several negative postmarketing studies, but was eventually reintroduced once the proper predictive biomarker to select patients who benefit from the drug was discovered. Bevacizumab in triple-negative breast cancer was withdrawn from the market after FDA hearings once the confirmatory trial failed to verify the clinical benefit in progression-free survival that led to the initial Accelerated Approval.

A recent effort by the FDA to address "dangling Accelerated Approvals" of immuno-oncology agents led to the withdrawal of four indications of PD-1/PD-L1 agents for refractory small cell and urothelial cancer due to failed confirmatory trials and a rapidly changing treatment landscape.[7] The FDA Oncology Office has tried to balance the tradeoff of the Accelerated Approval process to provide patients access to treatments when the ultimate benefit is uncertain. Overall, it has achieved such a balance and helped ensure patient access to promising drugs in the United States.

The FDA Oncology Office has also frequently used breakthrough therapy designation, initially implemented by the US Congress in 2012 for drugs for serious diseases that show preliminary clinical evidence of substantial improvement over available therapy. Breakthrough therapy designation was in part a reaction to the trials with BRAF inhibitors, such as vemurafenib in BRAF V600E mutant melanoma, where unprecedented responses in early clinical development led some to question the ethics of conducting further randomized trials against chemotherapy, which was known not to be effective in melanoma. Breakthrough therapy designation has spurred a rethinking of definitive trial design when preliminary clinical results are exceptional: it is a team-based mentality where the agency partners with the pharmaceutical company to ensure that the drug is developed as expeditiously as possible.

President Obama and then–Vice President Biden's "Cancer Moonshot" formed the FDA Oncology Center of Excellence, which harmonizes cancer efforts across the product centers at the FDA. Since its formation in 2017, the Oncology Center has advanced numerous innovations, including Real-Time Oncology Review, which is an iterative rolling review of cancer drugs that show great promise in clinical development, and Project ORBIS, which provides simultaneous submission and review of certain oncology drug applications between the US and Canada, Australia, Switzerland, Singapore, the United Kingdom, and Brazil.

Patient-Focused Drug Development

Patients now have a larger voice in the process of drug development. Since the days when HIV advocates protested at medical conferences, the White House, and the FDA for earlier access to promising therapies, patient advocates in oncology have learned from their HIV/AIDS advocacy counterparts and taken a more proactive approach. Patient advocates now have a seat at the tables where key decisions are made, participating in everything from venture philanthropy, to trial design of platform trials and master protocols, to key committees, including NCI steering committees and the FDA Oncologic Drugs Advisory Committee. While there has been some incorporation of Patient Reported Outcome measures and Patient Preference studies into drug development programs, this remains a key gap that novel tools, such as wearables and other digital technologies, may help address.

Major Issues in Cancer R&D

Redundancy

One frequent criticism of cancer R&D is the redundancy in drug development, with companies developing multiple "me-too" drugs rather than new molecular entities probing new targets. For example, five ALK inhibitors have been approved to treat advanced ALK rearranged non-small-cell lung cancer. There are certain advantages to having multiple agents developed and approved in the same class, even for rare patient populations, such as ALK-rearranged NSCLC. These drugs have different pharmacologic properties, some have better central nervous system penetration to treat brain metastasis, and some have greater specificity in targeting resistance mutations.

As discussed previously, there are also many PD-1/PD-L1 inhibitors in development, which raises the question—how many PD-1/PD-L1 inhibitors do we really need? Is it still ethical to enroll patients in trials where patients are randomized to more traditional chemotherapy in settings where PD-1/PD-L1 agents are now the standard of care and have definitively demonstrated improved survival? The questions of redundancy versus resiliency (having multiple marketed options) continues to riddle the field.

High Cost of Development

The cost of running clinical trials has steadily increased over time due to increased complexity, higher cost of cancer drugs and clinical care, and increased regulatory burdens. The mean cost per patient for clinical trials increased fourfold between 1989 and 2011, from $3,773 to $16,567.[8] In 2014, oncology clinical trial costs per study were estimated at $4.5 million for Phase 1, $11.2 million for Phase 2, and $22.1 million for Phase 3, with multiple studies occurring at each phase.[9] These might be underestimates and have increased since 2014. One study estimated that the median cost for all pivotal oncology clinical trials between 2015 and 2016 was a staggering $648 million, which also may be an under-estimate.[10] The number of procedures and steps to launch a trial and to run registration-enabling trials continues to increase. The high cost has been cited as one factor driving up the cost of R&D and ultimately the high cost of anticancer therapies.

The global COVID-19 pandemic may have forced some helpful change. Lockdowns restricted access to medical sites, spurring an acceleration of decentralized clinical trials. This shift, including remote patient visits with the investigator, remote monitoring of the patient and of the trial site, electronic or video informed consent, and decentralization of laboratory and imaging tests will likely continue once the pandemic subsides and could incrementally lower the costs of clinical development. Still, the costs of development remain considerable and may actually rise as therapies become ever more complex and the quantity and types of data collected (such as imaging and biomarker data) become more extensive.

Lack of Knowledge of Real-World Effectiveness and Safety

Critics of the current cancer drug development paradigm state that new agents are tested in highly controlled experiments with strict eligibility criteria, highly regulated monitoring and follow-up, and rigid endpoints. When the drug is finally authorized and reaches patients, oncologists have little insight into the safety or efficacy of these drugs for patients who were excluded or not adequately represented in the trials. This is especially true for elderly patients, pediatric patients, those from underrepresented minorities and ethnic groups, and those with other comorbidities.

Compounding the problem is the seemingly impenetrable wall between clinical research and clinical practice. Most electronic medical record (EMR) systems in hospitals and oncology practices are not designed to optimize clinical research questions. Most of the critical data collected on the typical oncology patient is highly unstructured and siloed within PDF documents in pathology and radiology reports. Thus, it remains a major challenge to understand safety and efficacy outcomes of drugs in the real world after they gain marketing authorization.

Several "real-world data/real-world evidence" ventures have arisen in the last decade to try to better curate and analyze this data. The 21st Century Cures Act mandated that the FDA develop the tools and guidance necessary to use real-world pharmaceutical effectiveness (RWE) in regulatory decision making. In 2018, the FDA released its RWE framework, outlining how RWE will be incorporated into therapeutic development.

Recalcitrant Cancers

Finally, despite great therapeutic advances in many cancer types, there are certain cancer types where very limited progress has been made in the twenty-first century. Such cancers as advanced pancreatic cancer, aggressive brain cancers, and some pediatric cancers remain—as all cancer used to be—a near-certain death sentence. National efforts, such as the Cancer Moonshot and novel adaptive platform trials, have attempted to address these cancers. For instance, the glioblastoma multiforme (GBM) AGILE trial and Precision Promise from the Pancreatic Cancer Alliance both study multiple agents in a single umbrella trial. But there still remains great unmet need in these and so many other cancer types. While we have made great progress in understanding the molecular and immunologic drivers of some cancers, in others the progress has been limited, and even when we do understand the drivers we still do not have good drugs to target the pathway. Further, such cancers as GBM and pancreatic cancer are often advanced at the time of diagnosis, when the delivery of therapies to the brain or to the pancreas can be quite challenging under the best of circumstances. New research needs both to find these cancers at an earlier stage and to locate novel mechanisms to deliver therapies, to make a demonstrable impact.

Future of Cancer R&D

Novel Therapies and Combinations

Despite the progress with targeted therapies and immuno-oncology agents, large unmet needs remain. This section highlights exciting new modalities, such as antibody drug conjugates, cell and gene therapy, and new small molecules that might better targeted recalcitrant cancers and be combined with existing therapies to enhance cure. The sharp uptick in new anticancer therapies in the past decade appears poised to continue, with an enormous amount of capital investment in new biotech companies studying new targets and new modalities and advances in older modalities. In terms of biologics, the FDA has approved many recent antibody-drug conjugates (ADCs), which are monoclonal antibodies armed with a warhead of cytotoxic chemotherapy to deliver the payload in a much more targeted fashion.

CAR-T therapies have seen huge investments, with several products targeting CD19 and BCMA FDA approved. In addition, pharmaceutical companies continue to research "off-the-shelf" allogeneic CAR-T products that would be easier and less costly to manufacture. Personal cancer vaccines, which use mRNA technologies similar to what was used with the Pfizer and Moderna vaccines against COVID-19, are also a new horizon of research. Personalized cancer vaccines might be able to identify the epitope or protein that might generate a strong immune response against the cancer. In the future, such a rapid synthetic personalized cancer vaccine could be paired with other immunotherapies, such as anti–PD-1 drugs, to enhance immune response against the cancer.

In addition to innovations in biologics, we are also seeing a great deal of promise for novel small molecules. One of the most challenging and common oncogenic drivers, the gene KRAS (Kirsten rat sarcoma viral oncogene homolog), had been an elusive target for scientists since the initial discovery of the gene in 1990. KRAS mutations are present in about 30 percent of patients with non-small-cell lung cancer (NSCLC), 40 percent of patients with colorectal cancer, and 90 percent of patients with pancreatic cancer. Dr. Kevan Shokat, of UCSF, first published work on covalent inhibitors of KRAS G12C in 2013. There are now at least nine of these KRAS covalent inhibitors in clinical development, with sotorasib receiving Accelerated Approval in refractory KRAS G12C mutant NSCLC in May 2021. Other promising small molecule approaches include targeted protein degradation and approaches to inhibit other previously undruggable oncogenes, such as mutant p53 and beta-catenin.

New Modalities

In addition to exciting new therapeutic approaches to treat cancer, there are new tools arising to detect cancer early, to profile cancers genomically, and to monitor cancer progression over time. New diagnostic companies have received large investments to develop platforms to detect circulating tumor DNA (ctDNA) in the blood. Companies such as Grail, Guardant, and Foundation Medicine have developed strategies to develop ctDNA for early detection, diagnosis, genotyping, and monitoring across solid and hematologic tumor types. Large-scale trials are under way to assess the clinical utility of ctDNA in early cancer detection. In addition, several ctDNA assays are being tested in clinical trials to assess their utility in detecting minimal residual disease (MRD) after surgical resection, which could help identify high risk patients who need more treatment and lower-risk patients who can get by with observation. Many efforts are under way to investigate whether measuring changes in ctDNA over time could be used as a surrogate marker for disease progression, recurrence, or death and could potentially be used as a reasonably likely surrogate for accelerated approval decisions.

Imaging technology will continue to improve and will replace more basic tools to assess tumor response. Radiomics—a method that extracts a large number of imaging features using data characterization algorithms—may become a powerful tool to predict which patients will respond to a therapy earlier than assessing changes in overall tumor burden. In addition, functional imaging will improve and greatly refine medical decision making as well as drug development decisions.

Patient-Centered Endpoints and Real World Data

The movement toward patient-focused drug development and increasing incorporation of RWE will continue to expand in the next fifty years. Patient-centered endpoints, more easily captured through sensors and wearables, will increasingly be deployed in clinical trials to better understand the benefit-risk profile of a drug. Increased use of RWE will require substantial public investments to upgrade and modernize EMR systems to be able to capture critical data necessary for clinical trial investigation. Such efforts as the ASCO mCODE project to standardize terminology within EMRs, including in pathology and radiology reports, will help to structure data and render RWD more interpretable. Use of more advanced tools such as artificial intelligence and machine learning algorithms will be increasingly deployed to incorporate diverse streams of high-volume and -velocity data to help patients and doctors and clinical investigators make better decisions on how best to treat the cancer and which trials are best to refer patients to.

Global Regulatory Harmonization

Delivering on all of the innovations and addressing the issues highlighted in this chapter will be predicated on developing and maintaining highly skilled, adaptive, and knowledgeable regulatory authorities. In this regard, the US FDA Oncology Center of Excellence is regarded as the gold standard, on the cutting edge of providing guidance on novel trial designs and experimenting with regulatory science pilots, such as Real-Time Oncology Review and Project ORBIS. Through Project ORBIS, there has been enhanced collaboration between health authorities to streamline reviews. This has led to faster approval in the ORBIS countries and, if adopted more broadly, will lead to more harmonization and more rapid adoption of global standards of care. Real-time review and ORBIS are both crucial new tools for regulators to expedite drug development for breakthrough therapies and ensure that ex-US regulatory authorities are keeping up with the pace and innovations set forth by the FDA.

A Vision for the Future

The COVID-19 pandemic provided prima facie evidence that the biopharmaceutical industry working in tandem with government agencies and academic centers can meet large challenges at warp speed. The public will expect similar results for cancers that remain nearly uniformly fatal fifty years after signing of the National Cancer Act. While drug development and regulation has always been of great public interest, the current pandemic has made the terms Pfizer, Moderna, and Emergency Use Authorization (EUA) household names. A recent proposal by the Biden administration to create a DARPA-like mechanism for cancer research to fund high-risk high-reward projects to augment the existing NCI-funding mechanisms would help de-risk efforts in certain hard-to-treat cancer types. This new agency would work with a variety of groups, including venture capitalists, academic researchers, and drug manufacturers to "de-risk" investments in future cures that otherwise may not be prioritized.[11]

In addition, we will need to take a hard look at the excessive bureaucracy and red tape within the clinical trials enterprise, which imposes needless burdens on patients and investigators and slows down the development process. For example, could we cut down on unnecessary reporting of adverse reactions that are known to be associated with the investigational drug or the underlying disease? We will also need to better incorporate modern imaging tools, plasma based circulating tumor DNA assays, and other biomarkers to better stratify patients using smarter adaptive clinical trial designs. Such a personalized approach will help us understand which patients need new combinations of drugs with different mechanisms of action and which patients might have great outcomes with less treatment. Earlier diagnosis and earlier intervention will lead to marked improvements in cure rates for patients. Meanwhile, national investments into our EHR systems and creating national networks of clinical trials will ensure the safety and efficacy of our drugs in the real world and guarantee that underserved populations can enroll in clinical trials. Our challenge for the next fifty years is in bringing together regulatory agencies, the pharmaceutical industry, and academic investigators to once again ally in this fight.

Notes

1. Joseph C. Del Paggio, "Evolution of the Randomized Clinical Trial in the Era of Precision Oncology," *Journal of the American Medical Association Oncology* (2021), https://jamanetwork.com/journals/jamaoncology/article-abstract/2777587.

2. Olivier J. Wouters, Martin McKee, and Jeroen Luyten, "Estimated Research and Development Investment Needed to Bring a New Medicine to Market, 2009–2018," *JAMA* 323, no. 9 (2020): 844–853, https://jamanetwork.com/journals/jama/article-abstract/2762311.

3. Ian Lloyd, *Pharma R&D Annual Review 2020* (New York: Pharma Intelligence Informa 2020), 14–27.

4. Lawrence H. Einhorn and John Donohue, "Cis-Diamminedichloroplatinum, Vinblastine, and Bleomycin Combination Chemotherapy in Disseminated Testicular Cancer," *Annals of Internal Medicine* 87, no. 3 (1977): 293–298, https://www.acpjournals.org/doi/pdf/10.7326/0003-4819-87-3-293.

5. Siddhartha Mukherjee, *Emperor of all Maladies: A Biography of Cancer* (New York: Scribner, 2011).

6. Julia A. Beaver et al., "A 25-Year Experience of US Food and Drug Administration Accelerated Approval of Malignant Hematology and Oncology Drugs and Biologics: A Review," *JAMA Oncology* 4, no. 6 (2018): 849–856, https://jamanetwork.com/journals/jamaoncology/fullarticle/2673837.

7. Julia A. Beaver and Richard Pazdur, "'Dangling' Accelerated Approvals in Oncology," *New England Journal of Medicine* (2021), https://www.nejm.org/doi/full/10.1056/NEJMp2104846.

8. Ernst Berndt and Ian M. Cockburn, "Price Indexes for Clinical Trial Research: A Feasibility Study," *Monthly Labor Review*, US Bureau of Labor Statistics (June 2014), https://www.bls.gov/opub/mlr/2014/article/price-indexes-for-clinical-trial-research-a-feasibility-study.htm.

9. Aylin Sertkaya et al., *Examination of Clinical Trial Costs and Barriers for Drug Development* (Washington, DC, and Lexington, MA: US Department of Health and Human Services and Eastern Research Group 2014), 3-3, https://aspe.hhs.gov/system/files/pdf/77166/rpt_erg.pdf.

10. Vinay Prasad and Sham Mailankody, "Research and Development Spending to Bring a Single Cancer Drug to Market and Revenues After Approval," *JAMA Internal Medicine* 177, no. 11 (2017) 1569–1575, doi:10.1001/jamainternmed.2017.3601.

11. Lev Facher, "In his biggest speech yet, Biden pitches a new health agency to help 'end cancer as we know it,'" *STAT* (April 28, 2021), https://www.statnews.com/2021/04/28/biden-pitches-new-health-agency-to-end-cancer/.

CHAPTER 16

US Federal Agencies

Advancing Cancer Research and Care Through Improved Coordination and Efficiency

Shelagh Foster, Shimere Sherwood,
and Richard L. Schilsky

The United States federal government has several agencies and departments that directly fund cancer research, oversee the way cancer research is conducted, regulate medical products used in cancer treatment, and govern the delivery of cancer care. The agencies and departments described in this chapter have significant impact on the outcomes of people with cancer as they either support, advance, and drive trends in cancer research, or have direct or indirect influence over coverage, reimbursement, or the overall provision of or access to cancer care. But the large number of federal agencies involved can also present barriers to advancing cancer care by imposing regulatory roadblocks, creating uncoordinated silos, or failing to keep pace with the breakneck speed at which cancer research is moving. In the first fifty years since the passage of the National Cancer Act, the US built an expansive infrastructure to

Shelagh Foster is Division Director, Policy and Advocacy, American Society of Clinical Oncology.

Shimere Sherwood is Associate Director, Science and Research Policy, American Society of Clinical Oncology.

Richard L. Schilsky is former Executive Vice President and Chief Medical Officer, American Society of Clinical Oncology.

support cancer care and research; the next fifty should address how best to harness all its power. This chapter will summarize the roles of key agencies that impact cancer care and describe areas where agency jurisdictions overlap, or where there may be opportunities for increased efficiencies and collaborations.[1]

To illustrate the federal government's complex and multifaceted role in the discovery, development, and delivery of critical therapies, we will trace how different agencies have impacted a groundbreaking immunotherapy—chimeric antigen receptor T-cell (CAR-T) therapy. Until now, cancer therapy has mainly relied on chemotherapy, surgery, and radiotherapy. Only recently has immunotherapy been identified as the "fourth pillar" of cancer treatment. The concept of genetically engineering a patient's T lymphocytes in a laboratory to produce a special receptor called a chimeric antigen receptor (CAR) that enables these now-modified cells to identify and attack cancer cells after infusion into the patient has so far, led to US Food and Drug Administration (FDA) approval of five CAR-T therapies for four indications, and the initiation of over two hundred CAR-T clinical trials that have been offered at a limited number of cancer centers with specialized expertise in cellular therapies.

Federal agencies have been essential to this story from the start. Basic research that led to key breakthroughs was funded by the National Institutes of Health (NIH) and the National Cancer Institute (NCI). Approval for human study and clinical use of CAR-T therapies was provided by the FDA, while access to this innovative class of therapies for Medicare beneficiaries is controlled by coverage decisions made by the Centers for Medicare and Medicaid Services (CMS). The Health Resources and Services Administration (HRSA) attempts to reduce inequitable access to CAR-T therapies, while the Office for Human Research Protections (OHRP) and FDA seek to protect patients participating in the clinical trials of these novel immunotherapies. By tracking the involvement of these agencies in a pathbreaking new treatment, a clearer picture emerges of the complex—sometimes overlapping and inefficient, at other times fragmented and siloed—ways in which the federal government impacts the present and future of cancer care in America. It also suggests pathways to reform as we look to the next fifty years.

Agencies in Action—The Role of Government Agencies in Cancer Care from Drug Development to Treatment at the Bedside

To better understand the federal role in cancer care, we begin by reviewing several major agencies whose responsibilities range from research funding to research oversight and care delivery. The agencies discussed here were established at different times, often to provide specialized expertise and management of the emerging issues of the day, leading to a patchwork of regulatory jurisdictions. The mission and authorities of these agencies are summarized at the end of this section in Table 16.1 and Appendix B.

Health and Human Services (HHS)

As the largest and most influential government agency in health care, HHS directs the critical functions of several agencies, many of which are described here, that can hasten or slow the pace of cancer research and promote or hinder access to care. Created in 1953 as a cabinet-level Department of Health, Education, and Welfare by President Dwight Eisenhower, it became HHS in 1980.[2] The secretary of HHS and its staff have direct access to the White House and can exercise that influence to prioritize or deemphasize cancer issues for an administration. Its subsidiary agencies follow HHS's strategic direction to implement policies and take actions that influence, even dictate, what cancer treatment is available to patients and whether it is affordable for a substantial segment of the US population.

National Institutes of Health (NIH)

Within HHS lies the NIH. Established in 1930 as the National Institute of Health out of the Public Health Service's Hygienic

Laboratory, its twenty-seven institutes and centers focus on specific diseases or body systems, and support discovery, clinical, and population research that contributes to advances in cancer care.[3] As the primary government funder of the basic biomedical research conducted in both public (including colleges and universities) and private laboratories around the country, the NIH arguably has the most critical role in supporting progress against cancer.

Cancer research, like most medical research, begins with basic research (often referred to as lab research), which seeks to answer fundamental questions that help us understand living systems and life processes. The NIH is not only a primary funder of basic research but also conducts intramural research that contributes to our understanding of health, aging, and disease. The NIH also supports and conducts translational and clinical research that seeks to transform the knowledge gained from basic research into solutions to medical problems through clinical trials and population research.

The NIH is funded through annual congressional appropriations and, as a result, does not have stable, predictable funding from year to year. Indeed, NIH funding is subject to the ebb and flow of political uncertainty, which can cause instability in the funding of biomedical research. For instance, the agency received flat funding or cuts from fiscal year (FY) 2004 to FY2015. However, from FY2016–19, "Congress provided the NIH with funding increases of over 5% each year," raising the budget "from $30.3 billion in FY2015 to $39.3 billion in FY2019."[4] The agency's funding level is currently $41.7 billion, an increase of 39 percent over the past five years. While this considerable investment in funding is positive, Congress could reassess its budget priorities and withdraw support at any time. Additionally, the recent increases have not been enough for the US biomedical research enterprise to fully recover from many years of funding that did not keep pace with inflation. This ebb and flow in funding can result in the slowing or stopping of laboratory research and clinical trials, delaying the delivery of potentially lifesaving new treatments to patients.

CAR-T THERAPY CASE STUDY:
FEDERAL GOVERNMENT AGENCIES' ROLES[5]

NIH Enabling Groundbreaking Therapies

- The NIH supports and manages large partnerships with biopharmaceutical companies to accelerate the development of new cancer immunotherapy strategies for more patients. Several NIH institutes, centers, and offices play a role in advancing the field of immunotherapy, including the National Center for Advancing Translational Sciences and the National Institute of Allergy and Infectious Diseases.
- Building on the understanding of the immune system to fight cancer, researchers in the NIH Intramural Research Program paved the way for modern cellular therapies for cancer through decades of painstaking basic research and innovative clinical trials culminating in the use of genetically altered immune cells that recognize the CD19 receptor protein present on some types of B cell malignancies, notably relapsed B cell acute lymphoblastic leukemia (B-ALL), chronic lymphocytic leukemia (CLL), and B cell non-Hodgkin's lymphoma (B-NHL).[6]

National Cancer Institute (NCI)

As the anchor of the nation's cancer research efforts, the National Cancer Institute (NCI), part of the NIH, is the largest public funder of cancer research in the world. Established by the National Cancer Act of 1937,[7] it manages a complex web of intramural and extramural research efforts. The NCI organizes and supports the National Clinical Trials Network (NCTN), with over 2,200 sites across the US, Canada, and other parts of the world. The NCTN is a collection of institutions and clinicians that conduct cancer clinical trials at these sites. The NCTN, and the related National Community Oncology Research Program, provide the primary infrastructure for NCI-funded therapeutic and advanced imaging trials, as well as cancer prevention and care delivery studies. NCI also confers recognition on cancer centers around the country that meet rigorous standards for transdisciplinary research focused on developing new and better approaches to preventing, diagnosing, and treating cancer. Recognized centers, known as NCI-Designated Cancer Centers, conduct basic cancer research, deliver cutting-edge cancer treatments to patients, and engage communities across the country in cancer control efforts.[8] These centers bring together scientists and clinicians from across an institution to focus on specific problems in cancer biology, conduct first-in-human clinical trials of promising new agents, organize multidisciplinary care teams to deliver broad-based expertise to patients, and engage the communities they serve in programs that aim to reduce cancer risk, improve cancer screening and enhance access to high-quality cancer care. The clinical trials conducted by NCI-Designated Cancer Centers, many supported by the Early Clinical Trials Network and the Specialized Programs of Research Excellence program, address critical questions and fill important research gaps that may not be addressed in other trials, such as those conducted by private industry.

CAR-T THERAPY CASE STUDY: FEDERAL GOVERNMENT AGENCIES' ROLES

NCI Enabling Groundbreaking Therapies

- The basic research that revealed genetic alterations in cancer has led to advancements in early detection, risk reduction, the use of more targeted therapies for cancer, and improved overall survival for patients with many cancer types. In particular, basic research funded by the NIH and NCI about how genes control the body's immune system have fueled the development of the novel adoptive cell therapy approach known as CAR-T therapy.
- The NCI has funded or cofunded much of the research that underpins the development of CAR-T therapy,

including research on the role of the immune system in cancer surveillance and progression, the introduction of monoclonal antibodies, and even the 1961 discovery by immunologist Jacques Miller of where T cells develop in the thymus gland.[9]

- The concept of genetically engineering a patient's T cells in a laboratory to produce a special receptor called CAR that enables these now-modified cells to identify and attack cancer cells after infusion into the patient has led to the initiation of over 200 CAR-T clinical trials that have been offered at a limited number of cancer centers with specialized expertise in cellular therapies.[10]

- In 2020, NCI initiated an effort to manufacture more CAR-T to improve access to this investigational therapy at multiple hospital sites.[11]

Food and Drug Administration (FDA)

Commercial or industry sponsored trials are regulated by the FDA, which was created in 1906 by the Pure Food and Drugs Act.[12] The FDA ensures that cancer therapies (submitted for review through a new drug or biologic licensing application) and diagnostic tests used in a cancer patient's care journey are safe and effective before market entry. Oncology drugs have accounted for 27 percent of all new drug approvals in the US since 2010.[13] Contemporary cancer care involves the use of drugs and biologics often guided by molecular tests used to identify patients most likely to benefit from treatment. The regulation of these diverse products has, in the past, been distributed across multiple centers, divisions, or offices of FDA, resulting in the application of different approval standards, review processes, and timelines.

To better organize these efforts, in 2017 the FDA created the Oncology Center of Excellence (OCE), which streamlined the approval process for oncology-related drugs, biologics, and devices by bringing multidisciplinary teams together across several FDA offices and programs. This new center demonstrated its effectiveness by bringing eleven oncology drugs to market in 2019,[14] utilizing various review and approval pathways, including breakthrough designation, accelerated approval, and priority review.[15] In addition to the FDA's regulatory role in approving new therapies, it also grants approval for trials to begin after receiving an Investigational New Drug (IND) application from the trial sponsor. This is one area that presents an opportunity for increased efficiencies in agency collaboration for NCI-sponsored trials.

The coordination of NCI and FDA review processes is essential to ensure that NCI-sponsored trials are launched in a timely fashion and not subject to redundant and sometimes discordant review processes. A 2010 report by the Institute of Medicine (now National Academy of Medicine) recommended NCI coordinate with the FDA for oversight of NCI-funded trials to ensure appropriate protocol design early in the process, reducing the number of revisions and re-reviews that may be required. It also recommended NCI defer review of protocols conducted under IND to the FDA.[16] It is not clear to what extent the agencies have implemented these recommendations.

FDA ADVANCING CAR-T THERAPIES

- In 2017, two CAR-T therapies were approved by the FDA, marking the first gene therapies approved for use in the US: one for the treatment of children with acute lymphoblastic leukemia (ALL) and the other for adults with advanced lymphomas.
- Using information learned from the clinical trials, the FDA required certification of any entity administering the therapy because of the risk of severe side effects and required a postmarket observational study by the manufacturer.
- The FDA also approved the launch of multiple new trials of CAR-T treatments that employ novel technologies and/or seek to expand approved uses.

Centers for Medicare and Medicaid Services (CMS)

Scientific advances are of little benefit unless they can reach the patients who need them. CMS plays an important part in enabling patient access both to clinical trials and approved treatments through its administration of Medicare, Medicaid, and the Children's Health Insurance Program (CHIP). Established in 1977 as the Health Care Financing Administration (HCFA) before taking its current name in 2001, CMS can redesign the landscape of practice and impact delivery of care through its coverage and reimbursement decisions. As the majority of cancer patients are aged sixty-five or older, CMS coverage decisions impact what diagnostic evaluations and treatments many cancer patients can receive and when they can receive them, following regulatory approval. Many newly approved cancer therapeutics are expensive, and CMS has to weigh the benefit of allowing coverage and reimbursement for a drug or service, both of which are necessary for patient access to FDA-approved therapies, against the budget it has available to support the needs of all its beneficiaries. While the FDA standard for drug/biologic approval is that the product is "safe and effective,"[17] CMS applies a different standard for reimbursement: that the product is "reasonable and necessary" for use in Medicare beneficiaries.[18] Application of these different standards can sometimes delay reimbursement of, and therefore access to, therapies newly approved by the FDA.

CMS policies can also impact patient access to clinical trials. Prior to 2000, coverage of routine clinical care costs for trial participants was not provided by Medicare or Medicaid, creating a significant barrier to clinical trial participation for many individuals. A 2000 executive memorandum issued by the Clinton administration required Medicare to cover routine clinical costs associated with trial participation, and this requirement was mandated by provisions of the Affordable Care Act as well. However, until very recently, Medicaid was not required to cover routine costs associated with clinical trials, thereby creating an obstacle to trial participation for patients with limited financial resources and contributing both to a lack of diversity in trial participants and disparities in cancer outcomes. However, with the passage of the Clinical Treatment Act in late 2020, Medicaid is now required to cover these costs.

Although Medicare coverage for clinical trials was a welcome development when first required more than two decades ago, it has not come without challenges. For example, trial sponsors must perform an analysis of clinical care costs prior to trial launch to delineate those trial procedures that may or may not be billed to Medicare. Performing such analyses is time-consuming and may contribute to delays in trial start-up times.

CMS CONTROLLING ACCESS TO CAR-T THERAPIES

- Coverage for CAR-T treatment is limited to FDA-approved (on-label or off-label with compendia) uses in certified institutions, which are few in number across the country. As experience is gained with this treatment, there are questions about whether that coverage can and should be expanded to additional institutions or physician-owned practices.
- The price of CAR-T therapy can exceed $300,000. CMS currently pays only a small percentage of that cost, leaving institutions to absorb the additional expenses.

Due to these two restrictions, access for patients to this potentially lifesaving therapy, while technically available, is limited.

Health Resources and Services Administration (HRSA)

To improve access to care for the underserved and reduce health disparities for vulnerable populations, HRSA ensures access to quality services and a skilled health-care workforce. Created in 1982, HRSA includes the Office of Rural Health Policy and the Office of Health Equity, and administers the 340B program, which mandates that manufacturers provide deeply discounted outpatient drugs, many of which are cancer treatments, to qualifying entities.[19] There has been much controversy around the 340B program, as it has expanded exponentially in the past decade and strayed from the original intent of the program to stretch scarce federal resources as far as possible, particularly to assist hospitals treating underserved patients. Although the deep discounts granted to 340B entities were intended to provide resources for care of underserved beneficiaries, it is unclear whether and how qualifying entities have used these funds for this purpose. There are concerns that some 340B entities have used the program to achieve stronger market presence by acquiring or more effectively competing with physician-owned practices that do not obtain the same discounted drug prices available to participating 340B hospitals. In so doing, some 340B entities effectively limit patient access to community-based cancer care.

HRSA ADDRESSING INEQUITIES OF EXPENSIVE NEW THERAPIES, SUCH AS CAR-T

- Because of safety concerns, CAR-T therapies can only be administered in certified centers, typically large urban institutions. HRSA's efforts to narrow the gap between the access to care in rural and more populated areas are critical when thinking about such groundbreaking therapies as CAR-T, which is not currently included in the 340B program.

CAR-T therapies cost hundreds of thousands of dollars and are often not fully reimbursed by payers. Expensive therapies like these exacerbate disparities in care and demonstrate a clear need for HRSA to address equity issues.

Office for Human Research Protections (OHRP)

Scientific progress through clinical research would not be possible without the participation of people in clinical trials and other research studies. However, with the potential benefits to patients of participating in a clinical trial also come risks, ethical considerations, and requirements for patient protection. Established in 2000 within HHS, OHRP replaced the Office for Protection from Research Risks that was established within NIH in 1972 to protect participants in biomedical research by requiring all federally sponsored clinical trials to adhere to the Common Rule requirements.[20] The Common Rule is the federal rule that stipulates the ethical standards for the conduct of government-funded research; outlines the provisions for Institutional Review Board (IRB) reviews; and mandates informed consent of study participants that clearly describes the risks, benefits, and alternatives of study participation. Notably, FDA, not OHRP, has authority regarding protection of human subjects who participate in clinical investigations that support applications for research or marketing permits for products regulated by the FDA. While regulations are generally similar between the two agencies, there are important differences including the definition of "human subject" and the circumstances under which exemptions from IRB review may be granted. The different regulatory standards applied by OHRP and the FDA risk creating confusion that may jeopardize patient safety when institutions participate in trials supported by different sponsors. A harmonized approach to human subject protections across all federal agencies would be preferred.

PROTECTION OF PATIENTS RECEIVING CAR-T THERAPY

- As a genetically engineered and personalized therapy, CAR-T therapy comes with a unique set of risks that make protection of participants in clinical trials, and adequate informed consent, even more critical.
- CAR-T therapies use different gene delivery methods that can pose some risk, and as each new gene delivery technology is moved into the clinics, the IRBs must be prepared to execute well-informed risk assessments.

- CAR-T therapy is a rapidly developing field. Each new advance in the technology requires appropriate oversight to ensure the safety of human study participants, including special considerations for institutional ethical and safety review of trials as well as understanding both the molecular and the clinical factors that inform the risk assessment for each protocol.

The promise of immunology to advance human health can only be fulfilled if the public maintains trust and confidence in the research. OHRP and the FDA play key roles in ensuring scientific and ethical integrity, safety, and public engagement in research. However, the different regulatory standards applied by OHRP and the FDA risk creating confusion that may jeopardize patient safety.

Office of the National Coordinator for Health Information Technology (ONC)

Interoperability of electronic health records (EHR) is an issue across health care but is especially important in oncology where patients need care coordinated by multiple specialists, sometimes across health systems. Currently, information exchange is limited because there is not a standard EHR format or mechanism to freely exchange specialized information specific to cancer care. Inconsistent access to clinical information or outcomes can result in fragmented care for cancer patients or other issues, such as duplicate screening and testing that increase the overall costs to the health-care system.

ONC was established to address this issue and coordinates with CMS to enforce its requirements through reimbursement penalties for providers who use technology that fails to meet ONC requirements. Created by an executive order in 2004, it was legislatively authorized in 2009 by the Health Information Technology for Economic and Clinical Health (HITECH) Act.[21] While

ONC has made some progress, for example, establishing criteria for certifying health information technology vendors, and defining and outlining penalties for information blocking, full interoperability has not been achieved. Continued barriers to interoperability include technical incompatibility, privacy concerns, financial costs, and in some cases intentional blocking of information by competitive entities.

ONC EFFORTS ON INTEROPERABILITY CRITICAL TO SURVIVORSHIP CARE FOR THOSE PATIENTS ON GROUNDBREAKING THERAPY

- Many patients receiving CAR-T therapy may be referred by their primary oncologist to large centers where it can be administered safely. It is important for patients to be able to convey records between physicians with ease and for providers to track the long-term health outcomes of CAR-T therapy.

Many patients will be cured by CAR-T therapy, some will have long-term side effects, and most will see various specialists and other providers over the course of their lives. The interoperability of EHRs will be critical to tracking their outcomes across multiple years of survivorship and multiple providers.

TABLE 16.1 US Federal Agencies Impacting Cancer Research and Care Delivery

Agency	*Mission*	*Key Cancer Facts*
Department of Health and Human Services (HHS) Created in 1953 as a cabinet level Department of Health, Education, and Welfare by President Eisenhower—became HHS in 1980.[a]	To enhance the health and well-being of all Americans, by providing for effective health and human services and by fostering sound, sustained advances in the sciences underlying medicine, public health, and social services.	Oversees 11 agencies and over 300 departments and programs with cancer-related research and care delivery, including NIH, FDA, and CMS.
National Institutes of Health (NIH) Created in 1930 as the National Institute of Health (later Institutes) out of the Public Health Service's Hygienic Laboratory.[b]	To seek fundamental knowledge about the nature and behavior of living systems and the application of that knowledge to enhance health, lengthen life, and reduce illness and disability.	Consists of 27 institutes and centers including the National Cancer Institute (NCI). Cancer research benefits from interactions across all institutes at NIH. Funded by annual congressional appropriations. Despite significant congressional support, funding for biomedical research lags behind inflation.
National Cancer Institute (NCI) Created in 1937 by the National Cancer Act of 1937.[c]	To lead, conduct, and support cancer research across the nation to advance scientific knowledge and help all people live longer, healthier lives.	Largest funder of cancer research in the world. The NCI Cancer Centers Program was created as part of the National Cancer Act of 1971. Consists of 30 divisions, offices, and centers that maintain a comprehensive cancer research agenda. Nearly a $6 billion budget with approximately 40% of funds being allocated for research project grants. Responsible for the $1.8 billion Cancer Moonshot initiative over 7 years.

Agency	Mission	Key Cancer Facts
Food and Drug Administration (FDA) Created in 1906 by the Pure Food and Drugs Act.[d]	To promote and protect the public health by helping safe and effective products reach the market in a timely way, and monitoring products for continued safety after they are in use.	Regulates many products that impact cancer patients, including drugs, biologics, cell therapies, devices, and tobacco. Fifty-five percent of the budget is through federal budget appropriations and 45% through user fees. Consists of 8 centers and 8 offices overseeing different aspects of food and drug regulation. OCE coordinates and expedites review of oncology drugs, biologics, and devices under one center by working with centers and offices across the FDA. Center for Tobacco Products regulates the manufacturing, marketing, and distribution of tobacco products. Oversees packaging, including warnings. The Office of Drug Shortages prevents, mitigates, and helps resolve shortages and works with the pharmaceutical industry and stakeholders to reduce the impact on patients and health-care delivery.

(continues)

TABLE 16.1 (*continued*)

Agency	*Mission*	*Key Cancer Facts*
Centers for Medicare and Medicaid Services (CMS) The Health Care Financing Administration (HCFA) was established in 1977 to manage the Medicare and Medicaid programs. It was renamed CMS in 2001.	To ensure that the voices and needs of the populations we represent are present as the agency is developing, implementing, and evaluating its programs and policies.	Oversight of Medicare and Medicaid programs. Makes national coverage decisions on critical cancer care services and reimbursement of cancer treatments. Can cover off-label uses of anticancer therapies, assuming the use meets specified criteria. It is estimated that approximately 55% of cancer treatment is off-label. Houses the Centers of Medicare and Medicaid Innovation, which is charged with testing innovative payment models, including the Oncology Care Model. Oversees clinical laboratory services through the Clinical Laboratory Improvements Act.
Centers for Disease Control and Prevention (CDC) Created in 1946 as the Communicable Disease Center.	To protect America from health, safety, and security threats, both foreign and in the US.	National Breast and Cervical Cancer Early Detection Program provides underserved populations access to breast and cervical cancer screening. National Comprehensive Cancer Control Program funds and guides the development of state cancer control plans. National Program of Cancer Registries funds state cancer registries. Colorectal Cancer Control Program funds and promotes colorectal cancer screening.

Agency	Mission	Key Cancer Facts
Agency for Healthcare Research and Quality (AHRQ) Created in 1989 first as the Agency for Health Care Policy and Research.[e]	To produce evidence to make health care safer; higher quality; more accessible, equitable, and affordable; and to work within the HHS and with other partners to make sure that the evidence is understood and used.	AHRQ's CAHPS Cancer Care Survey assesses the experiences of adult patients with cancer treatment provided in outpatient and inpatient settings. Invests and creates material to teach and train health-care systems and professionals to put the results of research into practice. Using AHRQ's research and tools, US health-care systems strive to prevent errors, save lives, and avoid wasteful spending.
Health Resources & Services Administration (HRSA) Created in 1982 through the merger of the Health Resources Administration and the Health Services Administration.[f]	To improve health outcomes and address health disparities through access to quality services, a skilled health workforce, and innovative, high-value programs.	Administers the 340B Program, which was created by Congress in 1992 and mandates manufacturers provide deeply discounted outpatient drugs, many of which are cancer treatments to eligible entities. Oversees the Federal Office of Rural Health Policy, which aids rural hospitals and promotes telehealth programs, which can be critical in connecting cancer patients in rural areas to appropriate specialists.
Office for Human Research Protections (OHRP) Created in 2000 to replace the 1972 Office for Protection from Research Risks under the Federal Policy for the Protection of Human Subjects, known as the Common Rule.[g]	To protect the rights and well-being of human subjects involved in research conducted or supported by the HHS.	Issues regulations and guidance on the protection of human research participants, including the Common Rule, and guidance for appropriate use of and elements included in informed consent for human research participants.

(continues)

TABLE 16.1 *(continued)*

Agency	Mission	Key Cancer Facts
Office of the National Coordinator (ONC) for Health Information Technology Created in 2004 by Executive Order and legislatively authorized in 2009 by the Health Information Technology for Economic and Clinical Health (HITECH) Act.[h]	To improve the health and well-being of individuals and communities through the use of technology and health information that is accessible when and where it matters most.	Leads the national effort to promote the use of EHRs. Issues guidance on how EHRs can be more inter-operable so physicians, hospitals, and patients can better exchange information contained in EHRs.

Notes

[a] US Department of Health and Human Services, "HHS Historical Highlights," retrieved from https://www.hhs.gov/about/historical-highlights/index.html.

[b] "About NIH," National Institutes of Health, accessed April 8, 2021, https://www.nih.gov/about-nihhttps://www.nih.gov.

[c] National Cancer Institute, "Important Events in NCI History," retrieved from https://www.nih.gov/about-nih/what-we-do/nih-almanac/national-cancer-institute-nci.

[d] US Food and Drug Administration, "When and Why Was FDA Formed?" retrieved from https://www.fda.gov/about-fda/fda-basics/when-and-why-was-fda-formed.

[e] Agency for Healthcare Research and Quality. "AHRQ Timeline." retrieved from https://www.ahrq.gov/cpi/about/20timeline.html.

[f] Health Resources and Services Administration, "About HRSA," retrieved from https://www.hrsa.gov/about/index.html.

[g] Office of Human Research Protections, "OHRP History," retrieved from https://www.hhs.gov/ohrp/about-ohrp/history/index.html.

[h] Office of the National Coordinator for Health Information Technology, "About ONC," retrieved from https://www.healthit.gov/topic/about-onc.

Addressing Fragmentation—Improving Cancer Care Through Increased Agency Collaboration

Each agency discussed in this chapter plays a critical role in the availability and access to therapies and how care is delivered to cancer patients. However, because of their distinct jurisdictions and varied technical expertise, there is a tendency for agencies to act in silos, merely completing their "step" in the process. This configuration can cause a disconnect in policies and procedures whereas increased collaboration between agencies would eliminate redundancies, reduce confusion amongst stakeholders, speed therapies to patients, and better support providers in their efforts to deliver quality and equitable care to patients. In the 2010 Institute of Medicine (IOM) report *A National Cancer Clinical Trials System for the 21st Century: Reinvigorating the NCI Cooperative Group Program,*[22] an expert panel recommended formation of a transagency task force to streamline and harmonize government oversight and regulation of cancer clinical trials. We recommend extending this vision beyond clinical trials to all aspects of cancer research and care delivery to create a highly coordinated, fully integrated, and efficient national enterprise to ensure that quality cancer care is available to all people with cancer.

The following are three examples where increased collaboration among federal agencies could mitigate current practices that slow or unnecessarily complicate the delivery of care to cancer patients.

Scenario 1

Key agencies that oversee facets of cancer clinical trials (NCI, FDA, OHRP, and others) should coordinate review across agencies during protocol development to increase efficiencies and reduce administrative burdens.

The 2010 IOM report recognized that the development of a clinical trial and the subsequent review process often requires the investigator to provide the same information to multiple agencies and then resolve disparate reviews and requirements. For example, the NCI funds and approves clinical trial protocols and reviews the progress of a study through the Protocol Review and Monitoring

System. However, if an NCI-sponsored study includes the use of an experimental agent, an IND application is required to be filed with the FDA. The FDA's role in clinical trials is to protect participants who receive investigational treatments and ensure that the trial design is appropriate for the objectives of the study and the intended use of the investigational product. Clinical trial results are an integral part of new product approval and are reviewed by the FDA before a product can be brought to market. OHRP provides oversight of the protection and privacy of research participants in federally sponsored clinical trials and ensures compliance with all HHS research regulations and alignment with ethical principles in research. While these various agencies and oversight bodies have different responsibilities, there is clear overlap and potential for redundancy in the review process that may contribute to the observation that, historically, the average time to design and activate a cancer clinical trial has been nearly three years. The IOM report proposed that the speed and efficiency of designing and launching a clinical trial could be improved by streamlining these regulatory roles. For example, the report recommended that NCI accept the FDA review of NCI-sponsored trials conducted under IND, instead of conducting a separate and independent review. Doing so would potentially greatly reduce the time spent between trial groups, NCI, FDA, and commercial sponsors in adjudicating and resolving multiple agency reviews. NCI took a major step toward reducing redundancy in protocol reviews with the creation of the Central Institutional Review Board (CIRB) in 2001 to review late-phase oncology trials in adults, thereby potentially replacing redundant local IRB reviews conducted at hundreds of institutions across the country that participate in NCI-sponsored trials. Initially voluntary, participation in the NCI CIRB program is now mandatory, and NCI has established four central IRBs that serve more than 2,700 institutions in all fifty states and Puerto Rico.

Scenario 2

The FDA and CMS collaborate on coverage and payment issues before approval.

The FDA and CMS each impact whether new therapies are available to patients in different ways. The FDA is responsible for evaluating the data submitted by a manufacturer to assess the benefits and risks of a medical product to determine whether it meets standards of safety and effectiveness prior to market entry. CMS, on the other hand, determines whether federal programs will reimburse the cost of the drug or device and, if so, how much will be paid for it. These are traditionally sequential steps, creating a gap in the availability of the drug or treatment to patients between approval and coverage determinations. Additionally, each agency uses a different standard to carry out their distinct roles. The FDA is focused on ensuring that a drug is "safe and effective"[23] so as to grant marketing approval, while CMS uses the standard of "reasonable and necessary"[24] when determining whether and how much to pay for a drug or device. While CMS generally covers FDA-approved drugs and devices, coverage is not automatic.[25] As outlined with the CAR-T example discussed earlier, CMS can add coverage requirements and determine payment levels that make it difficult for patients to access a therapy. This bifurcation of roles creates inequities in access to care whereby patients living near a certified site and with the means to make up the differential in payment are able to access a therapy, but others cannot even though it is deemed to be safe, effective, and available for use.

Ideally, determinations of coverage and payment would happen at the same time as approval, with regulators, payers, and manufacturers engaging in discussions about clinical and cost data. In this scenario, announcement of a new drug or device would include clear and consistent guidance on its use, and coverage and payment issues would be determined in advance. As federal partners within HHS, the opportunity and resources to do this are available. The agencies have taken some steps to increase collaboration, but more is needed. For instance, in 2010, the FDA piloted and later made permanent a parallel review process to shorten the amount of time between FDA product approval and CMS coverage decisions. If a manufacturer chooses this path, CMS can review clinical data pre-approval.[26] While a positive step that has yielded some improvement, it is not clear that this process has resulted in a reduced timeline for introduction of most products. Additionally, in 2019, the FDA, CMS, and CDC announced a tri-agency task force to enable deployment of diagnostic tests in a public health emergency. By standardizing collaboration efforts through a taskforce, the federal partners sought to address issues related to implementation of diagnostic tests authorized for emergency use under an Emergency Use Authorization, as well as other unmet needs and gaps in preparing and responding to global health threats. The task force also provides a forum for each agency to coordinate, consult on, and improve the availability of diagnostic tests during public health emergencies, such as the COVID-19 pandemic. Modeling this agency collaboration could assist agencies in refining and streamlining interagency approaches to assessing the safety and effectiveness of therapies.[27]

Scenario 3

Clinical and claims datasets and analyses are collected in a consistent manner and shared across a network of private and public stakeholders to advance understanding and knowledge of cancer in real-world practice.

Because cancer discoveries are reaching patients with unprecedented speed, many gaps persist in understanding their real-world effectiveness. Rigorous postmarket data collection could yield even more insight into the effectiveness and safety of new treatments, particularly in populations not represented in clinical trials. It could also help identify clinical trends and inform clinical guidance. Several data collection efforts and clinical registries seek to achieve these aims. For example, the Surveillance, Epidemiology, and End Results registries, run by NCI, collect population-based data on cancer incidence and surveillance. This network of registries has been operational since the 1970s and while they include important data for researchers, this data is of limited use because of its incompleteness and variable reporting. In the nonprofit sector, the American Society of Clinical Oncology (ASCO) created CancerLinQ to aggregate data from providers to yield clinically meaningful insights.[28] Inspired by the IOM recommendation for a rapid-learning health-care system, CancerLinQ enables real-time, practice-level data collection and analysis. Although CancerLinQ contains more than two million cancer patient records as of this writing, it is limited by a lack of integration with other data registries and the need for extensive manual curation of unstructured clinical data to extract meaningful insights. Both problems could be mitigated by widespread adoption of a universal data dictionary and coding system across EHRs, such as the Minimum Common Oncology Data Elements (mCODE) codeveloped by ASCO.[29] Both the ONC and CMS play vital roles in the potential adoption and use of mCODE by EHR vendors and health-care systems. A national initiative to share data across clinicians, researchers, government, and patients is likely necessary to stimulate such action. The cross-agency task force that released the Cancer Moonshot Blue Ribbon Panel Report envisioned much of this national infrastructure in its recommendation for a "National Cancer Data Ecosystem," as detailed in its 2016 report.[30] The Enhanced Data Sharing Working Group of the task force examined data collaborations across the country and concluded additional integration and coordination is necessary to allow for the contribution, sharing, and full analyses of datasets. At present, it is unclear if and how implementation of these recommendations is proceeding.

Bringing It All Together

The US health-care system has been criticized for not operating as a unified "system." Duplicative oversight caused by overlapping jurisdictions or lack of coordination can create obstacles for researchers and clinicians, slowing progress in the delivery of quality care to cancer patients. That said, meaningful reform aimed at breaking down silos is possible as demonstrated by the creation of the FDA's OCE that brings together scientists and clinicians with expertise in oncology drugs and devices from across the agency into a single center charged with organizing and conducting the review of all oncology products. Identifying opportunities for further innovation, including by better coordinating NCI and FDA review processes for clinical trials and harmonizing data collection across programs and agencies, is essential as we look to the next fifty years of cancer research and care in America.

The federal government has a critical role in supporting cancer research and ensuring care reaches the people who need it. Federal funding for cancer research has led to significant, life-changing advances, as demonstrated by the development, approval, and delivery of innovative CAR-T immunotherapy. As of 2019, advances in cancer prevention, detection, diagnosis, treatment, and quality of life for patients has led to 16.9 million survivors of cancer in the US. The ASCO National Cancer Opinion Survey found that 73 percent of Americans support the government spending more on finding treatments and cures for cancer.[31] The breakthroughs that have been made against cancer provide hope for the future and fuel public expectation for a continued, steady rate of progress to conquer cancer over the coming decades. Delivering on this promise requires reexamining the structure, functions, and relationships among the federal agencies charged with supporting and overseeing the nation's cancer care and research enterprise.

APPENDIX A.
TIMELINE OF US FEDERAL GOVERNMENT ROLE AND MAJOR EVENTS IN THE DEVELOPMENT OF CAR-T THERAPY

US Government Role in
Research, Development, and Care Delivery

Timeline of Major Events Utilizing the Topical Example CAR-T Therapy[32]
1906   Food and Drug Administration (FDA) created by the Pure Food and Drugs Act.
1930   National Institutes of Health (NIH) created in 1930 as the National Institute of Health out of the Public Health Service's Hygienic Laboratory.

1937 National Cancer Institute (NCI) created by the National Cancer Act of 1937.

1946 Centers for Disease Control and Prevention (CDC) created as the Communicable Disease Center.

1953 Department of Health and Human Services (HHS) created as a cabinet-level Department of Health, Education, and Welfare by President Eisenhower, becoming HHS in 1980.

1961 Origin of T cells discovered.

1971 National Cancer Act of 1971 becomes law.

President Nixon signs the National Cancer Act that leads to a major expansion of cancer research efforts in the US. The act provided unprecedented levels of funding for the National Cancer Institute and directed the NCI to expand federal cancer research facilities and award new research grants.

1973 First "immunotherapy" treatment using bone marrow stem cells to replace patient's blood cells after chemotherapy.

1977 What would become the Centers for Medicare and Medicaid Services (CMS) established as the Health Care Financing Administration (HCFA) to manage the Medicare and Medicaid programs. The HCFA was renamed CMS in 2001.

1982 Health Resources & Services Administration (HRSA) created through the merger of the Health Resources Administration and the Health Services Administration.

1986 National Cancer Institute team, including Steven Rosenberg, treated patients with tumor-infiltrating lymphocytes. These cells are removed from a tumor and expanded in the lab before going back into the patient. This demonstrated a patient's own immune cells can attack cancer cells.

1989 Agency for Healthcare Research and Quality (AHRQ) created, initially known as the Agency for Health Care Policy and Research.

1992   Massachusetts Institute of Technology immunologist
       Michel Sadelain and colleagues, funded by several National
       Cancer Institute research grants, begins T cell engineering
       using newly developed genetic engineering tools to
       introduce genes into T cells.

1993   T cells engineered with first chimeric molecule to become
       known as the first-generation chimeric antigen receptors
       (CARs).[33]

2000   Office for Human Research Protections (OHRP) created
       to replace the 1972 Office for Protection from Research
       Risks under the Federal Policy for the Protection of Human
       Subjects, known as the Common Rule.

2002   Memorial Sloan Kettering Cancer Center team, including
       Michel Sadelain, Isabelle Rivière, and Renier Brentjens,
       becomes CAR-T therapy pioneers by building the first
       effective CARs targeted against a prostate cancer antigen.

2003   Second-generation CARs built in mouse model
       demonstrating the effectiveness of human CD19-directed
       CAR-Ts to kill leukemia cells.

2004   Office of the National Coordinator (ONC) for Health
       Information Technology created by Executive Order.
       ONC was legislatively authorized in 2009 by the Health
       Information Technology for Economic and Clinical Health
       (HITECH) Act.

2013   Utilizing a National Cancer Institute R01 and several other
       federal research project grants, Memorial Sloan Kettering
       Cancer Center team has its first published study using
       CAR-Ts to treat acute lymphoblastic leukemia (ALL).

2014   The US Food and Drug Administration grants Breakthrough
       Designation to CD19-directed CAR-Ts to expedite the
       development and review of the therapy intended to treat a
       serious disease or condition.

2017   The US Food and Drug Administration approves CD19-directed CAR-Ts for the treatment of relapsed, refractory acute lymphoblastic leukemia in children and young adults.

2019   The Centers for Medicare and Medicaid Services national coverage decision to allow more patient access to CAR-T therapy for cancers.

APPENDIX B.
MAJOR FEDERAL GOVERNMENT AGENCIES INVOLVED IN CANCER RESEARCH AND CARE DELIVERY

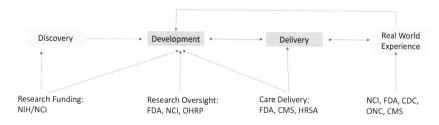

Major Federal Government Agencies Involved in Cancer Research and Care Delivery

Notes

1. The views expressed in this chapter are those of the authors and do not represent the views, positions, or policies of the American Society of Clinical Oncology.

2. "HHS Historical Highlights," HHS.gov, last modified January 21, 2021, https://www.hhs.gov/about/historical-highlights/index.html.

3. "About NIH," National Institutes of Health, accessed April 8, 2021, https://www.nih.gov/about-nih.

4. Judith A. Johnson and Kavya Sekar, "The National Institutes of Health (NIH): Background and Congressional Issues," Congressional Research Services report R41705, updated April 19, 2019, https://fas.org/sgp/crs/misc/R41705.pdf.

5. See Appendix A for additional major timeline events in the development of this cancer therapy.

6. "Foundation for CAR T-Cell Therapy Yescarta" National Institutes of Health Intramural Research Program, accessed April 8, 2021, https://irp.nih.gov /accomplishments/foundation-for-car-t-cell-therapy-yescarta.

7. "National Cancer Institute," NIH.gov, last modified November 27, 2019, https://www.nih.gov/about-nih/what-we-do/nih-almanac/national-cancer -institute-nci.

8. "NCI-Designated Cancer Centers," Cancer.gov, last modified June 24, 2019, www.cancer.gov/research/nci-role/cancer-centers.

9. Geoff Watts, "Jacques Miller: Immunologist Who Discovered Role of the Thymus," *Lancet* 378, no. 9799 (2011): 1290, https://doi.org/10.1016/S0140 -6736(11)61565-1.

10. Jessica Hartmann et al., "Clinical Development of CAR T-Cells— Challenges and Opportunities in Translating Innovative Treatment Concepts," *EMBO Molecular Medicine* 9, no. 9 (2017): 1183–1197, https://doi.org/10.15252 /emmm.201607485.

11. "NCI Initiative Aims to Boost CAR T-Cell Therapy Clinical Trials," *Cancer Currents* Blog, Cancer.gov, April 23, 2020, https://www.cancer.gov/news -events/cancer-currents-blog/2020/car-t-cell-nci-manufacturing-clinical-trials.

12. "When and Why Was FDA Formed?" FDA.gov, last modified March 28, 2018, https://www.fda.gov/about-fda/fda-basics/when-and-why-was-fda -formed.

13. Tufts Center for the Study of Drug Development, "Analysis and Insight into Critical Drug Development Issues," *Tufts CSDD Impact Report* 21, no. 5 (2019).

14. *Advancing Health through Innovation. New Drug Therapy Approvals 2019* (Silver Spring, MD: US Food and Drug Administration, 2020), https://www .fda.gov/media/134493/download.

15. "Fast Track, Breakthrough Therapy, Accelerated Approval, Priority Re-view," FDA.gov, last modified February 23, 2018, https://www.fda.gov/patients /learn-about-drug-and-device-approvals/fast-track-breakthrough-therapy -accelerated-approval-priority-review.

16. Sharyl J. Nass, Harold L. Moses, and John Mendelsohn, eds., *A National Cancer Clinical Trials System for the 21st Century: Reinvigorating the NCI Cooper-ative Group Program* (Washington, DC: The National Academies Press, 2010), https://doi.org/10.17226/12879.

17. Federal Food, Drug, and Cosmetic Act, 21 U.S.C. §§ 301–92 Suppl. 5, 1934, https://www.loc.gov/item/uscode1934-006021009/.

18. Social Security Act, 42 U.S.C. §§ 301–1305 Suppl. 4, 1935, https://www .loc.gov/item/uscode1934-005042007/.

19. "About HRSA," HRSA.gov, last modified October 2019, https://www .hrsa.gov/about/index.html.

20. "History," HHS.gov, last modified June 18, 2020, https://www.hhs.gov /ohrp/about-ohrp/history/index.html.

21. "About ONC," HealthIT.gov, last modified March 12, 2021, https://www .healthit.gov/topic/about-onc.

22. Nass, Moses, and Mendelsohn, *A National Cancer Clinical Trials System for the 21st Century.*

23. 21 U.S.C. §§ 301–92 Suppl. 5.

24. 42 U.S.C. §§ 301–1305 Suppl. 4.

25. James D. Chambers, Katherine E. May, and Peter J. Neumann, "Medicare Covers the Majority of FDA-Approved Devices and Part B Drugs, but Restrictions and Discrepancies Remain," *Health Affairs* 32, no. 6 (2013): 1109–1115, https://doi.org/10.1377/hlthaff.2012.1073.

26. Scott Gottlieb, "New Program with Payors Aims to Accelerate Patient Access to Medical Devices," FDA.gov, September 5, 2018, https://www.fda.gov/news-events/fda-voices/new-program-payors-aims-accelerate-patient-access-medical-devices.

27. "FDA, CDC, and CMS Launch Task Force to Help Facilitate Rapid Availability of Diagnostic Tests During Public Health Emergencies," FDA.gov, February 26, 2019, https://www.fda.gov/news-events/press-announcements/fda-cdc-and-cms-launch-task-force-help-facilitate-rapid-availability-diagnostic-tests-during-public.

28. Danielle Potter et al., "Development of CancerLinQ, a Health Information Learning Platform from Multiple Electronic Health Record Systems to Support Improved Quality of Care," *JCO Clinical Cancer Informatics* 4 (2020): 929–37, https://doi.org/10.1200/CCI.20.0064.

29. Travis J. Osterman, May Terry, and Robert S. Miller, "Improving Cancer Data Interoperability: The Promise of the Minimal Common Oncology Data Elements (mCODE) Initiative," *JCO Clinical Cancer Informatics* 4 (2020): 993–1001, https://doi.org/10.1200/CCI.20.00059.

30. Blue Ribbon Panel for the Cancer Moonshot, *Cancer Moonshot Blue Ribbon Panel Report 2016*, Cancer.gov, last modified October 17, 2016, https://www.cancer.gov/research/key-initiatives/moonshot-cancer-initiative/blue-ribbon-panel/blue-ribbon-panel-report-2016.pdf.

31. "Federally Funded Cancer Research," ASCO.org, accessed April 9, 2021, https://www.asco.org/advocacy/advocacy-agenda-initiatives/federally-funded-cancer-research.

32. American Society of Clinical Oncology, "Cancer Progress Timeline: Research and Guidelines Cancer Progress," retrieved from www.asco.org; Memorial Sloan Kettering Cancer Center, "CAR T-Cells: Timeline of Progress," retrieved from www.mskcc.org.

33. C. H. June et al., "CAR T-Cell Immunotherapy for Human Cancer," *Science* (March 23, 2018), 1361–1365.

CHAPTER 17

The Fifty States of Cancer

Cary Gross and Deborah Schrag

Under the Tenth Amendment to the United States Constitution, state and local governments retain the primary responsibility for public health. With advances in modern medicine and health systems infrastructure, states have assumed broad roles at the intersection of the War on Cancer and the promotion of public health, including vaccination campaigns against cancer-causing pathogens, surveillance and reporting of cancer epidemiologic data, public health education campaigns, and even major litigation efforts against menaces to public health, such as the tobacco industry.

At the same time, the federal government has gradually taken an ever larger role in health policy, particularly with regard to cancer. The federal government is an essential contributor to national cancer control efforts through supporting cancer research, collecting and publishing epidemiologic data, and directly funding and providing cancer care. Two federal insurance programs, Medicare

Cary Gross is Professor of Medicine (General Medicine) and Epidemiology (Chronic Diseases) as well as Director of the Cancer Outcomes Public Policy and Effectiveness Research (COPPER) Center at Yale School of Medicine and Yale Cancer Center.

Deborah Schrag is Professor of Medicine at Harvard Medical School, and Chief of the Division of Population Sciences and Medical Oncologist at Dana-Farber Cancer Institute.

and Medicaid, pay for the care of approximately 70 percent of new cancer patients each year.[1]

The federal government also plays a major role in cancer surveillance and prevention efforts (e.g., the Centers for Disease Control and Prevention [CDC] and the US Preventive Services Task Force [PSTF]). The National Cancer Institute (NCI), founded in 1937, has grown to support a nationwide network of seventy-one Cancer Centers and is the largest funder of basic and translational cancer research.

Despite these growing federal responsibilities, vast federal spending initiatives, and high-profile federal legislation, states play a central role in the cancer space. At the highest level, states build on the regulatory floor and priorities set by the federal government. However, some responsibilities, such as physician licensure, lie almost entirely with the states. Municipalities and localities also play a part in cancer prevention and control, such as establishing local ordinances and zoning restrictions on smoking. Additionally, even when federal regulations specify insurance coverage requirements, such as Medicaid, there can still be substantial variability across states. For example, states may apply for "State Innovation Waivers," waiving some Affordable Care Act (ACA) requirements and allowing for innovative health insurance regulation.

The question is not whether state leaders *can* impact the burden of cancer within their borders, but *how* they choose to exercise this power. States are given wide latitude to set cancer control priorities according to local needs, resources, and culture. The substantial variation across states with respect to the choice of levers used to address cancer, and the precise strategies pursued, lays a critical groundwork for success—or failure—in progress against cancer at the state level. First and foremost, intensive state engagement in cancer prevention and treatment have been found to decrease cancer incidence and mortality. Further, cancer treatments impose a substantial financial burden on state Medicaid budgets, reinforcing the need for providing effective, efficient care for state Medicaid populations. Additionally, states contribute millions of dollars to cancer research and public health surveillance initiatives.

This chapter contends that fully federalizing the landscape of cancer care in the US is neither possible nor desirable. The federal government can identify best practices, establish metrics, set standards, and develop resources to support states' cancer control efforts. What it cannot do, however, is efficiently address state heterogeneity in cancer risk factors, cultural norms, behaviors, and health-care delivery infrastructure. The states function as laboratories for innovation in and investigation of population-wide policy changes in cancer control. In the course of such innovation, states have made and will inevitably continue to make politically motivated health policy choices that are not in the interest of public health. While we acknowledge this ongoing problem, we argue both for ways to mitigate it by properly aligning state incentives, and contend that any remaining harm done by such choices is outweighed by the opportunities presented by allowing the states the freedom to innovate and tailor cancer care to local population needs.

State Involvement in Cancer Prevention, Screening, Diagnosis, and Treatment

The burden of cancer at the population level varies widely between states. For example, although colorectal cancer mortality rates have declined since the 1970s, the decline has been significantly more rapid in northeastern states than in southern states.[2] While the cause of this variation is multifactorial, the decrease in mortality is strongly correlated with uptake of colorectal cancer screening. Differential implementation of cancer prevention, screening, and treatment strategies between states underlies variations in cancer mortality. National analyses of cancer registry data reveal a "cancer belt" in the southeastern US where mortality from the most common cancers, particularly lung and colorectal, remain higher than in other parts of the country. These states have populations with higher rates of smoking, obesity, and uninsurance; lower uptake of screening; and were also less likely to expand Medicaid after passage of the ACA. To support health insurance expansion that would help eradicate the "cancer belt," the federal government

TABLE 17.1 State Laws Mandating Private Insurance Coverage of Various Cancer-Related Benefits

Benefit	Utah	Ohio	Florida	Texas	New York	California
Prevention						
Smoking cessation	-	-	-	-	-	Y
Human papillomavirus vaccine	-	-	-	-	Y	Y
Screening						
Cervical	-	-	-	Y	Y	Y
Colorectal	-	-		Y	-	Y
Mammography	-	Y	Y	Y	Y	Y
Ovarian	-	-	-	Y	-	Y
Prostate	-	-	-	Y	Y	Y
Treatment						
Oral chemotherapy parity	Y	Y	Y	Y	Y	Y
Clinical trials	-	Y	Y	Y	Y	Y
Infertility	-	-	-	-	Y	Y
Long-term care/ hospice	-	-	-	-	Y	Y

"Y" indicates "Yes."

should use economic levers to support states' public health efforts through provision of matching dollars and funds to support health insurance expansion.

Ideally, states reduce the burden of cancer by supporting policies in the realms of prevention, screening, and treatment. One of the most common levers used by states is the promulgation of laws requiring insurers to cover cancer-related benefits, otherwise known as "cancer mandates." Table 17.1 displays the variation in these laws for six large states representing different regions and policies.

Prevention

Cancer prevention efforts, particularly those related to tobacco cessation, are quite effective. States utilize many different levers in pursuing prevention efforts. To reduce lung and other tobacco-associated cancers, states leverage excise taxes, insurance coverage and direct provision of free care, and education campaigns. For the prevention of cervical cancer, a number of states use insurance mandates, and many rely on widespread education and public messaging campaigns.

Although the federal government plays a key role in identifying and recommending effective preventive strategies, largely through the PSTF, states are generally responsible for the implementation of prevention programs. Recognizing that it was insufficient simply to set national goals and leave it to states to determine whether and how to achieve them, the CDC began encouraging states to develop individual cancer control plans in 1998. Today, each state has such a plan. Although all states contribute to national priorities set each decade as part of the "Healthy People 2020 goals," each state sets an additional slate of cancer control goals and metrics based on its distinctive priorities. Cancer is unique in this regard, likely due to variability across states in willingness to address cancer risk factors (tobacco, environmental, dietary) and access to care, as well as the strong advocacy community in cancer, which provides local, grassroots ideas and energy to cancer control plans. Notably, this contrasts with cardiovascular disease policy, which tends to conform to national priorities set by the CDC.

State cancer control plans set benchmarks and prioritize specific cancers with high incidence, mortality, or rates of disparities based on data collected by the state's cancer registry. In addition, they rely on the Behavioral Risk Factor Survey System that tracks individual patients' tobacco use, alcohol use, weight, and participation in cancer screening and prevention. States set goals based on survey responses among their residents. However, there is no uniform federal framework for the content or evaluation of state cancer plans, making cross-state comparisons difficult. Centralizing this process in the federal government could enable states to retain some autonomy in prioritizing specific goals yet facilitate more nimble execution and enable states to learn from each other's experiences about which implementation strategies are most successful. The federal government should use policy levers to establish goals and benchmarks for state plans and to support data collection, measurement, and continuous performance feedback. This could eliminate the need for creation of redundant infrastructure, which is a particular strain on less affluent states. Moreover, more federally coordinated, systematic study of the effects of state-level policy innovations should allow for states to share knowledge about best practices.

Policies related to tobacco use reduction are key components of cancer control plans and have been tremendously successful. The CDC estimates that since 1990, roughly 1.3 million cancer deaths have been avoided because of a reduction in tobacco use alone.[3] The population of Americans smoking cigarettes declined by over 5 percent from 2005 to 2015, and state preventive efforts have been central to that progress. The federal government, states, and cities all control the amount of excise taxes placed on cigarette purchases, for a national average tax rate of $1.82 per pack. While the federal cigarette tax is $1.01 per pack, state taxes vary from $0.17 in Missouri to $4.50 in Washington, DC, with the highest combined state-local tax rate at $7.16 in Chicago, Illinois.[4] The 2020 Surgeon General's Report on Smoking Cessation found that a 20 percent increase in the unit price of tobacco products led to a 14.8 percent decrease in demand among young people aged thirteen to twenty-nine.[5] In addition to excise taxes, localities are also able to enact smoking bans, such as in restaurants and bars. Studies show that bans are most effective in preventing social smoking, and taxes are more effective at deterring heavy smoking.[6]

States also support tobacco-related cancer prevention activities. Every state maintains a tobacco quitline, which can help individuals stop smoking by offering counseling and medication. Qualification standards for these programs and the treatments offered vary widely by state. For example, Florida provides only nicotine patches free of charge via its quitline, and only to individuals aged eighteen and older. Texas, by comparison, covers nicotine gum and lozenges in addition to the patch.[7] Concurrently, states carry out mass-media campaigns driving smokers to quitlines and encouraging cessation. The Surgeon General's Report found that the benefit-to-cost ratio for these campaigns ranged from 7:1 to 74:1, with an estimated cost of $213 per life year saved.[8]

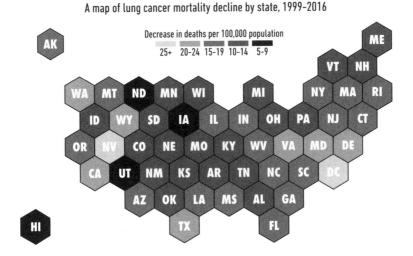

A map of lung cancer mortality decline by state, 1999-2016

Decrease in deaths per 100,000 population
25+   20-24   15-19   10-14   5-9

FIGURE 17.1 State Variation in Trends in Lung Cancer Mortality, 1999–2016

The impact of these public health efforts can be profound. For instance, the decline in lung cancer death rates during the first fifteen years of the twenty-first century varies as much as five-fold across states, as shown in Figure 17.1, and has largely been attributed to variation across states in antitobacco policies. Cancer control plans, with millions of health-care dollars at stake, should be viewed by states and the federal government as mission-critical plans, rather than aspirational frameworks. The federal government, or such agencies as the Department of Defense, Veterans Affairs, or the Patient-Centered Outcomes Research Institute (PCORI) should incentivize states to collaborate through the design, conduct, and reporting of systematic trials that compare alternative policies and approaches to cancer control. The federal government, via the CDC, should provide a clearinghouse to display state approaches and to enable states to benefit from both the successful and unsuccessful strategies adopted by other regions.

Human papillomavirus (HPV), which causes almost all cervical cancers, is another target of state prevention efforts. Only two of six surveyed states mandate private insurance coverage of HPV vaccines (see Table 17.1),[9] although these vaccines are associated with a nearly 100 percent reduction in cervical, vulvar, and vaginal disease related to the most common types of HPV. The ACA mandates coverage of the vaccines for private plans, but millions of Americans remain uncovered by the ACA. The federal government could accelerate cancer control efforts by providing infrastructure that would allow states to address fundamental pragmatic policy questions. For instance, a consortium of states could agree to systematically compare two alternative policies for controlling HPV. In this situation, some states could promote administration of HPV vaccines by school nurses, whereas others would require administration by physicians. Using pragmatic study designs, these alternative approaches could be compared to understand how they compare with respect to the incidence of HPV-associated cancers.

Increasingly, obesity is replacing tobacco as the most common modifiable risk factor for cancer. As is the case with several cancer-related risk factors and behaviors, the prevalence of obesity varies substantially across states. However, state-specific regulation of obesity is still in its infancy, and relatively few states have implemented taxes on sugar-containing beverages, a major contributor to the obesity epidemic. The ACA contained several measures to foster transparency in disclosure of nutritional content, but these have not been widely implemented. State policies that influence obesity rates include regulating the content of school lunches, the required amount of physical activity in the school day, and policies surrounding labeling menus with calorie counts. Some states have implemented mandatory disclosure of calorie counts on menus, whereas others have passed legislation specifically banning such disclosures as an infringement on free speech. Prevention of obesity is a new frontier in cancer prevention, and states will play an important role in developing policies that promote population health. The federal government should establish toolkits, longitudinal funding sources, and infrastructure for states while allowing them to appropriately tailor implementation to their populations' needs. States would benefit from shared expertise in data infrastructure, data management software, and visualization tools to help public health leaders track key metrics, such as the rates of obesity and tobacco use, as well as the uptake of screening.

Screening

Although states use a variety of levers to encourage uptake of cancer screening, mandated insurance coverage statutes again play a critical role. Other levers, many of which are laid out in detail in states' comprehensive cancer control plans, include education and outreach programs, targeted grant funding, and direct provision of free or low-cost screening services.

Most recommended cancer screening is covered by federal insurance law, such as the Breast and Cervical Prevention and Treatment Act of 2000. That act allows states to offer low-income and underinsured women access to treatment through Medicaid if they are diagnosed with cancer through the National Breast and Cervical Cancer Early Detection Program (NBCCEDP), which is administered by the CDC. Above the federal floor, state law provides key protections for individuals covered by many private plans. State laws mandating coverage of screening modalities are more common than those covering preventive treatment, with mandated coverage of mammography the most common benefit. States vary widely in their selection of mandated coverage statutes (see Table 17.1). For instance, Utah has no statutes mandating coverage of the surveyed screening modalities, whereas New York statutes mandate coverage of all of them.

Widespread education and outreach campaigns designed to further increase uptake of recommended screening, coupled with targeted grant programs, also form part of the bedrock of state screening efforts. The NBCCEDP helps states to fund patient navigators and community health workers to target nonmedical barriers to enhanced screening. On the Fond du Lac Indian Reservation in Minnesota, for example, the NBCCEDP partners with a clinic to send birthday cards to women who are due for breast cancer screening.[10] The CDC also provides targeted grants to states related to breast, cervical, and colorectal cancer screening, among other types of cancer. It works with states to develop cancer control plans that emphasize concrete actions to achieve enhanced adherence to screening guidelines formulated by the PSTF.

Studies suggest that such mandates are modestly effective at increasing screening rates.[11] Even the ACA, which required the majority of insurance plans to cover recommended cancer screening, had similarly modest results, indicating that the costs of screening may not be the primary barrier to wider uptake.[12] To discover the most effective ways to encourage screening, we need more opportunities for states to share best practices, and pragmatic trials that compare different interventions or program rollout across different states and regions, thus improving the evidence base for cancer control policies. The federal government can use its convening power to create a platform that allows states to learn from each other's successes and failures and incentivize states to innovate and set and achieve ambitious goals for reducing the burden of cancer population-wide.

Treatment

Whether and how much a person's insurance covers cancer treatment dramatically alters their experience and outcomes of cancer at the state level, as do laws related to the provision of care itself. State laws mandating coverage of certain therapies often offer broader coverage than that required by federal law and regulate insurance plans not reached by federal requirements, as discussed earlier.

Coverage of infertility treatment is a clear example of the influence of state insurance law. Both chemotherapy and radiation—common treatment modalities for cancer—have the potential to cause infertility in cancer patients. As a result, women of child-bearing age who undergo cancer treatment may wish to bank eggs or embryos prior to treatment or may require in vitro fertilization or other advanced fertility procedures after completion of treatment. However, treatment of cancer-related infertility is not one of the essential health benefits set under the ACA. As shown in Table 17.1, only two of the six states surveyed mandate coverage of infertility treatment by most insurance plans. The cost of infertility treatments, often over $10,000, keeps them from being a viable option for many patients in states without such laws.

Long-term care and hospice coverage are more complicated examples of state gap-filling. Medicare, Medicaid, and insurance regulated under the ACA generally cover long-term care and hospice, although with some limits on the length of stay. For the millions of Americans not covered under federally regulated insurance plans, options are more limited. Again, only two of six surveyed states mandate coverage of these benefits by most insurance plans. In states without such coverage, cancer patients under age sixty-five are generally forced to draw down their own assets until they qualify for Medicaid.

Although the ACA is federal law, state implementation choices underscore the importance of state cancer-related policy. Several studies have demonstrated that Medicaid expansion is associated with earlier stage at cancer diagnosis, improved access to cancer care, and better outcomes.[13]

Variations in state laws related to telehealth also create barriers to equitable access to care for cancer patients. One study found that 24 percent of Medicare patients with cancer travel longer than one hour to access their cancer care site.[14] Access to care is particularly burdensome for those living in states with high populations of rural residents. Expanding access to telehealth therefore brings the possibility of improving outcomes for patients in rural areas and reducing travel burdens on all patients, as recent systematic studies have suggested.[15] Despite this potential, as of November 2019, forty-nine states required that physicians engaging in telemedicine be licensed in the state in which the patient lives.[16] Although the Interstate Medical Licensure Compact has attempted to create an expedited licensure process for these states, many states—such as Florida and Texas—have not adopted the process.[17] Furthermore, only six states have parity laws requiring equal reimbursement by private insurers for telemedicine and in-person visits, a disparity that is likely to reduce access to the option. Many states loosened telehealth restrictions during the COVID-19 pandemic, which may lead to improved access to high-quality cancer care. For instance, some of the relaxation in telehealth reimbursement criteria may become permanent after the pandemic has subsided.

State Laws Supporting Patients with Cancer
and Their Families

A cancer diagnosis frequently leads to unemployment, both from the frequency and burden of treatment itself and the long-term consequences of the disease. Studies show that over 50 percent of cancer survivors lose their job or quit working.[18] For cancer patients, the protection of paid sick leave, antidiscrimination laws, and for many, unemployment benefits, is crucial. Three federal laws establish baseline employment protections for many workers, as seen in Table 17.2. However, these laws have significant gaps, giving states a uniquely important role in adding provisions that supplement federal legislation.

The Family Medical Leave Act of 1993, for example, only applies to private employers with over fifty employees, and does not require paid leave. As of January 2020, thirteen states and Washington, DC, provide for paid sick leave.[19] The second key federal law, the Americans with Disabilities Act of 1990 (ADA), prevents employers from discriminating against employees on the basis of disability caused by cancer. However, the ADA only covers employers with fifteen or more employees, leaving state law to regulate smaller employers. The majority of states have antidiscrimination laws mirroring the ADA that cover smaller employers, with a number covering employers with just one employee.

A third federal law, the Consolidated Omnibus Budget Reconciliation Act (COBRA), allows workers who are terminated, quit, or adopt reduced hours to continue their coverage under their employer-sponsored insurance, but employers are not required to cover the cost of insurance. Therefore, under federal law, many workers with cancer are required to pay the full cost of this transitional insurance themselves, plus a 2 percent administrative fee. As of 2018, forty-two states and Washington, DC, have expanded COBRA's protections with so-called mini-COBRA laws.[20] These laws often apply to smaller employers, offer longer periods of coverage, and apply to a broader subset of employees.

State laws, therefore, can provide important protections above the federal floor for both employed and unemployed individuals

TABLE 17.2 Federal and State Employment and Unemployment Benefits, and Availability of State Disability Insurance

State and Federal Legislation Germane to Support of Patients with Cancer

Federal

Family Medical Leave Act	Requires employers to provide certain employees with up to 12 weeks of unpaid, job-protected leave per year[a]
Americans with Disabilities Act (ADA)	Prohibits discrimination on the basis of disability caused by cancer
Consolidated Omnibus Budget Reconciliation Act (COBRA)	Gives employees and their families the right to choose to temporarily continue group health benefits after termination of employment or death of an employee[b]

State	*Utah*	*Ohio*	*Florida*	*Texas*	*New York*	*California*
Employment benefits						
Fair employment law prohibiting discrimination on the basis of disability	–	Y (4)	–	–	Y (4)	Y (5)
Paid sick leave	–	–	–	–	Y[c]	Y[d]
Paid family leave (wks)	–	–	–	–	Y (8)	Y (6)
Unemployment benefits						
Maximum weekly benefit	$580	$480	$275	$521	$504	$450
State maximum weeks	26	26	12	26	26	26
State disability insurance	–	–	–	–	Y	Y

[a] The FMLA applies to employers with 50 or more employees.

[b] COBRA applies to employers with 20 or more employees and extends insurance availability for 18 months in most cases.

[c] Under the FY2021 New York State budget, employers with between 5 and 99 employees and net income over $1 million must provide 40 hours of paid sick leave. Employers with 100+ employees must provide 56 hours.

[d] Minimum of 24 hours for full-time employees. Some cities, such as Los Angeles, have additional sick leave laws.

with cancer, and help to alleviate the burden of disease for a large number of Americans. Increasing protections for individuals is a crucial function of state law, but states also play a major role in cancer research initiatives and public health activities that target cancer at the population level.

State Support of Cancer Research

Although the federal government is the most substantial contributor of funding for cancer research, largely through grants administered by the NCI, state investment remains a major source of financing. A notable example of such investment is the Cancer Prevention and Research Institute of Texas (CPRIT). In 2007, Texas amended its state constitution to establish CPRIT and authorized the issuance of $3 billion in bonds to finance cancer research and prevention services. CPRIT funding has supported over one hundred clinical trials, encouraged twelve companies to move to the state, and resulted in $1.75 billion in follow-on investing by venture capital firms in start-up companies. In 2019, CPRIT was renewed by an overwhelming majority—64 percent of Texas voters supported it—and available funds were doubled to $6 billion.

Another major source of cancer funds for states was the Master Settlement Agreement of 1998 (MSA). The MSA was reached between the four largest tobacco companies and forty-six states after years of high-profile civil litigation relating to the harms caused by tobacco smoke. In exchange for annual payments to the states in perpetuity, the signing states agreed not to bring future legal claims against the companies. States have used these annual payments to contribute millions of dollars to research initiatives, screening and prevention campaigns, and the treatment of low-income uninsured patients. As of 2019, for example, Georgia has received over $3 billion under the MSA, and from 2015 to 2019, devoted 3 percent of these funds to expanding clinical trials in the state.

Unfortunately, state health needs appear to have little effect on the degree of funding allocated to tobacco-control programs, and funds under the MSA are an underutilized resource to prevent smoking-related morbidity.[21] States have great discretion in how tobacco settlement funds are allocated. California, for example, achieves 93.7 percent of CDC-recommended MSA fund spending.[22] In contrast, North Carolina achieves just 2.2 percent of its suggested allocation,[23] and the state has been widely criticized for its misuse of MSA funds.[24]

Finally, several states have required private insurers to reimburse patients for the routine care costs of enrollment in clinical trials. These mandates were associated with a significant increase in early-phase cancer trial enrollment, compared with states that did not require equivalent coverage.[25] Although there is again variation between states in the degree and targets of investment, state funding of cancer research allows for broader and more varied approaches to the disease, increasing the likelihood that successful treatments might be discovered. It also ensures that resources are allocated to understudied cancers and rare diseases.

State Activity Pertaining to Cancer Surveillance, Public Health Infrastructure, and Consumer Protection

States have historically retained primary responsibility for public health, and many of the population-level approaches to cancer surveillance and infrastructure are controlled at the state level. Although the federal government acts to set national priorities and contribute financial resources, implementation of many public health initiatives is driven by state agencies and local health departments, as seen in the earlier discussion of prevention and screening. As with the policies examined there, the federal government could assist state reforms by developing best practices guidelines, investing in interoperable health technology infrastructure, and incorporating successful state strategies into the federal floor.

One example of this cooperation is the collection of cancer data by state cancer registries, a process known as disease surveillance. The National Program of Cancer Registries (NPCR), administered by the CDC, provides funds to states to develop, improve, and standardize their cancer registries, which collect patient demographics, tumor characteristics, treatment modalities, and outcomes for all cancer patients. Before NPCR was established in 1992, only ten states had registries. Today, forty-six states have a cancer registry.[26] Each state administers its own registry and submits its data annually to the CDC. The data collected by these programs are used by stakeholders at the state and federal levels for tracking incidence and prevalence of disease, designing targeted approaches to prevention and screening and public health messaging, and enabling more accurate analysis of the impact of public health initiatives.

States also bear primary responsibility for establishing the form and distribution of health-care infrastructure. Many states—thirty-five as of December 2019—have Certificate of Need (CON) laws requiring state approval of the creation and expansion of major health-care facilities and technologies.[27] These laws attempt to control health-care costs by ensuring a uniform distribution of health-care services and restricting duplicative or unnecessary spending. The effectiveness of these laws is controversial, with some studies showing a potentially problematic reduction in the numbers of available hospital beds with only a modest reduction in expenditures.[28] In recent years, some states have attempted to use CON laws to limit access to novel, expensive, therapies, as Michigan did—unsuccessfully—for CAR-T therapy, a promising cancer treatment.[29] In 2008, Michigan's CON commission allowed only one proton beam center—a facility providing similarly expensive cancer treatments—to open in the state.[30]

State attorneys general (AGs) also play an important role in the layout of public health infrastructure, ensuring quality care, and protecting consumers. State AGs play a critical role in antitrust enforcement, including by preventing problematic consolidation of hospital systems or the use of anticompetitive contract clauses that would lead to increased prices for consumers.[31] Many AGs, including Massachusetts', maintain a consumer helpline dedicated to health care, through which they can receive consumer complaints related to concerns such as product safety, insurance fraud, and billing issues.[32] Mediators can then handle these complaints directly, or forward the complaints for investigation and possible litigation. AGs have returned millions of dollars to cancer patients, as Arizona's AG did in 2019 in an enforcement action against sham cancer charities.[33] They also frequently bring lawsuits against the manufacturers of products found to cause cancer, as they did against the tobacco industry in the 1990s.

―――――

MEANINGFUL PROGRESS AGAINST cancer over the next fifty years will depend in large part on the strength of the federal government's partnership with the states. We believe that an effective collaboration between the states and the federal government will ultimately prove more beneficial to American citizens than either complete federal control of the cancer care landscape or complete state control. The question is not *whether* states exert great control over cancer care in this country, but *how* they do so—and how the federal government might collaborate with the states most effectively.

State Innovation: Improving Care by Demanding Stronger Evidence of Value

States have the potential to be great laboratories of innovation for cancer care. For instance, states can ensure that the value of a cancer therapy is demonstrated before significant public funds are dedicated to its use. New cancer therapies are frequently approved through the FDA Accelerated Approval Program. Although drugs approved in this way are typically required to undergo additional study, there is often substantial uncertainty regarding the true impact of new therapies on clinical outcomes. This is an important challenge to payers and providers: after a cancer therapy is approved by the FDA and included in a "compendium" of approved and recommended treatments, Medicare is obligated to reimburse for the drug. In the US, there is no independent assessment of costs and benefits. In contrast, in the UK, the National Institute for Health and Clinical Excellence is tasked with making treatment recommendations to the National Health Service based on analyses of both the therapeutic effectiveness and the cost effectiveness of drugs. This practice, however, is prohibited within the US Medicare system, and cost-benefit analysis cannot be considered when determining Medicare coverage.

The use of cost effectiveness analyses in Medicare coverage decisions is unlikely to change. However, states are stepping in to fill this policy need and to address public expenditures on medication. In 2017, New York authorized a Medicaid Drug Utilization Review Board to narrow the discrepancies between the prices of prescription drugs and their therapeutic value by setting a drug spending cap on the state Medicaid program. When drug spending is projected to exceed the cap, officials are able to negotiate rebates with drug manufacturers. States can also use strategies, such as directing Medicaid managed care organizations to remove a drug from their formularies or instituting prior authorization requirements.[34] Just because a drug has received accelerated approval from the FDA does not mean a state needs to provide insurance coverage for it on its formulary. The advantage of this approach is that states have the opportunity to exert influence to curb the use of drugs with low benefit and high cost. The challenge is that states need to maintain an infrastructure that includes experts equipped to make these decisions and to handle an administrative appeals process. These bodies must be transparent, include patient representatives, and be capable of withstanding immense pressure. By experimenting with different approaches to formulary management and maximizing the value of prescription drug utilization, innovative state policy can meaningfully advance cancer care.

The Federal Role: Supporting States Through Funding, Standard-Setting Policies, and Consolidating Best Practices

While states are laboratories of health policy, they cannot act effectively without federal guidance and support. In the critical years ahead, the federal government should continue to support states using three key mechanisms. First, the federal government can use economic levers—such as matching dollars and funds to support health insurance expansion—to support states' public health efforts. Second, the federal government can use policy levers to establish benchmarks as well as to support data collection and continuous performance feedback. Third, systematically studying the impact of state policies could encourage states to learn from each other's experiences.

These approaches can be complementary. Providing generous cancer control resources to the states alongside accountability targets will not only support state innovation—it could also generate evidence about successful state strategies. This information could guide federal reforms and be disseminated back to the states through federal agencies, including the Agency for Healthcare Research and Quality, the CDC, PCORI, and the Center for Medicare and Medicaid Innovation, which provide strategic guidance, toolkits, and support for states to develop, test, and implement innovative cancer control policies.

Lastly, the federal government should play a much greater role in incentivizing state cancer control efforts, with clear accountability measures and resources to back them up. Approaches to cancer control can and should vary across states. Yet expectations of demonstrable progress—encouraged by the federal government setting high standards for improving cancer control—should apply to all states. Using federal dollars as a mechanism to reward states that make greater progress against cancer would provide resources and urgency to the cancer control cause. In the next fifty years, federal and state policy makers must work in tandem to treat cancer care as a core priority. Together, the "Fifty States of Cancer" might yet produce a healthier union.

Notes

1. Scott D. Ramsey, "How State and Federal Policies as Well as Advances in Genome Science Contribute to the High Cost of Cancer Drugs," *Health Affairs* 34, no. 4 (2015): 571–575, https://doi.org/10.1377/hlthaff.2015.0112.

2. Deepa Naishadham et al., "State Disparities in Colorectal Cancer Mortality Patterns in the United States," *Cancer Epidemiology, Biomarkers & Prevention* 20, no. 7 (2011): 1296–1302, https://doi.org/10.1158/1055-9965.EPI-11-0250.

3. "Cancers Linked to Tobacco Use Make up 40% of All Cancers Diagnosed

in the United States," CDC.gov, last modified November 10, 2016, https://www
.cdc.gov/media/releases/2016/p1110-vital-signs-cancer-tobacco.html.

4. Ann Boon, "State Cigarette Excise Tax Rates & Rankings," Campaign
for Tobacco-Free Kids, March 15, 2021, https://www.tobaccofreekids.org/assets
/factsheets/0097.pdf.

5. "Tobacco Control Interventions," CDC.gov, last modified June 8, 2017,
https://www.cdc.gov/policy/hst/hi5/tobaccointerventions/index.html.

6. Mike Vuolo, Brian C. Kelly, and Joy Kadowaki, "Independent and Inter-
active Effects of Smoking Bans and Tobacco Taxes on a Cohort of US Young
Adults," *American Journal of Public Health* 106, no. 2 (2016): 370–380, https://doi
.org/10.2105/AJPH.2015.302968.

7. "State Tobacco Cessation Coverage," Lung.org, last modified March 15,
2020,   https://www.lung.org/policy-advocacy/tobacco/cessation/state-tobacco
-cessation-coverage-database/states.

8. "Tobacco Control Interventions."

9. Jason P. Block, "The Calorie-Labeling Saga—Federal Preemption and
Delayed Implementation of Public Health Law," *New England Journal of Medicine* 379 (2018): 103–105, https://doi.org/10.1056/NEJMp1802953.

10. "Promoting Early Detection and Treatment of Cancer," CDC.gov, last
modified June 26, 2020, https://www.cdc.gov/cancer/ncccp/priorities/early
-detection-treatment.htm.

11. Marianne P. Bitler and Christopher S. Carpenter, "Effects of State Cervical Cancer Insurance Mandates on Pap Test Rates," *Health Services Research* 52,
no. 1 (2017): 156–175, https://doi.org/10.1111/1475-6773.12477.

12. Lindsay M. Sabik and Georges Adunlin, "The ACA and Cancer Screening Diagnosis," *Cancer Journal* 23, no. 3 (2017): 151–162, https://doi.org/10.1097
/PPO.0000000000000261.

13. Quyen D. Chu et al., "Positive Impact of the Patient Protection and Affordable Care Act Medicaid Expansion on Louisiana Women with Breast Cancer," *American Cancer Society* 127, no. 5 (2020): 688–699, https://doi.org/10.1002
/cncr.33265; Ying Liu et al., "Association of Medicaid Expansion Under the
Patient Protection and Affordable Care Act with Non-Small Cell Lung Cancer Survival," *JAMA Oncology* 6, no. 8 (2020): 1289–1290, https://doi.org/10.1001
/jamaoncol.2020.1040; Helmneh M. Sineshaw et al., "Association of Medicaid Expansion under the Affordable Care Act with Stage at Diagnosis and
Time to Treatment Initiation for Patients with Head and Neck Squamous Cell
Carcinoma," *JAMA Otolaryngol Head Neck Surgery* 146, no. 3 (2020): 247–255,
https://doi.org/10.1001/jamaoto.2019.4310; Jose Wilson B. Mesquita-Neto et al.,
"Disparities in Access to Cancer Surgery After Medicaid Expansion," *American Journal of Surgery* 219, no. 1 (2020): 181–184, https://doi.org/10.1016/j.amjsurg
.2019.06.023; Tong Gan et al., "Impact of the Affordable Care Act on Colorectal
Cancer Screening, Incidence, and Survival in Kentucky," *Journal of the American
College of Surgery* 228, no. 4 (2019): 342–353.e1, https://doi.org/10.1016/j.jamcoll
surg.2018.12.035.

14. Gabrielle B. Rocque et al., "Impact of Travel Time on Health Care Costs
and Resource Use by Phase of Care for Older Patients with Cancer," *Journal*

of Clinical Oncology 37, no. 22 (2019): 1935–1945, https://doi.org/10.1200/JCO.19 .00175.

15. Anna Cox et al., "Cancer Survivors' Experience with Telehealth: A Systematic Review and Thematic Synthesis," *Journal of Medical Internet Research* 19, no. 1 (2017): e11, https://doi.org/10.2196/jmir.6575.

16. "Telemedicine Policies: Board by Board Overview," Federation of State Medical Boards, last modified July 2020, https://www.fsmb.org/siteassets /advocacy/key-issues/telemedicine_policies_by_state.pdf.

17. Interstate Medical Licensure Compact, accessed April 12, 2021, https:// www.imlcc.org.

18. M. P. van Egmond et al., "Barriers and Facilitators for Return to Work in Cancer Survivors with Job Loss Experience: A Focus Group Study," *European Journal of Cancer Care* 26, no. 5 (2017): e12420, https://doi.org/10.1111/ecc.12420.

19. "Paid Sick Leave," National Conference of State Legislatures, July 21, 2020, https://www.ncsl.org/research/labor-and-employment/paid-sick-leave.aspx.

20. "Federal & State Mini-COBRA Chart," HR Knowledge, last modified February 6, 2018, http://www.hrknowledge.com/wp-content/uploads/2018/02 /Federal_and_State_Mini_COBRA_Chart.pdf.

21. Cary P. Gross et al., "State Expenditures for Tobacco-Control Programs and the Tobacco Settlement," *New England Journal of Medicine* 347 (2002): 1080–1086, https://doi.org/10.1056/NEJMsa012743.

22. "A State-by-State Look at the 1998 Tobacco Settlement 22 Years Later," Campaign for Tobacco-Free Kids, last modified January 15, 2021, https://www .tobaccofreekids.org/what-we-do/us/statereport/.

23. "A State-by-State Look."

24. Alison Snow Jones et al., "Funding of North Carolina Tobacco Control Programs through the Master Settlement Agreement," *American Journal of Public Health* 97 (2005): 36–44, https://doi.org/10.2105/AJPH.2005.070466.

25. Cary P. Gross et al., "Cancer Trial Enrollment After State-Mandated Reimbursement," *Journal of the National Cancer Institute* 96, no. 14 (2004): 1063–1069, https://doi.org/10.1093/jnci/djh193.

26. "About the [National] Program [of Cancer Registries (NPCR)]," CDC .gov, last modified July 1, 2018, https://www.cdc.gov/cancer/npcr/about.htm.

27. Robert A. Berenson et al., *Addressing Health Care Market Consolidation and High Prices* (San Francisco: Urban Institute, 2020), 46, https://www.urban .org/sites/default/files/publication/101508/addressing_health_care_market _consolidation_and_high_prices_1.pdf.

28. Berenson et al., *Addressing Health Care Market Consolidation*, 45–49.

29. Lindsay Killen and Naomi Lopez, "Cancer Therapy Dispute Highlights Need to Repeal CON Laws," November 16, 2019, https://thehill.com/opinion /healthcare/470316-cancer-therapy-dispute-highlights-need-to-repeal-con -laws.

30. Andrew Pollack, "States Limit Costly Sites for Cancer Radiation," *New York Times*, May 1, 2008, https://www.nytimes.com/2008/05/01/technology/01 proton.html.

31. Berenson et al., *Addressing Health Care Market Consolidation*.

32. "Health Care Resources at the Attorney General's Office," Mass.gov, accessed April 13, 2021, https://www.mass.gov/health-care-resources-at-the-attorney-generals-office.

33. "AG Brnovich Announces $2.5 Million of Sham Cancer Charity Funds Will Go to Real Cancer Charities," Arizona Attorney General, June 20, 2019, https://www.azag.gov/press-release/ag-brnovich-announces-25-million-sham-cancer-charity-funds-will-go-real-cancer.

34. Claudio Jommi et al., "Implementation of Value-Based Pricing for Medicines," *Clinical Therapeutics* 42, no. 1 (2020): 15–24, https://doi.org/10.1016/j.clinthera.2019.11.006.

CHAPTER 18

Cancer and Congress

Hon. Rosa L. DeLauro and Abbe R. Gluck

The past, present, and future of cancer is shaped by the government, and every actor in government has a unique role to play. The president is the convener in chief, uniquely positioned to galvanize industry and scientists to work together, set bold goals, and push a bureaucracy that might otherwise be reluctant to change. That bureaucracy plays an outsized role in prevention and treatment, comprising officials ranging from scientists to regulators overseeing every aspect of the cancer-treatment research and delivery process. The states have assumed central roles in the promotion of public health. And then there is Congress.

Many roads in Cancerland run through Congress. Access to insurance is key to receiving cancer preventative care and treatment, and the central insurance-reform laws that Congress has enacted—such as the Affordable Care Act, which dramatically expands access to cancer screening and treatment—have been transformative in the cancer space. Through legislation, including the 1971 National Cancer Act that launched the war on cancer, Congress has helped create the modern cancer research and care delivery landscape,

---

Rosa L. DeLauro is a United States congresswoman for Connecticut's 3rd Congressional District.

Abbe R. Gluck is the Alfred M. Rankin Professor of Law and the founding Faculty Director of the Solomon Center for Health Law and Policy at Yale Law School; she is also Professor of Medicine at Yale School of Medicine.

and subsequent laws impact issues ranging from access to health care to protecting patient data privacy and encouraging the expedited development of potentially lifesaving treatments. Sometimes, Congress highlights specific cancers; sometimes, it focuses on the general research mission. Advocates have a central role to play here; their lobbying efforts before Congress have led to laws that prompted breakthroughs in cancer care, such as the development of new pediatric cancer drugs and treatments for other rare diseases.

Perhaps most significant, Congress holds the federal purse strings—doling out funds at a level no other actor could hope to match. Its funding efforts help set priorities for the research community and, whether intentionally or not, what Congress funds tells the country what is "important." Basic research versus translational research? Drug development versus prevention? One cancer over another? And so on. This chapter looks back at Congress's overarching work in the cancer space over the past half century, and then turns its focus to its role as funder. One of us is a cancer survivor who has served in Congress for thirty years and is now chair of the House Committee on Appropriations—much of this chapter comes from that perspective.

Congress and Cancer in America: An (Abridged) Early History

Congress has defined the cancer space for decades. While presidents have at times received outsize attention for signing landmark legislation into law, it is often members of Congress who deserve significant credit for getting bills to the Oval Office in the first place. This proved true for one of the first seminal acts related to cancer.

On August 5, 1937—decades before the National Cancer Act of 1971—President Franklin Delano Roosevelt signed the National Cancer Act.[1] FDR's role in the establishment of the National Cancer Institute (NCI)—though important—was secondary to that played by two senators and a congressman. Matthew Neely, a senator from West Virginia, first took up the drive to address cancer in the late 1920s. Having noticed an uptick in deaths attributed to cancer—rising from 70,000 in 1911 to 115,000 by 1927—Neely pushed for congressional work in this area, culminating in the 1937 effort to establish a federal agency specifically dedicated to treating cancer.

The search for cancer research funds was central to Neely's mission, but so was institutional design—a vision of *how* the federal government should respond to cancer. In the years that followed, congressional advocates for cancer care pressed for research funding through the appropriations process and enacted innovative legislation that sought to bolster prevention efforts. To take just one example: An obscure late addition to the Food Additives Amendment of 1958—what became known as the Delaney Clause, after James J. Delaney, a Democratic congressman from Queens, New York—was the first use of consumer-safety legislation to guard against potentially carcinogenic additives.

Cancer advocates—such as Mary Lasker, a major philanthropist and chief architect of some of the most important cancer campaigns of her time, including the War on Cancer itself and the reorganization of the American Cancer Society—built relationships with key members of Congress to advance research and treatment. Their work paid off. Between 1955 and 1960, Congress increased the NIH budget from $81 million to $400 million. During the Eisenhower years, NCI funding increased from $18 million to $110 million.[2] By 1970, it topped $200 million.

What Congress failed to prioritize is just as striking. Throughout the 1960s, the NCI's budget set aside only small amounts for prevention efforts. By the late 1960s, it spent no more than $30 million on cancer control initiatives—around 15 percent of its overall budget. Tensions also flared between researchers and advocates, with scientists seeking Congress's support for basic biological research—arguing that the fundamental mechanisms by which cancer operated remained largely unknown—while the latter pushed for more applied research.

The National Cancer Act itself was the product of a compromise negotiated on Capitol Hill between Senator Ted Kennedy—who sought to create an independent NASA-inspired agency dedicated to cancer—and Representative Paul Rogers in the House, who proposed a sharp increase in cancer funding while keeping the NCI housed under the National Institutes of Health (NIH). Although Richard Nixon took center stage when the act was signed into law, it was members of Congress—urged on by advocates—who shaped many of its core features. In the decades that followed, Congress has continued to rely on several core levers to make its mark on cancer; most important, legislation and appropriations.

Legislation

Legislation has affected almost all aspects of cancer—ranging from the reorganization of agencies (such as the creation of the National Cancer Institute in 1937 and its renovation in 1971), to targeting individual cancers (through acts tailored to breast and other cancers) in addition to classes of ailments (including overlooked diseases, through the Orphan Drug Act, as well as types of cancer, such as those affecting the pediatric population). Legislation has also shaped the modern regulatory landscape (such as by streamlining the Food and Drug Administration [FDA] review process through the creation of breakthrough therapy designations) as well as the broader health-care system, governing who can get access to prevention, screening, and treatment through insurance reform (including through the historic enactments of our modern health insurance system, most notably Medicare and Medicaid in 1965 and the Affordable Care Act in 2010) plus the creation of various planks of the social safety net. A brief survey of some of the major legislation, including some examples covered elsewhere in this book, offers a sense of the role legislation has played in cancer policy.

Overlooked Diseases and Targeted Efforts

Congressional intervention has been key to addressing overlooked areas of cancer. The famous "fire alarm" theory of Congress emphasizes that this legislative body only acts when *pushed*—when people are shouting that the house is on fire. Cancer advocates thus have a critical role to play in spurring action—effectively, shouting "fire!"[3] As she details in Chapter 9, lawyer Nancy Goodman became a powerful advocate for pediatric cancer after losing her son to the disease. Realizing that promoting the commercialization of pediatric drug development is key to encouraging the pharmaceutical industry to invest in this long-overlooked population, Goodman drafted a bill herself and brought it to Congress—the Creating Hope Act. It became law in 2012. The act incentivizes companies to develop drugs for children with cancer and other life-threatening illnesses by offering companies that do so an FDA voucher upon approval of their drug, conferring rights to faster FDA reviews of future drugs. The legislation has led to the development of thirty new drugs for children, including four specific to pediatric cancers, as of May 2021. Goodman then drafted a second bill, the RACE for Children Act, which was passed in 2017, which addressed another oversight: companies had not been required to test promising adult cancer drugs on children, offering no way to determine whether the drugs are effective in this critical population.

Other rare diseases likewise offer drug manufacturers few incentives to invest money and time into developing treatments. Congress sought to solve this problem through the passage of the Orphan Drug Act in 1983.[4] The act targeted drugs developed for diseases that occur "so infrequently in the United States that there is no reasonable expectation that the cost of developing and making available in the United States a drug for such disease or condition will be recovered from the sales in the United States of such drug." Through the act, Congress established a system for granting seven-year marketing exclusivity to sponsors of approved orphan drugs—a key incentive that, alongside a tax credit covering 50 percent of expenses tied to human clinical trials, has had an impact. Between 1967 and 1983, 34 drugs were approved that would have met Congress's "orphan drug" designation. Between 1983 and 2016, 177 drugs have been approved for rare cancers—representing 36 percent of all approvals granted under the act.[5] Congress's intervention in this space addressed a gap only Congress could fill—galvanizing the pharmaceutical industry to help populations that would otherwise go overlooked with reliance on the private sector alone.

Legislating Specific Cancers—Congress as Priority-Setter

Both legislation and appropriations allow Congress to set priorities for the federal effort against cancer. A major form of congressional priority setting centers on money—specifically, where Congress directs funds and how an agency spends money through earmarks. Sometimes this takes the form of disease-specific legislation, which has occasionally stirred controversy. For instance, in 2010, both the House and Senate passed a bill called the Pancreatic Cancer Act. This bill would have created a stand-alone pancreatic cancer initiative, putting pancreatic cancer investigators in charge of spending money allocated to the NCI—something its then director, Harold Varmus, and others were opposed to. One major concern cited by Varmus was that the NCI's scientific leadership should judge how to distribute funds based on their expertise, rather than tilting the playing field toward any given cancer based on congressional directives.

Varmus and others helped shape a milder bill that eventually became law as the Recalcitrant Cancer Act. This calls for the NCI to create a "scientific framework" to address cancers with five-year survival rates under 20 percent that affect over thirty thousand people a year (criteria that apply only to pancreatic and lung cancers).

But the question of whether to fund specific cancers remains a perennial one. Many cancer-specific advocates have argued for either increasing funding that is earmarked for particular cancers or even establishing cancer-specific programs. Sometimes this can be effective. Through the committed work of the Ovarian Cancer Alliance, for example, funding for ovarian cancer research doubled rapidly. Congresswoman DeLauro has advocated for funding research specific to ovarian cancer at the Department of Defense (DOD) even as some opposed the DOD's involvement in cancer research in the first place. And coalitions focused on breast and prostate cancer have managed to secure significant victories in terms of both funding and legislation through dedicated organizing and advocacy. In the halls of Congress, those with the loudest voices get heard. Money follows closely behind.

Encouraging targeted research by Congress in this way can be helpful. However, there is a risk that compartmentalizing research around particular categories or cancers might create a harmful silo effect, balkanizing the research community. In the late 1980s, the Congressional Caucus for Women's Issues considered supporting the creation of a program centered on women's health within NIH. At the time, not everyone thought this was a good idea. By creating a stand-alone program, the critics reasoned, the initiative could be isolated, receive less money, and might actually serve to dissuade other institutes and centers from engaging in efforts related to women's health. They could always claim that research on women's health was being handled by the program created for women's health rather than trying to integrate or elevate those issues within ongoing work. That said, targeted programs can have a positive impact. Congresswoman DeLauro is very supportive of the Office of Women's Health Research (OWHR), which was created in 1990.

The future presents fresh challenges. The rise of precision oncology, as detailed in this book, suggests that it might not be useful for Congress to continue focusing on specific cancers. Thanks to breakthroughs in our understanding of cancer, researchers now see it not as one disease, or even dozens of diseases—but as thousands. Lung cancer alone has shifted from being defined around two major types—small cell and non-small cell—to a category containing many unique variations, each responsive to specific therapies. More broadly, new understandings of the genetic makeup of cancer mean that therapies targeting a particular mutation in a malignant cell may effectively treat cancers that appear across many parts of the body.

Earmarking in this context could become counterproductive—a bill dedicated to LKB1-deficient lung cancer might not be the best way for policy makers to support researchers and, ultimately, patients. And pharmaceutical companies might be disincentivized from developing ever more targeted treatments impacting increasingly narrow populations, while those suffering from these newly defined cancers might not have the numbers to effectively advocate for themselves. Congress has important levers—especially through how it funds cancer research—to help make sure that does not happen.

A Broader Lens: The System as a Whole

The 1971 act had a relatively narrow lens. Its primary focus was on strengthening the NCI. But, as the chapters in this book make clear, the future of progress in the fight against cancer requires a broader perspective—a 360-degree approach to the determinants of cancer in our system. That includes establishing a stronger safety net. As Otis Brawley notes, access to education has an enormous impact on cancer outcomes. The Family Medical Leave Act, which Congress passed in 1993, requires employers to give certain employees up to twelve weeks of unpaid, job-protected leave, vital for protecting patients and families going through cancer. It also means expanded legal protections for those in the cancer system. The Americans with Disabilities Act (ADA), enacted in 1990, prohibits discrimination based on disability caused by cancer. The HIPAA Privacy Rule was established in 1996, setting up guidelines for the de-identification and sharing of data; Congress amended it in 2013 to cover genetic information as "health information" subject to HIPAA protection, an important addition as cancer has moved further into genetics. Congress also prohibited the use of genetic information by health plans for underwriting purposes as part of an attempt to implement the Genetic Information Non-discrimination Act of 2008.

Health insurance coverage is a leading predictor of access to care and health outcomes. Medicare and Medicaid, established in 1965, dramatically expanded access to persons over age sixty-five and with low income. Medicare is the largest payer for cancer care in the United States. Together with Medicaid, these programs cover the care of approximately 70 percent of new cancer patients each year. And the Affordable Care Act of 2010 of course stands out as a landmark achievement, adding more than twenty million to the insurance rolls and expanding protection from health-plan discrimination for preexisting conditions, including cancer, throughout the health care landscape, benefiting more than 100 million Americans. The ACA also expanded access to cost-free preventative screening for cancer.

If Congress had failed to act with any one of the laws we have discussed, the impact would be devastating for countless Americans.

FIGURE 18.1 Select Survey of Major Legislation Impacting Cancer

1937   *National Cancer Act:* Establishes the National Cancer Institute

1958   *Delaney Clause of the Food Additives Amendment:* Prevents the use of substances as food additives if they are found to cause cancer in animals or humans

1965   *Medicare and Medicaid Act:* Establishes Medicare and Medicaid, which together cover the care of approximately 70 percent of new cancer patients each year

1970   *Clean Air Act:* Curbs air pollution—a significant contributor to many types of cancer

1971   *National Cancer Act:* Empowers the NCI while increasing research funding and creating a national network of designated cancer centers

1982   *Orphan Drug Act:* Encourages the development of treatments for "rare" diseases, including pediatric and certain types of adult cancers

1985   *Consolidated Omnibus Budget Reconciliation Act (COBRA):* Gives employees and their families the right to choose to temporarily continue group health benefits after termination of employment or death of an employee

1990   *The Americans with Disabilities Act:* Prohibits discrimination on the basis of disability caused by cancer

1993 *Family Medical Leave Act:* Requires employers to provide certain employees with up to 12 weeks of unpaid, job-protected leave per year

1993 *NIH Revitalization Act:* Requires NIH to include women in federally funded Phase 3 clinical trials

1996 *Health Insurance Portability and Accountability Act (HIPAA):* Protects employees from discrimination for preexisting conditions, including cancer, in employer-provided health plans

1998 *Women's Health and Cancer Rights Act:* Provides protections to patients who choose to have breast reconstruction in connection with a mastectomy

2005 *Patient Navigator Outreach and Chronic Disease Prevention Act:* Expands patient navigator programs through the NCI and cancer centers to increase access in communities of color and poor communities

2008 *Caroline Pryce Walker Childhood Cancer Act:* First pediatric cancer–focused stand-alone law, aims to advance treatments for pediatric cancers

2008 *Genetic Information Nondiscrimination Act (GINA):* Prohibits employment and health insurance discrimination on the basis of genetic information

2010 *Affordable Care Act:* Significantly expands insurance access while protecting Americans from discrimination by insurers on the basis of preexisting conditions

2010 *The James Zadroga 9/11 Health and Compensation Act:* Establishes health programs dedicated to 9/11 survivors, many of whom have been diagnosed and treated for cancer

2012 *The Creating Hope Act Pediatric Priority Review Voucher Program:* Gives priority drug vouchers to companies that successfully develop and have approved a rare pediatric cancer drug

2012 *Advancing Breakthrough Therapies for Patients Act:* Established the "breakthrough therapy" designation by which the FDA can accelerate access to promising treatments

2013   *The Recalcitrant Cancer Act:* Replaces efforts to create a stand-alone pancreatic cancer institute and calls for NCI to create a "scientific framework" to address cancers with a 5-year survival rate under 20%, causing at least 30,000 deaths per year

2014   *Gabriella Miller Kids First Research Act:* Tax legislation to reprogram savings to provide for a 10-year pediatric research initiative administered through the NIH Common Fund

2014   *Sunscreen Innovation Act:* Aims to accelerate FDA review and approval of sunscreens with new active ingredients

2016   *Child Nicotine Poisoning Prevention Act:* Requires the Consumer Product Safety Commission to promulgate a rule to require child safety packaging for liquid nicotine containers

2016   *The 21st Century Cures Act:* Commits $1.8 billion for cancer research over seven years

2017   *The RACE for Children Act:* Requires drug manufacturers to test targeted cancer drugs on pediatric patients

2017   *FDA Reauthorization Act:* Revises and extends the user-fee programs for prescription drugs, medical devices, generic drugs, and biosimilar biological products

2018   *Childhood Cancer STAR (Survivorship, Treatment, Access, Research) Act:* Supports the expansion of biospecimen collection from children as well as initiatives supporting pediatric cancer survivors

2019   *Henrietta Lacks Enhancing Cancer Research Act:* Requires federal agencies to report steps they are taking to improve access to federally funded cancer clinical trials from underrepresented populations

2020   *Further Consolidated Appropriations Act:* Raises the minimum age for buying tobacco products from 18 to 21

Cancer, Congress, and the Power of the Purse

Legislation is not Congress's only tool when it comes to cancer. Perhaps the most important one is money. The remainder of this chapter will focus on appropriations, beginning with Congress's role in funding the NIH budget before considering inadequate efforts to fund the Centers for Disease Control (CDC) and support prevention, the pitfalls of sequestration, and the need for better public/private partnerships.

Funding NIH

NIH, the nation's biomedical research agency, plays a pivotal role in supporting research that has led to major breakthroughs in cancer treatment. The unusual bipartisan support around funding NIH means that its budget has almost always gotten an annual raise—though the percentages vary—while consistently taking in about 20 percent of the funding in the overarching appropriations bill it is part of. No small feat, considering the broader bill also funds special education initiatives, Pell Grants, Head Start, the CDC, and hundreds of other important programs. Bipartisan support also translates to different approaches when deciding how to protect NIH funding. Republican support for NIH has been described by some as surpassing everything other than defense spending. Democrats are no less committed to NIH, but have generally been unwilling to slash education or other vital programs to pay for it. As a result, they are more likely to fight for a larger overall appropriations bill so that NIH increases do not compromise other priorities.

NIH is funded through annual appropriations—a cycle that presents a challenge for how it functions, specifically in relation to the multiyear grants it frequently awards. A somewhat volatile system has emerged, whereby NIH makes extended commitments to investigators while never quite being sure of what it can expect in the year (much less, years) ahead. It is often the case that when a new budget comes in, most of the NIH money is already committed to grantees from prior years. Predicting the funding that might be available for new initiatives becomes a difficult process as a result. Creating a more predictable funding structure is an important goal for the near future.

One possible improvement supported by Varmus, among others, would add a rolling five-year plan to the annual appropriations process specifying certain percentages by which the budget of an agency would increase per year over a set number of years. This would be modeled on the five-year plan included in the 1998 appropriation, which mapped out how NIH funding would be doubled over half a decade. A separate reform would make NIH funding mandatory, rather than discretionary funding as it currently is. This would lock in exactly how much money NIH will receive from year to year—for example, setting an automatic annual increase of 5 percent. This brings with it a variety of serious risks. First, the approach would almost certainly have to be time-limited as there would be no sure way to pay for automatic increases extending in perpetuity. Separately, making funding mandatory would take away any real control over the appropriations process from the congressional appropriators, which would allow Congress to further specify and make adjustments to accounts taking into account real-time issues, such as a global pandemic. Lastly, there are political considerations to bear in mind. Republican support for the Labor Health and Human Services appropriations bill largely hinges on NIH funding. Many things in Congress are connected by political deals. Removing NIH funding from the process could eliminate important levers for other programs.

While maintaining control over the funding process is important to appropriators, they walk a fine line when deciding *how* to disburse funds. They may seek to encourage NIH research on specific diseases—the report that accompanies the bill may encourage work on categories like pediatric cancers or a particular disease, such as ovarian cancer, ALS, or Alzheimer's—but historically, Congress has generally refrained from earmarking specific funding levels in the appropriations bill for individual diseases. Congressional deference to the scientific leadership has proven key to NIH's success and been a longstanding practice.[6] That said,

Congress has recently begun to specify sums tied to specific diseases, something we may need to guard against. In 2017, Congress told NIH to spend precisely $1.391 billion on Alzheimer's disease. Congress also directed NIH to spend exactly $50 million more on antibiotic research than it did the year before.

While Congress annually sets aside billions of dollars in funds for NIH, were one to look at the appropriations bill that supports the work of NIH—known as the Labor Health and Human Services and Education Appropriations Bill—one would find no single line listing the total amount set aside for NIH overall. Instead, specific amounts are listed for the various individual institutes and centers that make up NIH. While this might suggest that Congress has been prioritizing diseases by finessing funding levels among programs, traditionally the exact opposite has taken place. Appropriators would typically distribute the overall increase to the NIH budget—say, 3 percent—more or less equally across its twenty-seven institutes and centers, with each getting about 3 percent more in turn. Congress thus avoids prioritizing certain programs or diseases over others while pursuing an overarching goal, in this case increasing funding by a set amount. Observers have pointed to this as one reason for the bipartisan support NIH funding enjoys—consensus is easier to achieve among appropriators while advocates can have a greater impact by speaking with one voice.

Advocates have taken the same approach. Unlike any other agency in the appropriations bill, advocates for NIH funding typically lobby members of Congress for a total increase to the NIH budget rather than smaller sums dedicated to particular initiatives. Thus, rather than asking for tens of millions for a given cancer, advocates often end up pushing for a certain billion-dollar increase to the overall NIH budget. Speaking with one voice sends a message to appropriators they cannot miss. When hundreds of advocacy groups descend on Congress making the same request—doubling NIH's funding, for instance—Congress listens. And traditionally, everyone would stand to benefit—with an overall increase in NIH's budget shared more or less equally across all its institutes and centers.

This stands in stark contrast to piecemeal requests from advocates for other programs, including prevention. Advocates arguing for an increase to the budget for prevention control efforts at the CDC lobby for specific sums tied to individual projects, such as tobacco control or cancer screening. This makes it harder to reach consensus, forces Congress rather than experts to choose between programs, and splinters the focus of the broader prevention advocacy community. Whereas CDC funding is built from the bottom up—program by program, sum by sum, NIH funding flows from the top down.

The Effect of Budget Sequestration

The appropriations process has been shaped by a decade of budget sequestration, the result of a compromise around how to deal with the debt ceiling negotiated between President Barack Obama and Congress in 2011. Sequestration brought automatic spending cuts that caused deep damage to Congress's discretionary programs—so much so that it will take years, maybe even decades, to catch up to the progress that could have been made had research funding remained on its pre-sequestration trajectory. Indeed, current funding levels for NIH, the CDC, and other vital agencies are not where they should be because a decade of sequestration has scaled them back. Sequestration cut some trials off midstream—enrolled patients were abruptly disenrolled while some trials were canceled entirely.

Sequestration is, for now, a thing of the past—Fiscal Year 2022 is the first where sequestration-related budget caps do not apply and it will be important to see what happens going forward. Hopefully, this will empower Congress to provide the proper funding to NIH, CDC, and other agencies—ensuring that they need not choose between worthy projects that deserve their backing.

Underfunding Prevention and the CDC

While great sums of money have been invested in research for cancer treatments, prevention has been largely overlooked. Bolstering prevention with more CDC funding does not enjoy the bipartisan support that applies to NIH appropriations. All this despite our knowledge that prevention could save many lives and quite a bit of money in the long run. This is partly a problem that derives from Congress' obligation to give a "budget score" to all our actions. For all the lives and dollars saved through prevention, we cannot get prevention scored in a way that looks favorable in the usual ten-year budget window. It takes years to recoup the investment in prevention, so it "scores" as a big loss, even though in the end it will save us much more.

Another issue goes back to the "fire alarm" theory of Congress we mentioned earlier. Specific cancers and private organization have loud voices when it comes to funding research. Prevention is not as flashy and does not have the same kind of sustained or well-financed lobby. The COVID-19 pandemic has shown us how shortsighted we have been to undermine prevention and public health. But without the same pressure applied to funding prevention programs, we risk continued underinvestment.

To understand how underfunded the CDC is, just look at the numbers. The CDC's budget for the current fiscal year totaled $7.9 billion for the entire agency, whose responsibilities include pandemic preparedness, grants to state and local health departments, global health initiatives, cancer prevention programs, and much more. CDC's cancer prevention programs were allotted just $358.79 million in funding. The NCI's budget, by contrast, was $6.3 billion. Budgets reveal priorities, and the numbers here tell a simple story. Congress has not done enough to fund prevention partly because Congress does not prioritize prevention. This should not be a binary choice; we have the resources to fund both.

Partnering with the Private Sector

While public-private partnerships already exist in drug development, better guardrails are needed to prevent pitfalls. For example, when NIH engages in research that leads to a cancer drug, that drug will ultimately be licensed to a manufacturer. The drug company it is licensed to can then charge whatever price it wants, often resulting in charges that make the drug unaffordable for many if not most patients. When Representative DeLauro first came to Congress, she worked to put together a Cooperative Research and Development Agreement (CRADA) between NIH and Bristol-Myers Squibb for a breast cancer drug—Taxol—that was being developed at the time. The CRADA was created and the drug eventually reached the market. In the end, many hospitals did not offer Taxol because it was too expensive. This cannot be the case moving forward.

The US government invests significant sums in critical, lifesaving biomedical research in this country that never get recouped, while pharmaceutical companies can take financial advantage of the same investments. Public-private partnerships are essential, but the partnership currently goes one way. Several reforms could help correct the imbalance. For example, the cost of prescription drugs can be negotiated. Other initiatives supported by Representative DeLauro include the use of targeted "march-in rights"—whereby the government can grant additional licenses for a patented invention created using federal funds, thereby stripping exclusivity, when the invention is not made available on "reasonable terms"— and competitive licensing should negotiations fail.[7] The latter approach would allow the government to buy a generic or biosimilar version of a drug in cases where a fair price is not agreed to by the patent holder.

The COVID-19 pandemic invites a reassessment of the government's role in manufacturing drugs. High risk/high reward research—with strong private sector engagement galvanized by government support—can lead to breakthroughs in record time. Congressional reforms could improve the collaboration between government and industry while ensuring that taxpayer investment in research leads to better and more affordable drugs. One shining example has been the partnership between the federal government and Moderna in developing its COVID-19 vaccine; we need to do the same for certain unproduced antibiotics or drugs for rare diseases because there is no profit to be had.

At the same time, we want to emphasize the continuing importance of basic research. As noted, foundational work can lead to discoveries with far-reaching applications that could not have been anticipated when setting out on a particular research project. Indeed, that is a core virtue of basic research. If we narrow the scope of what we set out to discover too much, we risk losing the cross-cutting benefits that come from wide-ranging scientific inquiry. The stunning advances represented by precision medicine would not be possible without decades of basic science research backing them up.

Looking to the Next 50 Years

Recent Efforts: Lessons and Missed Opportunities

As we look forward, we should learn from the missed opportunities of recent reform efforts. The 21st Century Cures Act offers an example. In attempting to expedite drug and device approval, the act paid too little attention to those the science and clinical trials are meant to help—the patients. The act did not address predatory practices by the pharmaceutical industry; and it stripped away funding from the Public Health Prevention Fund, undermining our efforts to fight the diseases that are the leading causes of death and disability in the United States. And while the act authorizes an average $480 million increase to the NIH budget each year for the next ten years, that amount is minor compared to recent funding proposals that passed in the House—which have been nearly four times that amount each year. There is also no guarantee that appropriators will follow through and provide the funding each year.

The coming months and years will almost certainly involve the tragic consequences of the Trump administration's failure to take COVID-19 seriously. Congress should be guided by the knowledge that many Americans will be diagnosed with cancer at later stages because of missed or delayed screenings caused by the pandemic. Labs that were undertaking cancer research also were forced to close down for months or longer—delaying vital breakthroughs and discoveries. Congress must work to counter the adverse effects of the pandemic as much as possible by investing in public health infrastructure and the workforce, as well as prevention activities.

In considering the type of programs that should be prioritized going forward, translational research—which applies scientific discoveries to treatments that reach patients, bringing "the bench to the bedside"—should be at the forefront. Such initiatives as the DOD's Congressionally Directed Medical Research Program also have a role to play by supporting important translational and clinical research. Congresswoman DeLauro has been a longtime advocate for the DOD program in particular, leading the letter to the House Defense Appropriations Subcommittee that ultimately resulted in a record high funding amount of $35 million for ovarian cancer research in last year's DOD program. President Biden's recent proposal for an ARPA-H agency seems rooted in similar principles of prioritizing translational work that gets treatments and cures quickly and safely to patients, thereby complementing NIH's ongoing work. This is a promising vision.

At the same time, we cannot lose our focus on the vital basic research funded by NIH as well as the other critical initiatives it supports. Many fundamental questions about how cancer works remain—ranging from the molecular basis for tumor initiation and progression to a deeper understanding of what distinguishes normal cell growth from that of cancer cells. Basic research can get us answers that will spur future treatments, including in precision oncology. We must also ensure that the bulwark of cancer research—the R01 grant—is better supported through the allocation of more funds. Currently, we fund only 8 to 10 percent of NCI R01 applications. A harmful cycle has emerged: investigators spend inordinate time writing more grant applications, which creates more grants to be reviewed and a lower proportion of grants funded. The average age of a first R01 is now over forty-one years, which threatens to turn away young investigators and thereby limit the next generation of talent. We must break this cycle and increase funding for emerging talent by allocating more money to R01 grants.

And all our work must dismantle racial and gender inequities. While the National Institute of Minority Health and Disparities does exist, it is terribly underfunded. The 2020 spending bill provided a high of $390 million. But one program or institute is not enough, even were it properly funded. Equity should be woven into all aspects of cancer policy, whether clinical trials, access to health insurance and prevention, expanding the social safety net or providing options for where treatment is offered. One challenge for cancer policy in general, as many chapters in this book reveal in different contexts, is that policy thinking is siloed. We think of prevention in one bucket, and research in another. We view the safety net under one heading and research and development (R&D) under another. The War on Cancer legislation itself was narrowly confined to enabling one powerful agency to do important work; but it did not take a broader view of the patient experience and cancer's financial burden, equity, the economics of cancer institutions, incentivizing treatments for cancers that will not be lucrative, and so on.

So, even as eliminating disparities must be a central task for the near future of cancer, we caution against creating another silo. The Office of Research on Women's Health (ORWH), for example, has done commendable work in ensuring that NIH-supported research addresses issues that affect women, promotes the inclusion of women in clinical research, and develops and expands opportunities for women throughout the biomedical research career pipeline. However, funding for ORWH has lagged behind the total funding for NIH over the past several years. $43,925,000 was set aside for ORWH to expand its work in fiscal year 2021—an increase of $5,000,000 above the estimated fiscal year 2020 funding level. And efforts to fund women's research outside of the specific office dedicated to it risk claims that "we don't need to fund that here, we have a special office for that"—the result of a well-meaning strategy that may ultimately lead to less funding and less integration of women's health across the entire cancer space.

Conclusion: Looking Ahead

Future legislative efforts must take a holistic approach that is ambitious, urgent, and informed by past lessons.

Ending cancer in America requires achieving universal health coverage for all Americans. Congress must legislate to ensure that this comes to pass soon and consider equity in all of its cancer policy making, not just when the topic is "about" disparities. Future reforms must also work to bring down the cost of prescription drugs while increasing access to providers. Prevention should not be left behind in favor of funding for treatments—we must be able to walk and chew gum at the same time when it comes to supporting both. This includes continuing to provide robust funding for basic research through NIH. And workforce training must be expanded to meet shortages in critically needed oncologists, nurses, and others.

Congress can reshape what Siddhartha Mukherjee so aptly calls "Cancerland" at the start of this book, ensuring that fewer Americans have to enter it and that more can emerge with healthy years of life ahead of them. If Congress acts with vision, this may become a place future generations will only know through history books—or at least a place that becomes far less central and destructive to our lives—thanks to the tireless work of physicians, researchers, patients, and their families, as well as dedicated policymakers on Capitol Hill.

Notes

Special thanks to Caitlin Peruccio and Eugene Rusyn for their assistance with this chapter.

1. Siddhartha Mukherjee, *The Emperor of All Maladies: A Biography of Cancer* (New York: Simon and Schuster, 2011), 26.

2. James T. Patterson, *The Dread Disease: Cancer and Modern American Culture* (Cambridge: Harvard University Press, 1987) 183.

3. Matthew D. McCubbins and Thomas Schwartz, "Congressional Oversight Overlooked: Police Patrols versus Fire Alarms," *American Journal of Political Science* 28, no. 1 (1984): 165–179.

4. Matthew Herder, "What Is the Purpose of the Orphan Drug Act?" *PLoS Medicine* 14, no. 1 (2017): e1002191, https://doi.org/10.1371/journal.pmed.1002191.

5. Clemens Stockklausner et al., "Novel Treatments for Rare Cancers: The U.S. Orphan Drug Act Is Delivering—A Cross-Sectional Analysis," *Oncologist* 21, no. 4 (2016):487–493, https://doi.org/10.1634/theoncologist.2015-0397.

6. Susan R. Morrissey, "Pork-Barrel Science," *Chemical and Engineering News*, August 7, 2006.

7. Michael Liu, William B. Feldman, Jerry Avorn, and Aaron Kesselheim, "March-In Rights and Compulsory Licensing—Safety Nets for Access to a COVID-19 Vaccine," *Health Affairs* Blog, May 6, 2020, https://doi.org/10.1377/hblog20200501.798711.

CHAPTER 19

Cancer and the President

The Moonshot and Beyond

Greg Simon and Allison Rabkin Golden

In his final State of the Union address on January 12, 2016, President Obama asked Vice President Biden to lead a new Cancer Moonshot. Or, as he put it, he wanted "Joe in charge of Mission Control."

The Cancer Moonshot aimed not at the stars but at our cells. It set an audacious but realistic goal—to double our rate of progress against a disease that takes 1,800 lives a day. The impact of the Cancer Moonshot on human health continues to grow—most recently, investments in emerging cancer treatment technologies, such as immunology, helped shape the development of RNA-based COVID-19 vaccines[1]—underscoring its power as a model for future efforts to elevate quality of life.

From the beginning, the organizational challenge was how to focus an effort involving twenty federal agencies to make real progress within the year while at the same time engaging the nation in the effort to the greatest degree. Simply expanding existing programs would not be sufficient; merely spending more money

---

Greg Simon is Former President of the Biden Cancer Initiative at the Biden Foundation; and former Executive Director of the White House Cancer Moonshot Task Force.

Allison Rabkin Golden received her JD from Yale Law School where she was a Solomon Center for Health Law and Policy Fellow.

would not address the cultural issues at the heart of the Cancer Moonshot's mission, from data hoarding to poor coordination across agencies to the underrepresentation of women and minorities in research grants to the lack of patient involvement in drug design. The agencies confronted the Cancer Moonshot's guiding question: How do you touch patients in their journey from prevention through diagnosis, treatment, and survivorship, and how can you double the impact of that touch *now*?

The public involvement of then–Vice President Joe Biden and Dr. Jill Biden gave the Cancer Moonshot the momentum it needed to unite hundreds of cancer organizations to focus on a shared mission. The millions of patients, thousands of doctors and researchers, and hundreds of organizations provided the engineering needed to create a new system for the twenty-first century. And perhaps most important, the active leadership of the vice president and his authenticity as a parent who had lost his son to cancer led people and organizations to spend considerable time and money to be part of the most ambitious public effort to attack cancer in decades. As one doctor put it, "My peers will do for Biden what they won't do for each other."

The Cancer Moonshot achieved more in nine months than many thought possible: over eighty collaborations, from highly technical projects to support for caregivers and families; $1.8 billion in new cancer funding; the active and collaborative engagement of thousands of cancer patients, researchers, doctors, nonprofits, universities, and corporations; and a direct and successful assault on the cultural problems that slowed progress for years.

Origins of the Moonshot

This national mission to cure cancer, a leading cause of death worldwide, was personal to Biden. But it is personal to every American—every life is affected by cancer, whether it is one's own battle, or that of a family member, a coworker, a friend. Vice President Biden had been methodically laying the groundwork for the liftoff of the Moonshot for months prior to the national announcement, consulting with nearly two hundred of the world's leading cancer physicians, scientists, and philanthropists and identifying key challenges around which to build the Moonshot goals—from the fact that only 5 percent of cancer patients participate in clinical trials to the fact that local, community oncologists, who treat nearly 85 percent of Americans with cancer,[2] often lack access to the latest cancer treatments.

By the end of January 2016, President Obama formally followed up on his State of the Union call to action and, drawing upon the findings that Vice President Biden had gathered, released a presidential memorandum establishing the White House Cancer Moonshot Task Force. As the memorandum outlined, while funded by the National Institutes of Health (NIH), the leadership of the Moonshot would draw on the talents of people in agencies across the government. In addition to the National Cancer Institute (NCI) of the NIH, President Obama specifically called for the heads of thirteen different executive branch departments, agencies, and offices to get involved in the effort: the Departments of Defense (DOD), Commerce, Health and Human Services, Energy (DOE), and Veterans Affairs (VA), the Office of Management and Budget, the National Economic Council, the Domestic Policy Council, the Office of Science and Technology Policy, the Food and Drug Administration (FDA), and the National Science Foundation. In other words, from the outset, a recognition that this effort would succeed only with careful collaboration across agencies—a recognition that progress would necessitate expertise in not just science and medicine, but economics, policy, and technology as well—guided the process.

The NCI Blue Ribbon Panel

The Cancer Moonshot was deliberately launched at an "inflection point" in cancer research,[3] a moment at which the science, data, and technology had advanced enough to allow new and potentially revolutionary approaches. Immunology, once viewed as a pseudoscience, had become a promising approach for many cancers. The Human Genome Project's great promise was finally being realized, sixteen years after its completion. Artificial intelligence and machine learning were beginning to make improvements in our ability to diagnose cancer, predict the best treatments, and accelerate understanding of molecular pathways that could now be more easily modelled and manipulated.

But all the technology and scientific innovation threw into stark relief how little the culture of research had changed at the NIH. Where there should have been collaboration, there was competition that led to data hoarding and a hesitancy to work with other institutions. Women and minorities were underrepresented in the grants, which were awarded by review committees where they were also underrepresented. Researchers were rewarded by the number of, not the impact of, their publications. Patients were generally excluded from being involved in trial or drug design.

The NCI was asked to address scientific and technological issues while the White House Cancer Moonshot Initiative focused on those cultural issues that were holding the technological progress back from its full potential impact. Thus, to accelerate the technological breakthroughs on the horizon and define and focus the research directions of the Cancer Moonshot, a Blue Ribbon Panel ("the BRP" or "the Panel") was assembled to advise the National Cancer Advisory Board. Organized into seven working groups, the BRP reflected the Cancer Moonshot's focus on collaboration by drawing its membership from leaders from a multitude of backgrounds with a diversity of perspectives, from scientific subject matter experts to representatives across the private, public, and nonprofit worlds to patients who could speak directly to the experience of cancer and treatment side effects.

Each working group evaluated a distinct research area: clinical trials, enhanced data sharing, cancer immunology, implementation science, pediatric cancer, precision prevention and early detection, and tumor evolution and progression. Their charge: to identify one to three opportunities where additional funding and exploration with new tools and data just becoming available could double the rate of progress in cancer research and treatments.

Ideas flowed in from every angle from the cancer community, especially through a dedicated website created to accept proposals. In total, the seven working groups of the BRP collectively and carefully considered more than 1,600 ideas. Months of research and deliberation later, the BRP announced ten unified recommendations to guide the scientific research to be funded by the Cancer Moonshot and to transform the modern understanding of both the prevention and treatment of cancer.

These ten recommendations continue to shape the NCI's efforts today, with the NCI ultimately establishing one hundred subcommittees to implement the recommendations. The NCI's progress in funding and carrying out the BRP's recommendations is ongoing. The National Cancer Data Ecosystem developed in response to the BRP continues to facilitate data sharing, and established a now broadly used resource, the Cancer Research Data Commons (CRDC). The creation of the Immuno-Oncology Translational Network (IOTN) and Pancreatic Cancer Microenvironment Network (PaCMEN) led to the discovery of new immune targets for cancer treatments and continues to expand immunotherapy understanding, which served as the backbone for the development of mRNA-based COVID-19 vaccines. The work of the Pediatric Immunotherapy Discovery and Development Network (PI-DDN) and My Pediatric and Adult Rare Tumor Network (MyPART) to reduce childhood deaths due to cancer by leading preclinical immunotherapy research for children and advancing understanding of rare cancers is ongoing. Moreover, in response to the BRP, three new initiatives have since been launched to improve cancer prevention and early detection strategies: Accelerating Colorectal Cancer Screening and follow-up through Implementation Science (ACCSIS), Implementation Science Centers in Cancer Control (ISC3), and the Cancer Center Cessation Initiative (C3I). And these are just a few examples of the ongoing efforts.

To achieve these goals, the Panel embraced the power of networks. Indeed, its first recommendation was to establish a network for direct patient engagement. Creating a federated network of databases where patients could voluntarily provide their data for research would serve two critical aims. It would enhance the scientific community's ability to study which interventions work and for which patients, enabling the development of targeted treatments. By streamlining and democratizing the process by which patients enroll in clinical trials, this patient engagement network also promoted the inclusion of a more diverse patient population in clinical trials, aiming to increase minority and traditionally underserved patients' involvement in the trials upon which future treatments would be developed.

The Panel also recommended the creation of a second network: a cancer immunotherapy translational science network. This would enable tumor collection and comprehensive profiling, with the objective of creating a national, coordinated strategy for uncovering new immune targets and analyzing novel immune-based approaches to facilitate the development of vaccines for a wide range of cancers. Reflecting the inclusive and collaborative mission of the Cancer Moonshot itself, this immunotherapy translational science network would include both adult and pediatric tumor samples, cancers from diverse populations sensitive to immunotherapy, and the full range of cancers resistant to, or with the propensity to develop resistance to, existing immunotherapies.

An additional Panel recommendation drew on the Cancer Moonshot's ethos of transparency and collaboration to institute two entirely new ecosystems: the National Cancer Data Ecosystem for the collection and dissemination of large datasets and a first-of-its-kind human tumor atlas. The National Cancer Data Ecosystem would enhance the ability of researchers, clinicians, and patients both to contribute data as well as leverage existing data in a centralized network that would directly promote new discoveries to improve patient outcomes. At the same time, the human tumor atlas would consist of a dynamic, three-dimensional map of the evolution of tumors of all kinds. It would document the genetic lesions and cellular interactions that shape each tumor's evolution from a precancerous lesion to advanced cancer that metastasizes and develops resistance to treatment. This centralized, comprehensive picture of the events that shape cancer cell behavior would allow deeper understanding of the biological processes that lead to cancer and enable better prediction of cancer development as well as more accurate prediction of patient response to treatments.

Beyond these collaboration-accelerating systems, the Panel also focused its recommendations around key challenge areas. Addressing the issue of drug resistance and seeking to promote the development of novel therapies that prevent or reverse drug resistance, it recommended the institution of an interdisciplinary research program designed to uncover the genetic, molecular, cellular, and physiologic mechanisms behind certain cancer cells' development of resistance to previously effective treatments over time. It also highlighted the need to deepen our understanding of abnormal fusion proteins resulting from chromosomal translocations that underlie numerous pediatric cancers, recommending a coordinated research effort to develop novel therapeutic approaches targeting the mechanisms of fusion oncoproteins associated with pediatric cancers.

The Panel additionally took direct aim at addressing underserved patient populations through three recommendations to rethink long-established norms within the medical community. First, to elevate the patient's voice and leverage the insufficiently tapped value of the patient's perspective, the Panel proposed accelerating the development of guidelines for standardized monitoring and management of symptoms reported by patients across all health-care settings and all cancer patient populations. This new systematic approach to gathering patient outcomes data and evidence-based symptom management for patients from diverse backgrounds would in turn facilitate the inclusion of underrepresented voices in the cancer research process, promote the development of targeted interventions, and improve adherence to effective treatments by better tracking and addressing side effects. Second, the Panel sought to reduce inequities and better address medically underserved populations by conducting implementation science research to accelerate the development and introduction of new, evidence-based strategies with the ability to materially reduce cancer risk and health disparities. In particular, the Panel proposed prioritizing prevention and screening modalities with established efficacy, for example human papillomavirus (HPV) vaccination, colorectal cancer screening, tobacco control, and the identification of genetic predispositions to cancer. Third, the Panel proposed the retrospective analysis of biospecimens from patients treated with the standard of care. Specifically, it recommended the acquisition of thousands of tumor samples, in particular samples from medically underserved populations, so as to deepen understanding of which tumor features are predictive of clinical outcomes and treatment resistance.

Finally, the Panel embraced innovation in everything it did, and proposed supporting the development of new technologies with the potential to accelerate the testing of therapies and the characterization of tumors. Namely, it identified several promising innovations, including implantable microdosing devices for testing drug effectiveness directly in tumors; new patient imaging approaches, such as radiologic imaging; nuclear medicine imaging methods using new metabolic probes; and computational platforms that permit new methods of advanced data integration.

In this way, the BRP recommendations facilitated an unprecedented level of coordination and collaboration between cancer researchers, clinicians, and patients across the nation. They accelerated the implementation of existing effective interventions while at the same time powering the development of novel technologies with the potential to transform cancer prevention and treatment. They prioritized and promoted transparency of data and knowledge sharing by building new centralized and systematic networks for everyone in the cancer community, including patients, to contribute to and draw from. And throughout, they gave patients from all backgrounds and with all types of cancer an amplified voice.

Initiatives and New Partnerships

The initiatives under the Cancer Moonshot program ranged from single agency commitments to agency partnerships and public-private partnerships as well as initiatives designed and carried out by private companies, foundations, and universities.

Single-Agency Initiatives

Examples of single-agency activities include:

1. The NCI drug formulary that prelicensed compounds from pharmaceutical companies so researchers could do multicompound studies without the delay of negotiating licenses for each individual drug.
2. The DOD's commitment to studying over 250,000 biological samples from soldiers taken over the last 25 years to identify new linkages between prediagnostic biological markers and various types of cancer.[4]
3. The Patent Office's commitment to accelerating oncology-related patent applications at no cost, shaving a year or more off the traditional patent review time. In addition, the office launched the "USPTO Cancer Moonshot Challenge" to use intellectual property datasets to identify trending cancer technologies, enabling more precise funding and policy decisions regarding promising new treatments.
4. The FDA's creation of a new Oncology Center of Excellence to unite cancer product regulatory review to enhance coordination and leverage expertise across FDA centers.

Some programs started as single-site projects and evolved into partnerships with great effect. For instance, early in the life of the Cancer Moonshot program, the head of public health at George Washington University visited the Cancer Moonshot and offered to create a program utilizing social media to promote tobacco cessation and lung cancer screening in Washington, DC, which has a high percentage of tobacco users and people with lung cancer. Within a week, the head of the Case Western Reserve Cancer Center, accompanied by representatives of the Cleveland Clinic and the University Hospital, visited the Cancer Moonshot offices. They proposed to do a similar tobacco cessation/lung cancer screening program in Cleveland, another city with high smoking and lung cancer rates. After pairing the two efforts, this eventually became a twenty-city program funded by NCI.

Multiagency Partnerships

Multiagency projects are difficult to launch, coordinate, and fund, given the complexity of the budgeting process and the aversion most departments or agencies have to sharing resources with other agencies. We addressed this problem head-on by requiring each member of the task force to pick a partner and figure out a collaboration that made sense. Subsequently, new solutions were designed and implemented—leveraging interagency agreements, discretionary budgets, material transfer agreements, and more. Here is a sample of what happened:

1. The VA and the DOE entered into a joint agreement under which the VA would fund a dedicated data network to allow information to flow from the VA to the supercomputers at the DOE to analyze VA medical records from the Million Veteran Program, a cornerstone of the president's Precision Medicine Initiative. The VA transferred $3.5 million for the program to the DOE, since existing networks were not adequate to handle the flow of data.[5]

2. One of the biggest and most complex partnerships was launched by the DOD, the VA, and the NCI. Applied Proteogenomics Organizational Learning and Outcomes (APOLLO) was built on the success of the NCI's Clinical Proteomic Tumor Analysis Consortium (CPTAC) that pioneered the integration of proteomics (proteins) and genomics (genes) in clinical cancer research, termed "proteogenomics." APOLLO uses state-of-the-art research methods in proteogenomics to more rapidly identify unique targets and pathways of cancer for detection and intervention—a critical big data challenge. The initial

focus was on lung cancer, using data from the VA and DOD health systems—two of the largest in the country.

3. NASA and the NCI established a new collaboration to study the biological effects of particle beam radiotherapy, a novel technology that may deliver a more targeted dose of radiation to tumor cells. Currently, the NCI supports several efforts in this area, including comparing the efficacy of carbon ion therapy for the treatment of pancreatic cancer, and NASA is studying the biological effects of a wide range of heavy ions to develop countermeasures for protecting astronauts from the space radiation environment. Under this new partnership, agencies will share data and biospecimens to assess the biological effects of particle beam radiotherapy and evaluate its potential value as a new approach to fighting cancer.

Public-Private Partnerships

Public-private partnerships were especially successful in leveraging the strengths of each sector. The VA has long had a problem with doing genomic analysis of cancer patients since there is wide variation in its centers in terms of process and access. When the head of Walter Reed National Military Medical Center's genome sequencing laboratory visited the Cancer Moonshot offices, he noted that Walter Reed's sequencers were among the best in the nation but were underutilized. Could Walter Reed offer its services to the VA? Yes, it could, for free. Walter Reed recognized the opportunity to showcase its utility and wanted to be a part of the growing Cancer Moonshot movement. The VA and Walter Reed quickly developed a partnership for VA cancer patients to have their tumors sequenced at Walter Reed.

Similarly, a representative from the IBM Watson program visited the Cancer Moonshot offices and offered up Watson if there were a use for it. Could Watson analyze the results of the tumor sequencing from the VA patients and determine from its vast medical library which therapies are available and successful for different tumor types? Yes, it could, and for free. Indeed, once purchased, these technologies could operate at nominal cost, and there was a clear recognition of the value of deploying them for the Cancer Moonshot.

The Cancer Moonshot Summit

In June 2016, the Cancer Moonshot Summit convened to inspire a national conversation and announce 35 new initiatives across the public, private, and nonprofit sectors. The Cancer Moonshot Task Force also announced numerous locally generated initiatives. Alex's Lemonade Stand Foundation committed to doubling its investment in childhood cancer research and cancer care services by investing $150 million and launching a bioinformatics lab to analyze and interpret pediatric cancer data. Coding for Cancer, a Laura and John Arnold Foundation project, partnered with the Harvard Medical and Business Schools to design and execute prize-based challenges in cancer research. Sage Bionetworks launched a $1.2 million Coding4Cancer (C4C) Challenge: The Digital Mammography DREAM Challenge, to advance the accuracy of digital-image breast cancer detection. The University of California Office of the President, University of California Health, the Athena Breast Health Network, Quantum Leap Healthcare Collaborative, and Salesforce together developed an entirely new model for health-care delivery that evolves the point of care into a patient-centric data hub, enabling, for example, the application of clinical trial data toward the creation of technology that permits the personalization of cancer treatments. Creative Commons, acting on Vice President Biden's call to increase transparency and knowledge sharing in the cancer research community, committed to provide publicly available educational resources to support researchers, funders, medical professionals, and professors as they developed an open access, collaborative cancer research community. These and so many more initiatives addressed the goals of the Cancer Moonshot.

Cancer Moonshot Sidebars

BloodPAC (Blood Profiling Atlas in Cancer)

Lauren Leiman, head of External Partnerships for the Cancer Moonshot, built more than fifty Cancer Moonshot partnerships across the public, private, and nonprofit sectors.[6] Together with Dr. Jerry Lee, then the deputy director for Cancer Research and Technology for the Office of the Vice President, she began investigating why liquid biopsy testing technologies seemed to have stalled in development in spite of their initial promise. The more they dug into the problem, the clearer the answer became: "What happened to liquid biopsy testing by 2016 was not a science issue but a collaboration issue."[7] Liquid biopsy technology companies were not working together to advance the science and share their information in ways that would benefit patients, or even their own bottom lines. Leiman and Lee asked experts whether they thought sharing their data would accelerate the field forward. Each in turn agreed it would. Then, Leiman and Lee asked a much tougher question: Would they be willing to share their data? The ultimately unanimous answer indicated that they had heard Vice President Biden's call to action, recognized the stakes for patient outcomes, and appreciated the mutually beneficial nature of collaboration: "Yes." Thereby spurred to partner in ways that would have been unheard of prior to the Cancer Moonshot in an industry known for fierce competition over resources, an unprecedented partnership developed to launch a Blood Profiling Atlas. This new resource would aggregate raw datasets from circulating tumor cells, circulating tumor DNA, and exosome assays, as well as clinical data and handling protocols, from thirteen different studies across a group of twenty stakeholders. Critically, this new curated database was open access.

The energy that this new Blood Profiling Atlas generated under the Cancer Moonshot and the advancements it made possible did not halt at the end of Vice President Biden's term. Four years later, the Blood Profiling Atlas built under the Cancer Moonshot is now known as BloodPAC, and continues to promote the evidence generation required to bring liquid biopsy into routine clinical practice as well as operate BloodPAC Data Commons to serve all stakeholders in the liquid biopsy space. The BloodPAC consortium has grown to over thirty-five members who participate in eight working groups dedicated to promoting the technological development and navigating the regulatory approvals necessary to make liquid biopsies routine in cancer care.

In other words, to achieve progress in pushing liquid biopsy testing forward, the Cancer Moonshot did not invent a new blood profiling mechanism nor pour consistent funding into liquid biopsy research for four years. Instead, it transformed liquid biopsy technology by acting as a catalyst, bringing former competitors together as partners and demonstrating the way collaboration could move the field forward faster in the process.

Family Reach

Beyond its devastating health effects, cancer and all of its unexpected associated direct and indirect economic costs—from loss of income to travel expenses to meals outside of the home to parking to copays to deductibles—literally bankrupts families: cancer patients are nearly three times more likely to file for bankruptcy.[8] Further, the medical and financial impacts of cancer do not occur separately from one another. Patients who file for bankruptcy as a result of the economic burden of cancer have higher mortality rates.[9] Put another way, the financial blows that result from cancer affect survival.

After working with the Cancer Moonshot to expand Family Reach's impact, Carla Tardif, CEO of Family Reach, developed an entirely new approach to ensure finances did not impact cancer patients' treatments and prognoses, an approach targeting prevention. Family Reach pledged with the Cancer Moonshot to offer cancer patients early in diagnosis a "Financial Treatment Program" to supplement their medical treatment. First, the Financial Treatment Program consisted of a guidebook to educate newly diagnosed cancer patients on the role finances would likely play, and to "take away the shame and fear" of talking about finances from patients who worried about not being given the best treatment or being told about the latest trial were they to reveal their financial struggles.[10] Second, it offered pro bono financial planning by certified financial planners. Third, it offered a resource navigation program with social workers to help advocate on cancer patients' behalf. And fourth, it provided emergency relief grants by stepping in and paying bills for patients directly, lengthy application forms and wait times not required.

In this way, Tardif explains, the Cancer Moonshot "challenged Family Reach to come up with collaborative, innovative solutions and gave us the leap of faith we needed to launch services we had dreamt about for a long time."[11] It validated the financial issues cancer patients faced, and it opened the doors for Family Reach to develop partnerships with hospitals, health-care leaders, pharmaceutical companies, and more.

Family Reach's data, too, reveal the enduring impact of the Cancer Moonshot. In 2016, Family Reach served 2,700 families with finite emergency grants for patients.[12] By 2019, it had expanded to serve eight thousand families with a full suite of services in the Financial Treatment Program.[13] Over the same time period, Family Reach also experienced a 120 percent increase in grants given to patients.[14] And its expansion is ongoing. Most recently, Family Reach added another new resource for cancer patients, a debt consolidation program, and it is piloting additional programs with Tufts University. As Tardif describes it, "The Moonshot was game-changing, I don't know any other word to say it."[15]

Specialty Care Center in the Navajo Nation

In January 2017, Kim Thiboldeaux, CEO of the Cancer Support Community and leading psychosocial oncology expert, was working with the Cancer Moonshot to expand cancer care support in medically underserved communities. Following a fruitful White House Cancer Moonshot session, two strangers approached her at the podium as she packed up her papers. "Did you know that there is not any cancer care offered on any Native American reservation across America?" they asked.[16] The Indian Health Service provided primary care services, but for specialty care, Native American patients needed to travel outside of the reservation, often hundreds of miles away from their homes. The two people were Brandy Tomhave and Dr. Johanna Dimento, and this fortuitous meeting became the beginning of their work with Thiboldeaux, who would subsequently spend years working with the Cancer Moonshot to change this reality.

The devastating effects of long-distance travel requirements go well beyond inconvenience. Not all cancer patients can travel hundreds of miles for their appointments. As a result, many were forgoing their needed medical treatments to instead work or care for family members, with severe health consequences as a result. In other words, in many cases lack of a local cancer care center translated into lack of cancer care altogether.

On May 22, 2019, with funding from the Tuba City hospital, contracted with the Indian Health Service, and donations and grants, including fund-raising by the Navajo Hopi Health Foundation, the doors of the Specialty Care Center opened in Navajo Nation, Arizona, becoming the first ever cancer center on a Native American reservation. Navajo Nation President Jonathan Nez and its First Lady, Phefelia Nez, welcomed Second Lady Biden, Thiboldeaux, and cancer care leaders who traveled from across the United States to the occasion to witness the historic moment that would improve the lives of Native Americans living with cancer. Currently, more than one thousand Native American cancer patients receive treatment at Specialty Care Center.[17]

The 21st Century Cures Act

Establishing these norms and putting this engine into motion required an initial investment. The 21st Century Cures Act provided that financial commitment. Passed by a Republican Congress in December of 2016 at the dusk of the Obama administration, it authorized $6.3 billion in funding, $4.8 billion of which was allocated to the NIH and $1.8 billion to the Cancer Moonshot.[18] Appropriated annually, the Cures Act allocated the Cancer Moonshot funding over a period of seven years.

At the public signing ceremony of the act, one of the guests of honor on stage with President Obama was a young woman named Stephanie. She was in her early twenties when she was diagnosed with colon cancer, a rare virulent kind that attacks people long before they would normally be screened. She had been headed for hospice when her sister found a clinical trial at Johns Hopkins University using a "new" kind of therapy—immunotherapy. This "new" therapy used the body's own immune system to fight the cancer, rather than chemotherapy to kill the cancer. (Immunotherapy had actually started at the turn of the twentieth century but was abandoned after the advent of chemotherapy. It continued to be thought of as an outlier science until the last decade. It has now become the most important approach to fighting cancer.) Stephanie's tumors melted away once she started the immunotherapy in the clinical trial at Hopkins, and she continues to be healthy and active to this day. Her presence onstage signified the hope underlying the Cancer Moonshot and the movement it generated.

The Next Chapter

A common question the Moonshot team received was, "How much can you really get done in just nine months?" Nine months is half the life span of a person diagnosed today with glioblastoma, a deadly form of brain cancer. Nine months is a quarter of the life span of people born with certain kinds of multiple myeloma. When you consider the lives of people with cancer, nine months may not be long enough to finish the work you need to do to make a difference, but it is more than enough time to get started.

The COVID-19 pandemic response demonstrated that when we work together with a sense of urgency, we can develop a vaccine in *nine months* when it used to take years. When we coordinate the NIH and the FDA, we can remove barriers to rapid development and testing of new therapies.

That is what the Cancer Moonshot meant to millions of cancer patients—a sign that the government and the nation were willing to start a movement to solve the vexing problems of this awful disease, a movement that will not stop until we have changed the face of cancer forever.

What should the Biden administration do to build on the legacy of the Cancer Moonshot? The focus of the original Cancer Moonshot was on changing the culture of research that seemed to be stuck in the 1970s. And we have seen that cultural inertia can be overcome at a rapid pace if leaders and public figures, such as Joe and Jill Biden, elevate the issue and convene people around a common cause.

The events since the Cancer Moonshot was launched in 2016 now point to one inescapable conclusion—it is time to change the culture of the *nation* to reap the full benefit of our progress in cancer research, treatments, and care.

Culture eats strategy for lunch. And unfortunately, we have learned from COVID-19 that it is lunchtime. Despite everything we know about the science of infectious disease, and despite the public health officials' warnings, we saw that political culture defeated our public health strategy, with the result that the United States lost nearly 600,000 lives to the virus. What are we to make of the fact that our culture is so hard to change?

The Cancer Moonshot focused on the culture of cancer—the lack of data sharing, the lack of diversity in clinical trials, the need to fund riskier research, the need to operate as if we were all in it together. That was our goal. And now we have to ask, what is COVID-19's impact on cancer and cancer culture, and how should we respond in designing the next Cancer Moonshot?

On the good side, the pandemic propelled us into a future we knew was coming, with telemedicine, virtual care, clinical trials that come to you, and the acceleration of novel therapeutic approaches. Creating vaccines in nine months is a miracle in modern medicine and has demonstrated that we are capable of far more innovation than we thought.

Further, COVID-19 showed that many of the critical elements of the Cancer Moonshot, such as data sharing, collaboration, and better surveillance of cancer trends and outcomes, are not "nice-to-haves" but "must-haves" if we are to successfully address grave threats to public health such as pandemics and cancer. The system of investigator-initiated research that is the hallmark of the NIH is insufficient to meet the needs of a health emergency. As he has done with COVID-19, President Biden will need to use his leadership to galvanize the nation's resources and deploy them as needed to address the challenge of cancer as well.

The Cancer Moonshot was noteworthy for creating inter-agency cooperation necessary for a complete response to cancer. The next Moonshot needs to expand on this theme to make inter-agency collaboration the norm, not the exception as it has been for years. Presidential leadership is the only way this will happen given the budget and administrative structures of each department and agency that reward competition rather than collaboration.

But on the bad side—we know that the pandemic highlighted all the cracks in our society. We know that the vulnerable, the poor, people of color, people in communities that are health deserts, suffered more casualties and more infections from COVID-19 than did people who were well off. We know that just as there will be a gap year in our education of young children that will follow them throughout their educational career, we will have a gap year in improving cancer outcomes.

Fewer people got tested for cancer. Therefore, fewer cancers were detected. That does not mean there were fewer cancers. We will have a surge in deaths from preventable cancers because we took our eyes off the ball during the pandemic. And we also know that if you were in therapy with cancer, this was a very difficult year.

Then there is the ugly, in addition to just the bad, about COVID-19. The racial disparity in outcomes of this virus is the same as the racial disparities in outcomes in every disease and in health generally. Indeed, the focus of a new Cancer Moonshot should be to address such racial inequities in cancer outcomes. There is nothing that would save more lives quickly than to bring the benefits of our cancer progress to all communities of America equally. This was always one goal of the Cancer Moonshot—now it needs to be *the* goal. Policy makers must provide expanded access to insurance, access to care for earlier and more effective diagnoses, access to clinical trials, and access to treatments, all of which will lead to better outcomes.

The clear failing of our public health system to anticipate this pandemic is evident in the lack of preparedness and the failure to use the Defense Production Act early in the pandemic to provide the masks, the ventilators, and all the other supplies we needed. And what was especially troubling was the lack of common cause in our society to follow the science and care for each other. Now we can envision the end of COVID-19 as a pandemic. But when we lower the death toll of this virus, we will still be losing 1,800 to 2,000 people a day to cancer. And that is unacceptable. Where do we go from here? What should the Biden administration focus on in creating the next Cancer Moonshot?

First, we need accountability. How did the Cancer Moonshot actually affect people's lives? How did the $1.8 billion get spent? Did it fund new researchers? Did it fund revolutionary, risky ideas? Was it spent in all of our communities, and not just on the East and West Coasts? Did we include everybody in the promise of a new approach to changing the culture of cancer?

Second, we need continuity and commitment to continue changing the culture of the cancer establishment. We still are not funding enough young people and people of color. We still give money primarily to the traditional institutions. We still are using a research system that came from the 1950s and 1960s.

There are many ideas for how to change and modernize our research system. For example, the proposal for the creation of an advanced research projects agency for health, just the way we have one for defense. After all, we are losing more lives every week to cancer than we have lost to any terrorist attack.

In addition to accountability and continuity, we have to cancel the culture of neglect that has allowed for racial disparities and racial injustice in our health system. Even when we acknowledge racial inequities, we address them by making solving inequities *one* of the goals of all of our cancer organizations, just as it was *one* of the goals of the Cancer Moonshot, and *one* of the goals of the Biden Cancer Initiative.

This can no longer be a bullet point. This has to be the headline in bold, huge font. It is unacceptable that Black women with breast cancer are 40 percent more likely to die than white women.[19] All of the work in immunology that is saving lives today, all of the work in childhood cancers that is giving people a full lifetime when they may have had only three or four years on this planet, all of that science will continue. But racial injustice has kept us from distributing it equally to our population. And that has to change.

Everything that we would do to achieve racial and social justice in cancer outcomes would help *everybody* in the system. We have to increase access to early detection, and then treatment. One of the Cancer Moonshot's first projects was in Washington, DC, and Cleveland to take lung cancer detection technologies into housing projects where smoking rates were high, insurance coverage was low, and lung cancer rates were well above the national average. But those were projects. We need to make that the centerpiece of our work. We need to make sure that patient-reported outcomes and evidence from communities of color and other minorities are available to physicians, and to cancer centers designing trials.

We have to provide social services. We need to ensure people have the ability to pay for their care, the ability to get a ride to the hospital, the ability to show up to the clinical trial, the ability to make it to the pharmacy. The absence of social support is one of the reasons people fail to take their medicines, fail to get checked, fail to get tested, and fail to get treated. It is not for lack of trying; it is for lack of the opportunity or lack of ability.

There is no one answer to how to address health disparities. The answers will come from all of us involved with the cancer enterprise and our health-care system. And while there are many innovations we can talk about in cancer—the advent of CRISPR, and mRNA vaccines that will soon be adapted, we hope, to cancer vaccines—these technological and imaging breakthroughs and home-care advances will not matter if we leave entire segments of our populace behind.

We each must think about what we can do to bring the benefits of the world's greatest cancer research enterprise in history to everybody in our nation, and eventually, to everybody around the globe.

Notes

1. See Morgan Brisse et al., "Emerging Concepts and Technologies in Vaccine Development," *Frontiers in Immunology* 11 (2020): 583077, https://doi.org/10.3389/fimmu.2020.583077.

2. Mehmet Sitki Copur, "Inadequate Awareness of and Participation in Cancer Clinical Trials in the Community Oncology Setting," *Oncology* 33, no. 2 (2019): 54–57, https://www.cancernetwork.com/view /inadequate-awareness-and-participation-cancer-clinical-trials-community-oncology-setting.

3. Joe Biden, "Inspiring a New Generation to Defy the Bounds of Innovation: A Moonshot to Cure Cancer" (Washington, DC: White House, Office of the Vice President, January 12, 2016), https://obamawhitehouse.archives.gov /the-press-office/2016/01/12/inspiring-new-generation-defy-bounds-innovation-moonshot-cure-cancer.

4. *Cancer Moonshot: Report of the Cancer Moonshot Task Force* (Washington DC: White House, 2016), 8, https://obamawhitehouse.archives.gov/sites /default/files/docs/final_cancer_moonshot_task_force_report_1.pdf.

5. *Cancer Moonshot: Report of the Cancer Moonshot Task Force*, 11.

6. Interview with Lauren Leiman, July 28, 2020.

7. Interview, Leiman.

8. Scott D. Ramsey et al., "Financial Insolvency as a Risk Factor for Early Mortality among Patients with Cancer," *Journal of Clinical Oncology* 34, no. 9 (2016): 980–986, https://doi.org/10.1200/JCO.2015.64.6620.

9. Ramsey et al., "Financial Insolvency."

10. Ramsey et al., "Financial Insolvency."

11. Ramsey et al., "Financial Insolvency."

12. Ramsey et al., "Financial Insolvency."

13. Ramsey et al., "Financial Insolvency."

14. Ramsey et al., "Financial Insolvency."

15. Ramsey et al., "Financial Insolvency."

16. Interview with Kim Thiboldeaux, July 30, 2020.

17. Interview, Thiboldeaux.

18. Sheila Kaplan, "Winners and Losers of the 21st Century Cures Act," *Stat News*, December 5, 2016, https://www.statnews.com/2016/12/05/21st-century -cures-act-winners-losers/.

19. *Cancer Disparities*, NIH (November 17, 2020), https://www.cancer.gov /about-cancer/understanding/disparities.

Acknowledgments

This book could not have come to fruition without the tireless and brilliant contributions of Eugene Rusyn, the senior fellow at the Solomon Center for Health Law and Policy at Yale Law School. Eugene helped lead this project from conception through completion. He played an integral role in shaping its content and attending to every detail. Our gratitude to and admiration for him are boundless.

This book also would not have been possible without the tireless efforts of a remarkable team of student research assistants who supported our authors during critical periods in the drafting process. We are deeply grateful for the contributions of Chaaru Deb, Tomeka Frieson, Deepen Gagneja, Carolyn Lye, Arjun Mody, Matt Nguyen, Allison Rabkin Golden, Blake Shultz, Jackson Skeen, and Evan Walker-Wells. Additional invaluable student support was provided early in our process by Eric Brooks, Matt Butler, Eamon Duffy, Jade Ford, Sandra Lynne Fryhofer, Rita Gilles, Alice Gu, Isabelle Hanna, Ivona Iacob, Mitchell Johnston, Rachel Kogan, Ike Lee, Ted Lee, Sophie Lipman, Joe Liss, Dan Listwa, Vishakha Negi, Tracy Nelson, Nicholas Oo, Adam Pan, Bina Peltz, Nicholas Sauder, Daniel Strunk, Veena Subramanian, Isra Syed, Erica Turret, and Camila Vega.

We are also grateful for the support we received from Yale University, our home institutions during this project. The Solomon Center for Health Law and Policy at Yale Law School is at the forefront of studying how cancer in America is shaped by law, policy, and the practice of medicine. We thank Yale Law School Deans Robert Post and Heather Gerken, the Solomon family, Yale School of Medicine Deans Robert Alpern and Nancy Brown, Solomon Center Executive Director Katherine Kraschel, Solomon Center Program Coordinators Jessenia Khalyat and Kathryn Mammel, and Senior Administrative Assistant Lise Cavallaro for their support of our work. Solomon Center Senior Research Fellows Laura Hoffman and Ryan Knox offered outstanding editorial assistance. We are also grateful to the Yale Cancer Center and Smilow Cancer Hospital for their invaluable support of our efforts, including their cosponsorship of a major conference hosted at Yale Law School in February 2018 on "The Policy, Politics, and Law of Cancer" that led to this book. We also owe appreciation to the Oscar M. Ruebhausen Fund and the outstanding team of dedicated staff at Yale, including James Barnett, Janet Conroy, Barbara Corcoran, Renee DeMatteo, Daniel Griffin, Debra Kroszner, Mike Thompson, and Lisa Yelon, for their support of the conference.

We thank Clive Priddle and the fantastic team at PublicAffairs for recognizing the value of assessing how policy, politics, and law influence cancer in America on the fiftieth anniversary of the War on Cancer.

Finally, we thank our all-star list of contributors for their insights and commitment to the project and, more importantly, for the work they have done and continue to do to address the challenges cancer poses and to chart a path—a New Deal for Cancer—toward a better future for all of us.

Index

AACR (American Association for Cancer Research), 176, 179, 227
ABC network, 175, 181
academic cancer centers (AMCs), 230, 232, 236
See also specific centers
academic research centers/care
accessibility, 37–38
economic challenges, 38
mission, 36
overview, 36
research, 37
services, 36–37
See also specific centers
Academy of Nutrition and Dietetics, 145
Accelerating Colorectal Cancer Screening/Implementation Science (ACCSIS), 362
Accountable Care Organizations (ACOs)
description, 61–62, 91
evaluations, 64
ACCSIS (Accelerating Colorectal Cancer Screening/Implementation Science), 362
acquired immunodeficiency syndrome. *See* HIV/AIDS
"acquired vulnerabilities," 192
ACS (American Cancer Society), 117, 118, 126, 127, 143–145, 338
Advancing Breakthrough Therapies for Patients Act (2012), 345
advocates/cancer
effects on oncologists, 217–219
NCI (National Cancer Institute), 218
piecemeal requests, 350
reasons for becoming an, 158, 173
roles, 218–219

"speaking with one voice," 349
See also specific individuals/ organizations
advocates/pediatric cancer
bringing treatments to market, 162–164
future work, 169–170
inverting funding paradigm, 159–162
novel treatment needs, 160–161
policy/legislation work, 159, 166, 167–169, 167–170
social media/storytelling, 164–166
traditional methods, 158–159
treatment toxicity issue, 160
trials/speed problems, 161
"Valley of Death" management, 159
See also specific diseases; specific individuals/organizations
Affordable Care Act (2010)
cancer screening, 58–59, 323
Center for Medicare and Medicaid Innovation (CMMI), 62
clinical trials, 292
coverage expansion/reform, 58–59
dependent coverage expansion (DCE), 58–59
disparities reduction, 69
expansion of insured, access, 344, 345
financial hardship reduction, 69
generic/biosimilar agents, 251
insurance as utility, 98–99
Medicaid expansion/need, 58–59, 63, 118, 119, 129–130, 324
Medicare Part D donut hole, 59
payment/delivery system reform, 58, 59–60
politics/undermining, 59
preexisting conditions, 54, 59, 345
preventive services, 59
State Innovation Waivers, 315

About the Editors

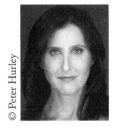

Abbe R. Gluck is the Alfred M. Rankin Professor of Law, the founding faculty director of the Solomon Center for Health Law and Policy at Yale Law School, professor of internal medicine at Yale School of Medicine and the faculty director of the Yale Medical-Legal Partnership. She is one of the nation's most cited scholars in the field of health law and policy, is an elected member of the leadership body of the American Law Institute, and is the chair of the Healthcare Committee of the Uniform Law Commission. She is a graduate of Yale College and Yale Law School, and a former law clerk to US Supreme Court Justice Ruth Bader Ginsburg. Her most recent book, *The Trillion Dollar Revolution: How the Affordable Care Act Transformed Politics, Law and Health Care in America*, with Zeke Emanuel, was published in 2020.

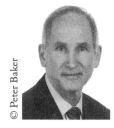

Charles S. Fuchs was director of Yale Cancer Center and physician-in-chief of Smilow Cancer Hospital from 2017 to 2021 and previously served as chief of the gastrointestinal oncology division and the Robert T. and Judith B. Hale Chair in Pancreatic Cancer at Dana-Farber Cancer Institute and Harvard Medical School. He is currently senior vice president and global head of oncology and hematology drug development at Genentech and Roche and adjunct professor at Yale School of Medicine.

PublicAffairs is a publishing house founded in 1997. It is a tribute to the standards, values, and flair of three persons who have served as mentors to countless reporters, writers, editors, and book people of all kinds, including me.

I. F. STONE, proprietor of *I. F. Stone's Weekly*, combined a commitment to the First Amendment with entrepreneurial zeal and reporting skill and became one of the great independent journalists in American history. At the age of eighty, Izzy published *The Trial of Socrates*, which was a national bestseller. He wrote the book after he taught himself ancient Greek.

BENJAMIN C. BRADLEE was for nearly thirty years the charismatic editorial leader of *The Washington Post*. It was Ben who gave the *Post* the range and courage to pursue such historic issues as Watergate. He supported his reporters with a tenacity that made them fearless and it is no accident that so many became authors of influential, best-selling books.

ROBERT L. BERNSTEIN, the chief executive of Random House for more than a quarter century, guided one of the nation's premier publishing houses. Bob was personally responsible for many books of political dissent and argument that challenged tyranny around the globe. He is also the founder and longtime chair of Human Rights Watch, one of the most respected human rights organizations in the world.

·　　·　　·

For fifty years, the banner of Public Affairs Press was carried by its owner Morris B. Schnapper, who published Gandhi, Nasser, Toynbee, Truman, and about 1,500 other authors. In 1983, Schnapper was described by *The Washington Post* as "a redoubtable gadfly." His legacy will endure in the books to come.

Peter Osnos, *Founder*